i

Body Image

Sarah P. Condor-Fisher

8.5" x 11.0" (21.59 x 27.94 cm)

Black on White paper.

589 pages

ISBN-13: 9798851067174

Imprint: Fisher Publishing Inc.

Fisher Publishing also publishes its books in a variety of electronic formats. Some content that appears in print may not be available in electronic books.

Library of Congress Cataloguing in Publication Data: A catalogue record for this book is available from the Library of Congress.

Library of Congress Publication Data
        Condor-Fisher, Sarah, P. (1972-   )
Genre: Nonfiction – Psychology – Education & Training

Date of first publication: July 4, 2023
Date of effective registration: July 13, 2023
TX 9-296-018 1-10653409831

10 9 8 7 6 5 4 3 2 1

Printed in the United States of America

Contents

Dedicated to

Gregory T. Fisher, M.D., F.A.C.S.

My Father, Mentor, and Lifelong Inspiration

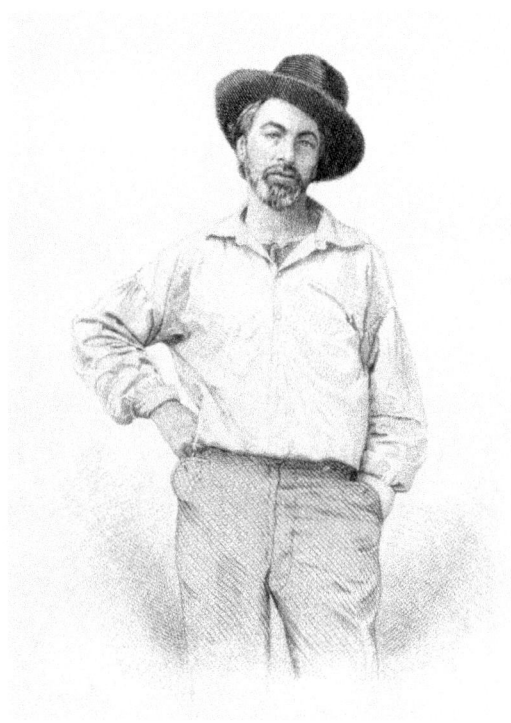

Apart from the pulling and hauling stands what I am,
Stands amused, complacent, compassionating, idle, unitary,
Looks down, is erect, or bends an arm on an impalpable
certain rest,
Looking with side-curved head curious what will come next,
Both in and out of the game and watching and wondering at
it.
Backward I see in my own days where I sweated through fog
with linguists and contenders,
I have no mockings or arguments, I witness and wait.

Walt Whitman
The Song of Myself
(*Leaves of Grass*)

Preface

The goal of this book is twofold: to acquaint the reader with the various aspects of body image, its history and development, philosophical and psychological aspects thereof, as well as with the intricacies of body image dysmorphic disorders and associated conditions; and to offer helpful practical advice, to the extent that such can be provided on a non-individualized basis. The chapters dedicated to the former (theoretical aspects) are naturally more scholarly and academic.

Therefore, the reader is in no way obligated to read the book from cover to cover, in order to understand the issue that concerns him the most. On the contrary, the author hopes that the book will be used as an occasional reference, and even a form of pastime, for those who are interested in this topic, for whatever reason. It is highly recommended that the reader thoroughly peruse the Contents of this book, and look up the chapters that might interest him first.

Nevertheless, the topic of body image is complex and multifaceted. A thorough understanding can only be achieved by those who, with patience and dedication, examine the chapters on its historical origins, its cultural and social aspects, as well as its sundry psychopathologies and associated comorbidities. Certain aspects of body image formation and function are still unsettled or have been variously contested by researchers and experts in the field. This book, albeit among the most comprehensive available, does not claim to resolve all issues or tackle all quandaries.

The APA format is used in citations. This means that the first time a technical term is introduced, it is italicized and abbreviation provided in brackets, where such is in common usage. Subsequent use of the same may be limited to the abbreviated form. The reader is advised to refer to the Glossary of Technical Terms and Phrases Used in the Text which, along with several useful appendices, can be found at the end of the book. To facilitate the reading of acronyms and abbreviations, a list of frequently used abbreviations follows this Preface.

Finally, as to the title of the book, the term *Body Image* is generally not hyphenated. Hyphenation may be desirable in the adjectival sense, such as *body-image issues*, or where the author separates the body from the image, in which case the body is a technical "preposition" to the image, akin to the "self" in *self-image* and *self-esteem.* These latter terms are almost always hyphenated. Quirk et al. (1985/2003) note that hyphens are available when the first word is used "to link syntactically-related premodifiers of noun phrases" (p. 1615). Therefore, it would be justifiable to avail oneself of this rule when discussing the body as a "premodifier" to the image. Syntax, however, is not ruled by philosophy.

Even if it were so, philosophically, the modern reader still operates in the Cartesian world of body–mind dichotomy, which may be why the absence of hyphenation in *body image* is the rule, not vice versa. The opposite might disturb the natural flow of the language, as the Editor poignantly observed. By logical extension, the absence of hyphenation may be linked to the concept of body-image dissonances and various forms of dysmorphic disorders which constitute the core of the matter discussed here. The disunity between the body and (its) image is reflected in the language used in their depiction and, perhaps, as long as such is the case, neither the powers of the individual nor of the expert, alone or in synergy, will suffice to unite the two in harmony. The problem is more than linguistic or philosophical. Therefore, where the *body* is spoken of as being in opposition to the image, the *em*-dash "–"is used (body–image).

Sarah Condor-Fisher

Frequently Used Abbreviations

AA: Alopecia Areata
AAS: Androgenic Anabolic Steroids
ABCD: Assessment of Body Image Cognitive
                Distortions
ABISS: Adolescent Body Image Satisfaction Scale
ACTH: Adrenocorticotropic Hormone
AD: Atopic Dermatitis
ADHD: Attention Deficit Hyperactivity Disorder
ADP: Adenosine Di Phosphate
AN: Anorexia Nervosa
ASI: Appearance Schemas Inventory
ATP: Adenosine Tri Phosphate
AU: Action Units
BAI: Beck Anxiety Inventory
BBAT: Basic Body Awareness Therapy
BD: Body Dysmorphic (feelings)
BDD: Body Dysmorphic Disorder
BDI: Beck Depression Inventory
BDNF: Brain-Derived Neurotrophic Factor
BED: Binge Eating Disorder
BESAQ: Body Exposure during Sexual Activities
                Questionnaire
BFOQs: Bona Fide Occupational Qualifications
BHB: Beta Hydroxy Butyrate
BIAS-BD: Body Image Assessment Scale–Body
                Dimensions
BICSI :   Body Image Coping Strategies Inventory
BID: Body Image Disturbance
BIS: Body Image Scale
BISS: Body Image States Scale
BMI: Body Mass Index
BN: Bulimia Nervosa
BNST-dspm: darkly staining posteromedial component
                of the Bed Nucleus of the Stria Terminalis
BPD: Borderline Personality Disorder
BPI: Body Perception Index
BPS: Body Prominence Score

xvii

BRT:	Bounded Rationality Theory
BS:	Barrier Score
BSQ:	Body Shape Questionnaire
BSQR:	Body-Self Relations Questionnaire
BST:	Bed of Stria Terminalis
CBF:	Cerebral Blood Flow
CBI:	Cutaneous Body Image
CBT:	Cognitive Behavioral Therapy
CSFQ:	Changes in Sexual Functioning Questionnaire
DMS:	Drive for Muscularity Scale
EAT:	Eating Attitudes Test
ED:	Eating Disorders
EPOC:	Excess Postexercise Oxygen Consumption
FACS:	Facial Action Coding System
fMRI:	functional Magnetic Resonance Imaging
FMS:	Fibromyalgia Syndrome
FRS:	Figure Rating Scale
FT:	Fast Twitch (muscle fiber)
FtM:	Female to Male (transsexual)
GD:	Gender Dysphoria
GDD:	Gender Dysphoric Disorder
GDS:	Gender Dysphoria Syndrome
GID:	Gender Identity Disorder
HFD:	Human Figure Drawings
HIT:	High Intensity Training
HIIT:	High Intensity Interval Training
HPA:	Hypothalamic-Pituitary-Adrenal (axis)
IBS:	Ideal Body Size
IFBB:	International Federation of Bodybuilding
INBA:	International Natural Bodybuilding Association
IPL:	Inferior Parietal Lobules
LOrF:	Left Orbito-Frontal cortex
MBSRQ-AS:	Multidimensional Body-Self Relations Questionnaire Appearance Scales
MD/MDD:	Muscle Dysmorphia, Muscle Dysmorphic Disorder
MPFC:	Medial Prefrontal Cortex

MS:	Multiple Sclerosis
MST:	Medial Superior Temporal
MtF:	Male to Female (transsexual)
MT:	Medial Temporal
NES:	Night Eating Syndrome
NPD:	Narcissistic Personality Disorder
OCD:	Obsessive-Compulsive Disorder
ON:	Orthorexia Nervosa
OSFED:	Other Specified Feeding and Eating Disorder
PBQs:	Professional Beauty Qualifications
PCC:	Posterior Cingulate Cortex
PKD:	Polycystic Kidney Disease
RCTs:	Randomized Controlled Trials
RPFC:	Right Pre-Frontal Cortex
SB:	Self Boundaries
SDH:	Succinate dehydrogenase
SoO:	Sense of Ownership over the Object
SPP:	Somatoparaphrenia
SRS:	Sex Reassignment Surgery
SSD:	Somatic Symptom Disorder
SSD:	Short Stature Dysphoria
SSRIs:	Selective Serotonin Reuptake Inhibitors
SSSS:	Sexual Self-Schema Scale
ST:	Slow Twitch (muscle fiber)
TAT:	Thematic Apperception Test
TNB:	Transgender and Non-Binary
TPJ:	Temporoparietal Junction
TRF:	Time Restricted Food Intake

Body Image

Body Experience, Body Schema, and Representation

The term *body image* commonly refers to the perception of "body size, body parts, and the proportion between them," as well as to the emotions associated with one's appearance that we tend to recognize as attractiveness or repulsion, frustration, and even self-hate (Freedman, 1990, p. 273). In turn, such feelings and physical experiences reflect and shape our body image (Shani-Sela, 2000). Austrian psychiatrist and psychoanalyst Paul Schilder (1886-1940) defined body image as the "image of the human body" that we "form in our mind" making ourselves "part of our body-surface" while perceiving a "unity" which we call a "schema of our body" or "body schema" (Schilder, 1950, p. 11). This schema is our cognitive construction as well as a "reflection of wishes, emotional attitudes, and interactions with others" (Fisher, 1990, p. 8).

Linguistically, the term body image is a compound composed of a "body" and an "image," two apparently equal entities which, as noted in the Preface, are not always understood and projected on equal planes. The *body* is something tangible and palpable. It develops naturally, as the human being grows and ages. Interestingly, note the use of the word "body" in phrases such as a "body of work" or the "idea embodied in…" or "the main body of the text" where the connotation is that of something stable, anchoring and stabilizing. On the other hand, the word "image," immediately evokes associations with the derivative verb, to imagine, an act which not only indicates malleability of the purportedly "stable" image, but also adds an extra layer to the concept of body image as a "body which is imagined" – thus not real. What becomes real is not the body itself but the perception of it, which is constantly mediated, deconstructed, and (re)interpreted.

1

Indeed, that which is imagined always craves substantiation and recognition: the most secret dreams wish to be realized and, as the famed American folklore has it, they do so, provided that one works hard enough and *makes* them *come true.* In body-image context, one may ask: what good would my *body-experience* be if my body was only imagined? One's living identity must be constructed from the image, which bears such relationship to the world as is *mediated* which, in brief, means projected, communicated, and founded on consensus and subject-object re-construction with *the other* human being in the given environment.[1] The human body is as material as the world surrounding it, in constant contact with the world, participating in existence. The attribution of this bipartite division into a body and an image is not unique to the human being albeit, even among the human race, is not equally perceived and mediated – like animals and even inanimate objects, some people are more "environmentally-dependent" than others.

Body image has three components: anatomical (relating to body shape), functional (e.g., powerlessness or its opposite, gastrointestinal, sexual function, etc.), and psychological, i.e., satisfaction with appearance (Koide et al., 2003). Anatomical and functional components may be termed *physiological.* When taken together, physiological and psychological components create human *body experience* (Sakson-Obada et al., 2016).

Body experience may be a better, all-embracing term for body image, because it can be interpreted as a sense of body unity in space and time, limited by physical boundaries and capacities, as well as psychological barriers (consisting of both the abilities to perceive, and to self-interpret, thus be perceived). When a child first begins to perceive the Self, it is via stimuli and their integration in the form of

---

[1] For a more detailed definition of *mediation,* see the following chapter.

sensorimotor representations. As soon as verbalization begins, the interpretation of the stimuli leads to "desomatization" and "symbolization of affect" (Krueger, 2002; Krystal, 1979; Sakson-Obada, 2016).

Apart from the direct sensorimotor input, feedback is provided to the child by the caregivers. Feedback information contributes to the formation of the individual's body image. Here is where body-image mediation begins. The caregiver assesses and defines the internal states of the child which the child learns from her (Stern 1985). Self-recognition, reflection, and self-regulation are thus inextricably intertwined, and what has been termed *human body experience* begins practically as soon as the human being emerges from the womb. Some studies even indicate that individual's body image is formed prior to birth, as the unborn human's tactile and sensory receptors become aware of its body-parts (Dijkerman & de Haan, 2007; Mitchell, 1997; Myowa-Yamakoshi & Takeshita, 2006). Price (2006) collated the accounts of *aplasic phantoms* (people who were born without a limb, yet present a complete body image as if the limb was present), and concluded that body image is "learnt from experience during both pre- and post-natal development" (p. 311).

Schilder's (1950) psychological insight into the operations of the body as (an) image (one of many) comports to such conclusions, as Schilder noted and emphasized the constant mediation between the "surface" and the "interior" of the body:

> The body contracts when we hate, it becomes firmer, and its outlines toward the world are more strongly marked... We expand the body when we feel friendly and loving... We expand and we contract the postural model of the body; we take parts away and we add parts; we rebuild it; we melt the details in; we create new details; we do this with our

3

body and with the expressions of the body itself...
When even so the body is not sufficient for the
expression of the playful changes and the destructive
changes in the body, then we add clothes, masks,
jewelry, which again expand, contract, disfigure, or
emphasize the body image and its particular parts.
(1950, pp. 210-211)

Since neither human faculties nor capacities for
evaluation are capable of perfect and undistorted detection,
and because the *body experience* is *mediated* through the
external environment, distortion occurs and is present at all
stages of human development. Such is the case in particular
during childhood when the child's abilities to interpret the
observed and perceived stimuli are in formative stages and
the human mind is not yet capable of fully grasping its
mortal, material self: from falling off the bicycle to being
punched when fighting over a toy, to being scorned for what
one wears or how one laughs, the brain is overwhelmed by
data inputs related to the body, its shape, form, condition,
and modes of perception.

Consequently, from earliest childhood, human
beings form a self-image which is best defined as a
representation. This representation is fluid and unstable – it
accretes and erodes with age and under the pressure of
circumstances. In order for the body image to become one
whole (unite), the process of *mediation* is necessary. As
noted above, mediation means communication of the image
and its interpretation. Ideally, this *mediation* should
correspond to one's *body schema*.

Body schema is more than a mere likeness (image).
The description which is sometimes applied to the body
image as a "perceptual identification of body features" as
represented by sensory and motor input to the brain, overlaps
with the definition of the *body schema* as the "location of
different body parts" in a sensorimotor map of body-space,

4

not always accessible to consciousness (Paillard, 1999). Dijekerman and de Haan (2007) also note that other authors distinguish a third representation "containing conceptual and semantic knowledge about the body" (p. 195). Marcus (1977) defined *self-schemas* as "cognitive generalizations about the self, derived from past experiences that organize and guide the processing of self-related information contained in an individual's social experience" which coincides with the definition of body image mediation applied here (p. 65).[2]

The most fundamental aspect of the body image is that it is not stable. The word "image" suggests something stable, immovable, and firm, such as a painting in a gallery. However, the human body constantly changes, develops, renews and transforms itself. All that the mind can do is to direct this transformation to positive, natural ends, while trying to comprehend, absorb and adopt the mediated *body experience.*

Body Image Mediation

The word mediation has three core meanings (MerriamWebster, 2021):

(1) intervention between conflicting parties to promote reconciliation, settlement, or compromise;
(2) indirect conveyance or communication through an intermediary; and
(3) a transmission by an intermediate mechanism or agency.

In medical context, experts often speak of a "mediated role" of a particular (e.g., physical) process in

---

[2] Cf. also *Body vs. Image,* below. *See* Johnson (1987).

reaction to a drug, injury or intervention. All of these meanings are applicable in the context of a *mediated* body experience, albeit the means, parties, intermediaries, and agencies may vary in different microspheres (Bronfenbrenner & Morris, 1998).

Padfield et al. (2017) conducted a study of body image best described as a *triangulation* of the pain-image between the patient and the physician, assuming that chronic, psychosomatic pain of indeterminate causation is pain formed by self-reflection and self-definition. The image could thus be viewed as "potential" and "transitional" because it is being constantly mediated (p. 1290). Patients in this study were given cards with pain images and asked to select those that best described their pain. The image themes were those of "loss, anxiety, fear, shame, disintegration, and even suicidal feelings" (p. 1290). For example, one image contained large letters "LOSS" printed in randomly scattered newspaper clippings. A patient selected this image but said no more. During the next session, he spoke the word "loss" out loud and added that there were "things missing in one's life" (p. 1291). The possessive "one's" (as opposed to the possessive "my") and the vagueness of "things" indicated a slow, still impersonal stage of self-portrayal. In the subsequent narrative, he described how he was avoiding "those issues" and avoidance was a way of adaptation and coping. Interestingly, avoidance has been marked as one of the conflict resolution methods and noted to be of some use in resolving interpersonal conflicts resulting in body-image distortions, and should certainly be explored here, if only because it is among the most frequent methods of "dealing" with what is commonly referred to as "body-image issues" (Condor-Fisher, 2021, p. 260).

Much like the image of "loss," the body image is still an image, and all images are open to interpretation. Representations are not only visual. Conversely, a visual representation (image) may convey non-visual sensations.

For example, visualize a perfectly cut athletic male body with a female face.[3] When the interpretation is so incongruous, dissonant and divergent from aesthetic and normative grounds that it defies immediate psychological synthesis, the initial reaction is commonly fear and apprehension. When the onlooking human bystander is unable to integrate and mediate the image, the bystander will react instinctively. Instinct demands rejection, and immediately invites the fight-or-flight reaction. Alternatively, when the observer is in a crowd, thus ostensibly safe, laughter functions as a protective, self-affirming mechanism.

The underlying psychological mechanics are not important at this point. What is important, however, is that in neither case will the image be mediated. It will not be subjected to mutual correction and understanding. Is mediation invariably not what the individual displaying the image of the self is looking for? What if the clashing sensations and anti-normative projection of the self make it impossible to mediate the body image? What if, save for affirming "the difference," there is no other response? What if the only response is ignorance? What then is a representation without interpretation? An empty gesture, a painting without audience, a story without a listener, a play in an empty theatre.

The all-important point Padfield (2017) makes is that the process of interpretation is always a process of mediation, manifestation, and sharing. Experience is detection and reflection which must be mediated and renegotiated – with one's self as well as the other – in order

---

[3] A real-life situation: a bodybuilding association presented this problem to an attorney, asking what their legal rights were either way – whether they permitted this athlete compete, risking potential resignation of judges or outrage from the audience; or, on the other hand, if they did not permit him to compete, which might expose the Association to potential legal liability under the Fourteenth Amendment.

to achieve validation and utility. In the previous example, the letters LOSS assumed a symbolic meaning, almost like a statue, painting, or a poem – they became a work of art which enabled the victim/sufferer to create and co-create human experience (a generic *loss* as part of human experience) and thereby one's identity and belongingness (the individual *loss* as a form of separation not only from the loved one but also from the rest of the society represented by the loved one).

The sensory apprehension creates the emotional one, and the self-image is the result of this body-mind mediation which, however, is nowhere permanently anchored. In other words, human beings are space-time phenomena which is perhaps why, while constantly seeking freedom, we can neither ever be entirely free nor do we truly want to be so, because absolute freedom requires dissolution of self-identity in *the other*. The moment this threat occurs as an actual potentiality, not even an actuality, freedom turns into anarchy and the bargained-for safety disappears in the flames of the first street "demonstration." Each such demonstration is essentially a manifestation of a representation craving for – superficially – self-affirmation, but, inherently, for a mediation of the body-self-experience.

The mediation starts with detection. Once the image is detected, the human being consciously locates the body, constructs and deconstructs it along various symbolic norms. Schilder (1950) was Freud's student and adopted Freud's symbolic assignations of ergogenic zones in the body as "major landmarks" that structure the human being (p. 124). These "genitalized" areas have been described as "interchangeable" – the nose symbolizing the phallus, cavities (the mouth, anus, vagina, ears) being ranked in "the same group" (p. 127). Schilder (1950) also noted that (the experience of) "almost every neurosis" has at some point intersected with the experience of "one's own body as strange and alien" (p. 139). Such psychopathology has been observed with schizophrenic patients, but may occur wherever there is "hostility against the self" (Cash & Pruzinsky, 1990, p. 11). Hostility against the self may result from abuse, trauma, or other environmental conditions and circumstances (PTSD). The body constitutes a protective boundary which ordinarily shields the human being from a potential traumatic invasion. Once the invasion takes place, one's trust in the body's defensive abilities is diminished or altogether undermined. This is noticeable in individuals who act in self-destructive ways, often without consciously realizing it; or in those who compensate (or, rather, overcompensate) for bodily deficiencies (such as bodybuilders or people addicted to various forms of cosmetic surgery "enhancements").

Body Ego: Body as Protective Barrier

Adler at al. (1917) emphasized that the ego is primarily a *body ego* and ego experiences are body experiences. "Organ inferiority" directly projects upon the ego and the resulting compensation may be that of the body or a body-part (Fisher & Cleveland, 1968). A clear "ego boundary" is necessary for healthy psychological development of every individual (Federn, 1952). Federn proposed a "complex link between the individual's personality conflicts, the expression of these conflicts in patterns of muscle tonus, and the impact of these tonus patterns upon the individual experiences of self and others" (Cash & Pruzinsky, 1990, p. 14). The body image takes on the symbolic and actual form of an armor which the individual wields against the perceived enemy: one may unconsciously tighten or loosen one's muscles depending on perception of danger, one may shrink and shrivel when recalling a traumatic situation. Clearly, someone who does not feel confident, competent, and content with their body image – not to mention the body itself – will be severely disadvantaged in such circumstances.

9

Similarly, a smile indicates pleasure, while a frown is interpreted as displeasure vis-à-vis some experience or percept. The face is the most readily observable body ego representation. Throughout history, the face has been identified as "the character mask of the concealed self" (Belting, 2013). It was Descartes in his *Meditationes de Prima Philosophia* (1641), who first identified the Ego and distinguished it from the body image: "The 'I' that has a face" belongs "to the machine of flesh and bones such as one finds upon a corpse and which I call body" (II.6, as cited in Belting, 2013, p. 28). Was this dysmorphic philosophy imbued in Humanism before Hobbes? Classical Humanism of Protagoras ("Man is the measure of all things."), Socrates ("Know thyself."), Aristotelian ethics, and Epicurean *eudaimonia* (happiness, welfare) considered Man (a generic human) to be a complete whole, mortal in substance, immortal in essence. Even so, Socrates claimed that we should treat our bodies as houses and homes for our souls that we have been granted to rent for a lifetime, and treat them accordingly. Socrates would likely have associated *the image* with the soul, but… *the body*? Well, the body is just a body, he would likely say, throwing a knowing wink at Freud.

Body Ego Formation: Sensory Inputs

It has been stated that body image has three components: anatomical, functional, and psychological (Koide et al., 2003), and that those components create our body experience (Sakson-Obada et al., 2016) through which body ego is created. Nonetheless, if human experience is mediated and takes place outside the Self, then body image and self-image cannot be identical, and the ego is not altogether the individual's. The Self is more than the body because it lies in part outside of the body and, conversely, if the body is not altogether in the possession of the Self, one may wonder, whose body is it?

Returning to the illustration of the image of LOSS referenced above: the individual suffered a loss which he refuses to accept. Everything reminds him of the one he loved. It is not just that the deceased loved one used and wore the things the surviving spouse dumbly touches and looks at now, but that she had lived in part through him – her smell, her touch, her *Being* made these things special and precious to him. Granted, the body that wore them is no more. The body image he loved is a photograph, a fast-fading memory. Nevertheless, the Self-image of his Beloved survives because it is a construct mediated by him in space and time which his own self-image also occupies. Therefore, he can hear her, feel her presence, and she will never quite disappear – as long as he preserves her image and continues to mediate, recreate, reconstruct, and restore it. That is love, and that is also why love can be immortal.

By the same token, however, it should be noted that one's care and emotional pain, which the individual senses through the body, are as real as any physical pain. MacDonald and Leary (2005), and Eisenberger and Lieberman (2005) found that the same centers of the brain are activated when one is hurt by physical pain as when the hurt originates in social-relational bullying (e.g., ostracism). Merely a threat of emotional pain is sufficient to cause not just mental, but physical pain.

It is impossible to live insulated from sensory inputs that cause and trigger emotional reactions, nor would it be desirable, for that would turn the human being into an automaton, or worse – a sociopath. A sociopath does not care for any body-experience mediation, feels no emotional pain, but also feels no happiness, because the converse is true as well – positive emotions reflect on the body-self positively, and it is well-known that balanced posture, correct breathing, and exercise improve mental stability and foster balanced emotional life.

The happiness which flows from a positive body-experience can be characterized as an achievement which results from choice and transformation of negative emotional inputs into positive ones – every loss is an opportunity for new growth and, just as the healing process starts immediately following a physical injury, so does emotional healing begin instantly upon an emotional injury. What is more, this process will remain stultified, unless the body-experience (both physical and emotional injuries) is mediated. The system of psychotherapy, from Mesmer to Freud to Rogers, is founded on the same principle.

Body experience and various forms of body representation discussed above suggest that the reasons why many people have "body image issues"[4] and related psychological conditions have to do with the fact that there is a certain "mental construct" of the body (often referred to as *body-self* or *body ego*) which has to be reconciled with the environment.

Mental Construct of the Body

Petrucelli (2016) discusses the emotional states that are created by negative experiences of one's body image. When an average girl "feels fat," her entire emotional structure is affected by the perception of her body image. She is not objectively fat, her BMI is within the norm. In fact, she is very pretty. Nevertheless, her self-perception is everything to her, all the reality there is. What is more, such feelings and perceptions are "contagious" and take place

---

[4] Terms *issues* and *disturbances* are used interchangeably here. The former is a more general term, with possible legal implications; the latter is a term used in psychology and psychiatry, with direct diagnostic implications. Sometimes, the term *dissonance* is used, appealing to a more holistically-minded body image warrior.

among girls when they are engaged in "fat talk" (Petrucelli, 2016, p. 18). What starts as a seemingly innocuous "talk" may take insidious roots in the person's psyche, cause them pain, and reflect adversely on their body image, creating a perception of impairment.

It follows that the concept of body image is a mental construct incorporating not so much the actual appearance as, rather, the experience of such appearance in how it relates to others, how others perceive it, as well as to the normative cultural ideal (Aron 1998; Baker-Pitts 2015; Bloom et al. 1994; Bulik 2012; Halsted 2015; Krueger 2002; Levine & Smolak 2008; Maine & Kelly 2005; Orbach 2009). This mental construct is neither stable nor does it rest solely within the mind of the perceiver. What is more, it may be distorted by the forces of the environment, such as bullying or drills. Petrucelli (Id.) points out that attempts at integration of such forces may be disruptive and create body image vulnerability, especially where there exists a misunderstanding between the cause (impulse) and effect (impact).

Ogden et al. (2006) observed that people who have suffered traumatic experience (such as childhood abuse, severe bullying, PTSD) tend to avoid their inner sensations and feelings because they feel "disgusted" with their negative body image, hoping that turning away will alleviate their suffering. In such cases, the therapist must approach the problem from the opposite side, looking at what the patient refuses to see, and filling in the lacunae with facts that will connect the body and the image (Levenson, 1982, 1987, 1988).

As a mental construct, the body image is composed of the optic images that correspond to the localization of different body parts, and the relations among those body parts, but also of the "imagination" which emphasizes "tactile similarity of symmetrical points" (Schilder, 1950, p. 21). Localization is "built up by optic and kinaesthetic [sic]

13

impressions," by "bringing the single impression into connection with the postural model of the body," but "the postural model of the body is a product of the gestalt creative powers of our psyche" (p. 21). Schilder (Id.) further notes that we perceive both conscious and unconscious images, as well as images which we do not "use" to formulate or interpret the body image. Even a blind person or a person with optic agnosia[5] has a body image of the self, and creates the body image of others via tactile and facultative means.

As shown by Stratton, Wooster, and Scholl, optical input is of utmost importance to the formation of body image (Schilder, 1950). Scholl subjected himself to an experiment in which he lived for eight days in an "upside down [sic] world" (p. 108). He wore a blindfold over his left eye and his right eye was covered with a "system of lenses which turned everything upside down and from right to left and *vice versa*" (Ibid.). The observation that when he raised his hands, they disappeared in his stomach, and similar oddities, produced the feelings of nausea and a "nervous disturbance" in him at first but, in two days, he remarked that he felt "more at ease" and, on day four, felt "no further discomfort" (p. 109).

Schilder (1950) summarized that it is through movement that we form our body image and that the "knowledge of our own body is to a great extent dependent upon our action" (p. 113). Literally, our body image is constructed by us and, even more interestingly, "the perception of our own body is not very different from the perceptions of any other outside objects" (p. 113).

One of the foremost experts in body image and corrective surgery, Gregory T. Fisher (1945-2020),

---

[5] Optic agnosia is an associative defect where the stimulus, acquired through fully functional sensory-motor means of perception, fails to be meaningfully interpreted. Such a failure is characterized as *agnosia* if it is not caused by an intellectual impairment, or associated with *aphasia* (inability to describe and name things).

conducted numerous surveys of cleft-palate children and how they perceived their body image before and after the corrective surgery he performed on them. He observed that children would first (usually before the age of three) touch themselves (tactile perception of the body image), perceiving no abnormality (even if such existed). Soon thereafter, however, they would begin to form their body image in response to the image mediated (presented back to them) by the environment which often included scorn and rejection. Importantly, it was not until their body image was mediated and perceived by others as an object-in-the-world that it was thrown upon them as deformed that feelings of embarrassment and shame were evoked in them (i.e., a result of the scorn and rejection by others). Dr. Fisher observed that such shame dissipated and disappeared almost immediately upon the correction of the perceived defect – not so much as a result of self-awareness of the new body but, rather, as soon as the individuals in their microsphere who mediated their body image ceased to show rejection, scorn, and abhorrence.

In numerous experiments, researchers found that people who were judged by others to be more attractive had a healthier self-concept and were more satisfied with their body image than people who were perceived by others as plainer or homely (Cash & Pruzinsky, 1990). What is more, the way individuals in these experiments saw themselves was found to have *causally* corresponded to how they were seen by others. Nevertheless, the appearance of the body and its image to others was deemed by Cash and Pruzinsky (1990) to be only one component of the mental construct of body image which, they concluded, is a *de facto* attitudinal construct, composed of three somatic domains: 1) physical appearance, 2) physical fitness, and 3) physical health or illness. These three domains supplant one another. What is more, the latter two domains are more important for healthy body-image than the former one (appearance). For example, a homely-looking athlete who excels in her sport will not

15

suffer from an inferior body image, because the two latter domains (physical fitness, and physical health) far exceed the first one in the composing of the body image as a self-construct, and are more fundamental for survival (which include social dominance and prestige).

Therefore, while physical appearance constitutes a significant part of the body image formation, it is not sufficient and may not even be overriding. On the other hand, even if the latter two domains consist of physical and material, that is to say tangible, factors – are they not as much mental constructs as appearance itself? After all, to the individual, body image means the experience *as subjectively perceived*, not objectively analyzed.

Cognitive and Affective Functions

To summarize what has been stated above, the body image consists of these components:

- Anatomical: body shape.
- Functional: body, and bodily functions.
- Psychological: perception of the body, and satisfaction with one's appearance.

These components are of two-fold nature: cognitive, and affective. The Anatomical Cognitive perception is how we see our anatomy. The Anatomical Affective perception is how we feel about it. Similarly, we may cognitively recognize our bodily functions, and affectively feel a particular sensation related to these functions (such as infliction or cessation of pain). The Psychological Cognitive function relates to our understanding of causation and environmental influences on us, while the Psychological Affective function is displayed in our emotions (e.g., anger, self-hate, etc.).

The *body experience* is formed by all of the above. It is also placed into the environment, limited by our body boundaries (skin, dress), continuity in space (air/room displacement), time (aging), and perception of unity or, conversely, derealization and depersonalization. The latter, depersonalization means disjointedness of the mind and the body: "an alteration in the perception or experience of the self so that one feels detached from, and as if one is an outside observer of, one's mental processes or body (e.g., feeling like one is in a dream)" (DSM-IV, cited in Berrios & Sierra-Siegert, 1994, p. 214). Derealization is a separate concept which imports an "alteration in the perception or experience of the external world so that it seems strange or unreal (e.g., people may seem unfamiliar or mechanical)" (Ibid.). Distorted cognitive and affective perceptions often result in depersonalization; whereas derealization is less common.

Researchers exploring the body image connection to various mental diseases often first approach the image and its affective evaluation, that is how the individual feels about their body (Cash 2011; Schilder 1935), and then inquire about the cognitive evaluation, which means how the individual comprehends and understands their body experience (Allport, 1960; Barsalou et al. 2003; Krueger 2002; Stanghellini et al. 2014). Many body image researchers follow this division for practical reasons. For example, it may be easier to treat a person suffering from eating disorders by first compartmentalizing their feelings, then analyzing their understanding of their feelings, or guiding them to such understanding.

However, it is virtually impossible to separate the cognitive from the affective function. For example, schizophrenia patients often suffer from body identity disorders in the form of "severe disturbances in perception, interpretation, and ability to cope with sensations, emotions, and body states" (Sakson-Obada, 2016, p. 398). Abnormal body experience is differentiated by Sakson-Obada (Id.) from "body image disturbances" on the grounds that there is no negative appearance-focused psychopathology in schizophrenia patients. Some signs of early schizophrenia may, nevertheless, be indicated by distorted body experiences, which "may be initially regarded as caused by physical conditions" (p. 399).

Petrucelli (2015) suggests that these body experiences may be accompanied by behaviors that are both adaptive (making the feelings go away) and maladaptive (such that interfere with the development or management of the body). Various eating disorders could be cited here as examples of maladaptive behaviors. Even in the absence of a more serious psychopathology, the internalization of an external body image may lead to inner vulnerability, dissatisfaction, and dissociative states. Such states are often accompanied by alexithymia which, in lay terms, may be described as the inability to verbally describe how the person feels.[6]

Therefore, the above-mentioned compartmentalizing of the body image distortion may not always lead to the achievement of cognitive comprehension, and the stage of confronting one's *body-experience* turns into avoidance caused by perceived incompetence because the human being is unable to cognitively confront what he or she cannot describe and verbally express. La Rose (2011) notes that such feelings are common to both sexes and may be triggered by seemingly innocuous environmental inputs, such as a gym wallpapered with posters of bodybuilders in their peak condition, perhaps intimidating the male visitors and imbuing in them feelings of weakness or inadequacy. At the same time, it is interesting how the opposite sex

---

[6] Alexithymia can be characterized as a dissociative disorder because its primary symptoms are the inability to identify and describe emotions, acquire social attachment, and distinguish emotions in others (Feldman et al., 2013).

perceives the same image. Women rarely perceive professional bodybuilders as attractive, balanced, or ideal. In both instances, however, it is the body which conveys the message. This message is the image, and the image is variously re-presented. It is mediated onto the self, akin to one standing in front of a mirror trying new clothes or a different hairstyle: How will I look? Is the new me a better-looking me?

Developmental Function: Body-Self

Researchers into schizophrenia speak of *body-self* as a "conceptual framework" or "concept" used to "build a bridge between different conceptual approaches to the body-mind issue" (Sakson-Obada, 2016, p. 391). The *body-self* concept is defined as twofold. It consists of the *body image* on the one hand (meaning the body as "the object of perception and affective evaluation"), *body-experience* on the other, defined as "the core dimension of identity... or cognition" (p. 392). This division is borne out by extensive research and observation (Allport 1960; Barsalou et al. 2003; Krueger 2002; Stanghellini et al. 2014). The argument in favor of this division lies in that the *body-self* concept "builds a bridge" between the body-object (image) and the mind-body as a "core aspect of self-experience" (Sakson-Obada, Id.). This twofold concept is subdivided into: (1) functions, (2) the sense of body identity, and (3) representations of sensations, body states, and body characteristics – in other words, into pragmatic, descriptive, and representative functions.

A great deal of normative discontent appears to underlie these divisions, as many researchers have been attempting to differentiate between the mind and the body. Several points ought to be made in this context. First, the key difference to be made is that between *dualism* and *monism*, the former holding that there are two fundamentally opposed forces in the universe, Good vs. Evil, or material vs. spiritual expressed in a variety of theologies and teleological principles, which are opposed to *monism*, a philosophy founded on one fundamental principle or category. Both *dualism* and *monism* are then to be distinguished from *pluralism*, a belief which espouses multiple categories (Robinson, 2020). Fundamentalist dualists believe that the two principles (the mind and the body) stand in direct opposition. By logical deduction, this would mean that the mind is not of the material world, hence the cognitive experience of the human body (whether ours of another's) is intangible, impalpable, and ineffable.

While seemingly absurd, this view cannot lightly be dismissed, for, as has been mentioned above, many human maladies of the mind originate from the inability to describe and interpret the body-state in which the person finds himself – arguably because the individual is unable to connect the body-state to the mind-state. Body dysmorphia or gender dysphoria come to mind in this context.

However, even such everyday phrases as "I don't want to talk about it" or the Garboesque "I want to be alone" and the like, may indicate that the mind has encountered an ineffable "body-problem" and cannot align the body-state and the mind-state. This suggests the conclusion that body issues are less likely to be grounded in the body as in the mind. Most of the time, the human body is a perfectly healthy organism but the body-mind pathway and body-self mediation processes do not function as they should. Unable to alter the mind, modify the synapses, accommodate the image, the sufferer then reaches for the modern means of altering the body, such as cosmetic surgery.

Historically, it should be noted that ever since the concept of the body as a "schema" had been introduced (by Bonnier in 1905), researchers argued over whether the body image is to be distinguished from the body schema or whether the two are identical. Schilder (1935, 1950) asserted that the body schema must be distinguished from the body image because only the experiential aspects of body awareness should be understood the body image proper. Head and Holmes (1911) opined that body-schema is the true body image because it requires the awareness of spatial coordinates, which would make body image largely a product of involuntary cortical mechanisms. The concept of body-self makes no such distinction, which is why it is considered a "bridge between different conceptual approaches" to body image related issues.

The arguments about what exactly are the cognitive, affective, and developmental functions of the body image may appear overtly philosophical. That is because they are. They go to the essence of how the individual defines their being. Some individuals are more oriented toward sensory inputs and easier to manipulate by the environment, while others are more structurally-founded and therefore able to use depersonalization as a facile modus operandi under stress. The former category is more image-driven, the latter more body-driven. Operational aspects of each individual should be used when addressing their peculiar body-image concerns.

Historical Development of Body Perception

In depicting the development of the body image, Fisher et al. (1984) emphasized the symbolic reconnection of the daily events to the human mind and the effect they have on the survival of the individual. Survival is directly related "to the way an individual sees himself as well as how society sees him" (p. 2). In other words, the individual is under constant pressure not only to survive but (as survival requires the human being to be seen and accepted by society) also to adapt one's physical and mental characteristics in response to the environment. These characteristics are in turn communicated by the person's body movement and sensory stimuli via a highly complex system grounded by neural pathways in the brain. A cacophonous sound or incoherent sight may produce an instinctive revulsion in the perceiver, resulting in an instantaneous withdrawal, which may lead to a decrease in adaptation and adaptability, and thus also to diminished chances of survival. Conversely, from the cognitive perspective, body image disorders may develop from irrational thoughts, unrealistic expectations, and incorrect explanations for sensory phenomena (Cash, Melnyk, & Hrabosky, 2004).

The first reports of body image perceptions were provided by Ambroise Paré (1510-1590) and René Descartes (1596-1650). Apart from his numerous accomplishments (which included innovations in wound management, arterial ligation for the prevention of hemorrhage during limb amputations, and the treatment of war-related head and spine injuries), Paré influenced the future development of neurosurgery, including his descriptions of phantom-limb pain and peripheral nerve injury, and is also remembered for his "innovations in neurotraumatology" (Splavski et al.,

2019, abstract).[7] Flor (2002) observed that 50 to 80 percent of amputees suffer from peripheral limb pain. Ambroise Paré first described this pain in 1552 and postulated that "peripheral factors" as well as a "central pain memory might be causing the phenomenon" (par. 4).

Subsequent to Paré, René Descartes (1596-1650) used the phantom limb phenomenon in his dualist theory of mind, to support "the unity of the mind in comparison to the fragmented nature of bodily sensations" (Id.). Descartes' "I think therefore I am" was almost immediately attacked by Baruch Spinoza (1632-1677). Spinoza rephrased the famous *cogito*[8] as "I feel therefore I am," thus foreshadowing our modern-day neuroscientific "affect revolution" (Eakin, 2003, par. 1).

More than a century later, in Scotland, William Porterfield (ca. 1696-1771) wrote about his experiences after having undergone a leg amputation. Porterfield was an optometrist and, as such, focused not on undermining the veracity of the senses (as Descartes had done) but, rather, on the integration of "sensory function" into human perception:

> The Connection betwixt our Ideas and the Motions excited in the Retina, Optic Nerves and Sensorium is unknown to us, and seems to depend entirely on the Will of God, who causes these Ideas or Sensations of which the Motions in the Sensorium are only the occasional Cause, . . . The Mind does not itself produce our Sensations, and consequently they

---

[7] Splavski (2019) further mentions that Paré served four consecutive French monarchs (Henri II and his 3 sons François II, Charles IX, and Henri III) and that, as a Huguenot (a Reformed Protestant), he "lived in an environment dominated by Catholicism" which implies that "his practice and life were sometimes hindered by political circumstances and religious prejudice" (Ibid.).

[8] "Cogito, ergo sum" – "I think, therefore I am." (Descartes, 1641/1990, Meditation II, 7:25; 7:140).

must be produced either by God himself, or some subordinate active Intelligence, according as the Sensorium is moved by Objects. . . . Sensation must therefore be produced by some immaterial active Cause, and consequently either by the Mind itself, or by the power of God, or of some other intelligent active Being acting under him. (Chance, 1936)

When Porterfield speaks of "ideas or sensations" here, he does not mean senses. What he means is our interpretation of our perceptions how our self-image changes in reaction to these inputs. He asks: *Whence does the output arise? How come I feel the way I feel about my body image?* For all the modern technology, MRIs, advances in neuroscience and psychology, such questions still remain largely unanswered.

Subsequent rise of phenomenology, in our minds associated with Edmund Husserl (1859-1938), further contributed to the interest in the phantom limb, in association with stimulus-based theories of perception, treatment of pain, and even the examination of out-of-body experiences (OBEs).

One may opine that pain also takes place "out-of-body" where the part of the body in which the pain is felt is no longer attached to the person. Although phantom limb pain is more common after the amputation of a limb, it may also occur after the surgical removal of other body parts, such as a breast, the rectum, the penis, the testicles, an eye, the tongue, or the teeth. It has also been described subsequent to lesions of peripheral nerves or the central nervous system, such as in brachial plexus avulsion or paraplegia (Andreotti, 2014; Marbach & Raphael, 2000; Ramachandran, 2008; Sörös et al., 2003). Ramachandran (2008) conducted an interesting survey of the phenomenon of phantom sensations, and concluded that "around 60% of men experience a phantom penis post-penectomy" (p. 1).

This number corresponded to (postoperative) female-to-male transsexuals, but was twice as high as in (postoperative) male-to-female transsexuals, which indicates that the body (somatic gender) need not correspond to the image (the gender in the brain). Ramachandran (2008) explained the "absence/presence of phantoms" here by "postulating a mismatch between the brain's hardwired gender-specific body image and the external somatic gender" (Id.). This conclusion is fully consistent with the 300-year-old contentions made by Porterfield.

Smith (2018) argued that phenomenology is probably as old as humanity, going back to the Hindu and Buddhist reflective states of meditation. He also connected Descartes', Hume's, and Kant's emphasis on "states of perception, thought, and imagination" to "practicing phenomenology" (par. 4). While we cannot credibly attribute to these philosophers the interest in the phantom limb phenomenon, we may contend that they would have been aware of this phenomenon, and that, even today, it is subsumed in the "body loop" theory, which unifies body-sensation and mind-perception.

The mechanics of mind-perception and body-sensation were studied by John Hughlings Jackson (1835-1911) who "opened up a rich seam of research into the pathologies of orientational body images" and the process of "assimilation and integration that went into the maintenance of a normal postural self-consciousness" (Ferguson, 2000, p. 57). This integration, said Hughlings, takes place at different "levels" at which the *body experience* is being integrated (Taylor, 1958). Hughlings' studies into epilepsy and aphasia opened the door not only to the neurological understanding of the body image, but also to the formation of the concept of "normalcy" – posing the question of what is a "normal" body image, if such a thing even exists, for, as Hughlings surmised, the body image is subject to a constant "presentation, re-presentation, and re-re-presentation," which means it is a "living form through which the self, organic processes, sensations, emotional life, and the world are experienced in their immediacy and continuous transformation" (Ferguson, p. 58).

Silas Weir Mitchell (1829-1914) and Jean Martin Charcot (1825-1893) revived the clinical interest in the phantom limb as a neurological phenomenon in the 1870s (Fisher, 1984). Charcot, the first European professor of clinical neurology and head of the celebrated School of the Salpêtrière, credited Mitchell in his research into neuropathic arthropathies (Charcot joints). Conversely, Mitchell made references to Charcot in his investigations of the fragility of bones in locomotor ataxia[9] (Goetz, 1997). They were both empiricists who based their papers on findings in clinical medicine. Silas Weir Mitchell is considered the "founding father of American neurology" (Biederman and Herman, 2003). The fact that Mitchell was also widely considered to be an "outstanding psychiatrist" indicates the proximity of the fields of neuroscience and psychiatry, without which the subject of body image cannot be successfully analyzed.

In 1920, the English neurologist Henry Head (1861-1940) suggested an explanation for the phantom limb phenomenon based on the "mental representation of the self" which is grounded in past experience and "capable of overriding the perception of reality" (Fisher, Id., p. 3). Henry Head and his colleague, Gordon Morgan Holmes, termed the concept "postural schema" (Head & Holmes, 1911). This schema referred to the spatial representation of patients

---

[9] *Ataxia*, from Greek "a" (without) and "taxis" (order), means without coordination. People with ataxia lose muscle control in their limbs, which leads to disbalance, lack of coordination, and tremors. Ataxia affects the body, but also one's speech, and eye movement. It may be caused by a stroke, MS, tumors, alcoholism, nerve damage, severe vitamin deficiency and metabolic disorders. Genetic predispositions are a key factor, however.

following damage to the parietal lobe of the brain. Head concluded that the parietal lobe is where the "crossover of sensory and memory tracts occurred" and where, therefore, the body image (or *schema*, as he termed it) resided (Fisher, 1984, p. 4). To add to the confusion between the body image and body-representation, the term *body schema* still survives in modern-day research (Haggard & Wolpert, 2005).

While many researchers use these terms interchangeably, body schema ought to be distinguished from body image because, pursuant to Head and Holmes, the former consists of the sensory-motor encoding of the body in the brain, thus achieving the capacity to control the posture and body movement, while the latter, body image, refers to the perceptions and beliefs about one's body.[10]

However, as has been elucidated in the previous chapter, and shall be further elaborated here, the image must be mediated, before it is adopted as a "belief" – where belief is to be understood as a conviction of reality, realization of an idea; thus, until the image is interpreted and realized, it cannot be "believed." The human mind (of the observer as well as the one who is observed) is the mediator between the picture-image and belief. On the other hand, body schema requires neural encoding and control which can take place, arguably, without interpretation – such as when one walks on the sidewalk and avoids a person without really noticing them or in any way mediating their body image. Ideally, the body schema corresponds to the body image where the body corresponds to the image (Ramachandran, 2008).

The concept of *body image* was further expanded by Paul Ferdinand Schilder (1886–1940), an Austrian psychiatrist and psychoanalyst who also conducted research in neurophysiology and neuropathology. Schilder's definition of body image included "both the sociological and the psychological meaning of the environment, emotions,

---

[10] For detailed analysis, see pp. 4-5, 21 above.

social relations, and bodily processes such as thinking, imagination, and visceral sensation" as "transmitted though the senses" (Fisher, Id., p. 4). Schilder did not use the term "mediated" but did apply it *de facto*, as a process of body image interpretation. He incorporated Head's postural model and Freud's "body ego" idea in portraying body image as a 1) self-relation, 2) relation to the other, and 3) existential "thrownness" – all of these being not states but, rather, processes.[11]

In his central work on body image, The Image and Appearance of the Human Body, Schilder argues that body image is the "nucleus from which all elements of the personality arise" (Fisher, Ibid.). This may be an overgeneralization, considering that some major personality traits, such as steadfastness, seriousness, persistence, reasonableness, etc. are either immutable or subject to life-long drills and education (McCrae & Costa, 2008; Soldz & Vaillant, 1999). However, since these personality traits relate to our "sensory impulses," they do contribute to the schemata of the self-concept, i.e., organized models of the self (Schilder, 1950, p. 11).

Conceptually, even more problematic is the assertion that all human beings have a number of body images, which may play different roles at different times (Ferguson, 2000). Berne (1964) explored these "roles" (also termed "ego states") in his eponymous best seller *Roles People Play*.

---

[11] *Thrownness* (German: *Geworfenheit*) means that an individual is "thrown" into the world without having power to change circumstances. Martin Heidegger (1889–1976) is understood to be the founder of this existential angst in philosophy, but we may clearly detect it in art even before philosophers began to voice their thoughts on the subject, as artists have always been much more poignant in expressing this human predicament than philosophers. One may think of Rabelais or Laurence Sterne in this context and, indeed, it is not surprising that Sterne stood at the birth of the Enlightenment, which stems from Renaissance Humanism, extolling the human being on the one hand while handing him the mirror with the other: The image never is what it seems.

Body image-wise, each such role represents a personality feature, which leads to the logical conclusion that multiple body images reflect multiple personas, much like the actor of the classical Greek theater changing his masks on the stage. Belting (2017) equated expression with action, and observed that since the "faces" portend the "roles we play," when the role is normatively posited to people, they have to put on a mask, which deprives them of "any free choice of their role" (p. 23).

Consequently, body image representation, of which the face is a primary functional part, has serious ethical ramifications pertaining to veracity, truth, and deception. It is a seemingly banal observation to state that whenever people try to deceive through their body image, they are opening themselves to being deceived by the very same image. Nonetheless, it is an observation which has to be made.

Apart from the ethical implications of a multifaceted body image, there are purely pragmatic concerns related to our perception of reality and the impact on the human psyche. Sullivan et al. (1956) underscored that it is "easier to act yourself into a new way of feeling than to feel yourself into a new way of acting" (Petrucelli, 2015, p. 32). Both feeling and thinking should be viewed pragmatically. In controverting Cartesian[12] dualism, Spinoza's "I feel therefore I am" led him to the perception of a "substance" with independent attributes (Nadler, 2020). This substance may be multi-faceted but, as Kernberg (1984) emphasized, it should be unifying, not diffusing, because such is the natural circumstance of our existence. The reverse would lead to a swift surrender to entropy. For Spinoza, the

---

[12] The mind-body dualism is also referred to as *Cartesian dualism,* after René Descartes (1596-1650). Baruch Spinoza (1632-1677) was one of the most important early modern philosophers, author of *Ethics,* and a critical exposition of Descartes's *Principles of Philosophy* (completed in 1663).

substance included the body *and* the mind, but not as separate and independent entities.

Fisher et al. (1984) underscored that Spinoza's argument is more relevant to the sociological understanding of this problem than the Cartesian view. Body image affects not only the individual who are is direct or indirect contact with the body, but society at large, and the human ability to understand and influence the process of body image interpretation (mediation) may have serious evolutionary consequences. Fisher et al. (Ibid.) provided an interesting example of how the Ubangi people in Africa[13] altered their tribe's female appearance, to prevent the women from being enslaved – they began to place plates in the mouth, in order to grossly distort their lips. This indubitably painful deformity was duly seen by the European slave-raiders as atrocious and disgusting. It had the immediate desired effect – no women "mutilated" in this way were taken into slavery. However, it also had a clearly foreseeable, though not clearly foreseen, secondary effect: children, who naturally continued to perceive their mothers as warm, nurturing and loving individuals, began to associate their mothers' "distorted appearance with love and comfort" and the "plated lip" eventually came to be seen by the tribal men as a much sought-after sign of beauty (p. 7). This leads to the conclusion that not only is there no stable body image, but that the body itself is malleable, and a multifaceted representation of it, which includes societal input and transformation, is the only truthful representation that can be made.

Charles Darwin (1872) conducted a survey of body image perceptions in various cultures, and concluded that the criteria of beauty vary from culture-to-culture and that "there

---

[13] Specifically the Bana tribe of the Masai People, inhabiting the region around the Ubangi River (also spelled Oubangui), which is the largest right-bank tributary of the Congo River in the region of Central Africa. Burton (2001) imputes the same practice to the Suri tribe in Ethiopia.

31

is no single standard of beauty with respect to the human body" (Cash & Pruzinsky, 1990, p. 82). What diverse cultures do have in common, however, is the fact that the human body is viewed as an "object and target of power" (Foucault, 1995, p. 136). Power, especially social power, is thus inextricably tied to beauty, which is represented by the body.

Konrad Lorenz, Jane Goodall, Harry Harlow, Irven Devore, and others have provided descriptions of the "body image" and behavior among animals, showing that (self)identity and its recognition are crucial to the well-being of every individual. Burton (2001) observed that the human body has always functioned as a sociological anchor and mediator, much as it does in the animal world. However, unlike in the animal world, in the human world, the body has always been targeted for mutilation and laid on the altar of social values and norms – in order to gain power, one must first be subjugated and subjected to power.

For example, consider circumcision or castration: in 1870, a physician, Dr. Sayre, delivered a paper before the American Medical Association, arguing for castration, both female and male, in cases of masturbation, hysteria, epilepsy, or nymphomania (p. 41). Circumcision was prescribed as a cure for epilepsy (19th century), STDs (1940s), cancer (1950s), and AIDS (1980s). Female mutilation (not just genital) has been practiced in all societies on the planet. The Western practice of facial and cosmetic surgery pales in comparison to the Bana custom described above (lip plating), the scarification of the chest among the Karo men in Ethiopia, the mutilation of the feet of little girls in China and Japan, widespread facial tattooing and piercing among various South American tribes (interestingly, corresponding to the decorative patterns found on local pottery), or the wearing of neck rings among the Karen (Kayan) and Padaung tribes of Myanmar, and others.

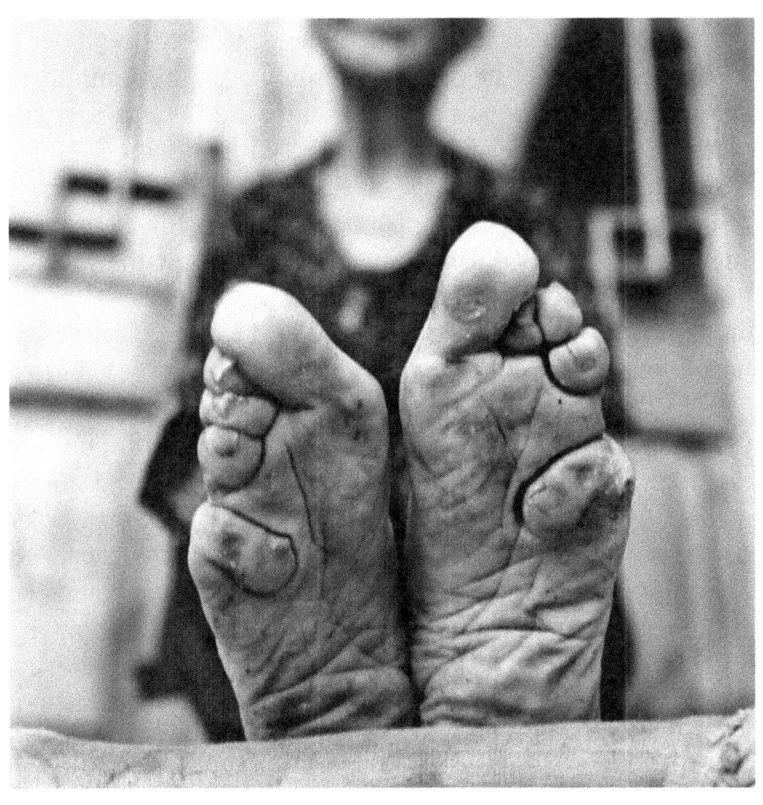

The feet of Zhao Hua Hong (Russon, 2014).

Permanent mutilation and scarification poses a deeper philosophical quandary: does the proverbial Grecian Urn[14] become more real – but also more ephemeral – by being imprinted on the body, or does the body acquire more enduring permanence by displaying the inner "truth" as a paradigm of outer "beauty?"

---

[14] *See* John Keats' *Ode on a Grecian Urn* (1819) wherein the author extolls the beauty of the figures depicted on an ancient Grecian urn: even though they remain petrified in their beauty in time forever, they also forever speak to the observer.

Yet, perhaps philosophy – and, by extension, poetry – arrogates to itself the prerogatives in the sphere completely devoid of such divagations. Akin to the Masai and Suri lip-plates, the neck rings had originally had pragmatic reasons, allegedly protecting against attacks by lions on the persons' necks, as well as distorting the girls to prevent them from "being taken by rival tribes" but, as was noted with the Bana people, the protective and pragmatic facets of these ornaments gradually gave way to the decorative purposes, becoming symbols of beauty and elegance (Senseney, 2019).

The history of the human race has been peppered with transformations of the useful into the beautiful, but not the other way round. True, no such tribes and local ethnic practices go to the extreme of, for example, a gender reassignment surgery, though it is certainly not for want of desire – rather, it is because of the lack of means and the ability, as instances of castration (even self-castration) by crushing or removing the testicles, and cutting off the penis with "swords, knives, shards of glass, razors and red-hot pokers" were fairly common in the ancient world (Jonckheere, 1954).

Nihil sub sōle novum. Johnson et al. (2007) noted a growing trend to genital self-mutilation and self-castration among the modern youth. Such acts will have been premeditated for many years in these individuals. Johnson et al. (Id.) identified four factors that may promote castration ideations: (i) abuse sustained during childhood, including parental threats of castration; (ii) homosexuality; (iii) exposure to animal castration during youth; and (iv) religious condemnation of sexuality. They further conclude that all such instances were accompanied by Body Integrity Identity Disorder and Gender Identity Disorders.

While far from uncommon in the general populace, body dysmorphic disorders can be extremely debilitating and incapacitating, preventing the sufferer from participating in ordinary life and human existence. Cash and

Pruzinsky (2002) further note that BDD thwarts intimacy in human relationships, and even in its milder forms (such as an excessive preoccupation with one's appearance) may lead to "antipathy and disparagement, salience and envy, and manipulativeness and competition" (p. 281) inducing prejudice and gender stereotyping.

Rather than imputing body modifications to a psychological illness, ignorance, or torture stemming from war, revenge, or religious intolerance, each particular instance of such mutilation should be considered in the peculiar social milieu which contributed to it or caused it (Bronfenbrenner, 1979). This necessarily begs the question what the human body and its transformation symbolize sociologically, ethnically, and culturally in a given context. Why would someone undergo such incredible physical pain (not to mention associated financial expense and potential health risk), subjecting themselves to multiple facelifts, breast augmentations, fat removal (sometimes only to be reinserted at a different place on the same body), or sex reassignment surgery, all extremely painful procedures with significant potential side-effects and medical risks? Why indeed, but that the individual body image must be subjected and subjugated to the social imposition of normative constraints and social mediation before it can bring the "owner" satisfaction in the form of acceptance – the acceptance which is invariably associated with social and economic advancement and satisfaction of the person's basic needs, because these needs can only be satisfied by and through the body, and without their satisfaction the person is unable to achieve any peak experiences, including *the flow*,[15] and often even fails to meet other "lesser" needs, such as belongingness and self-esteem (Bandura, 1997; Condor-Fisher, 2021; Maslow, 1965).

---

[15] Concentration of psychic energy on a task without any burdening consciousness of the self (Csikszentmihalyi, 1990).

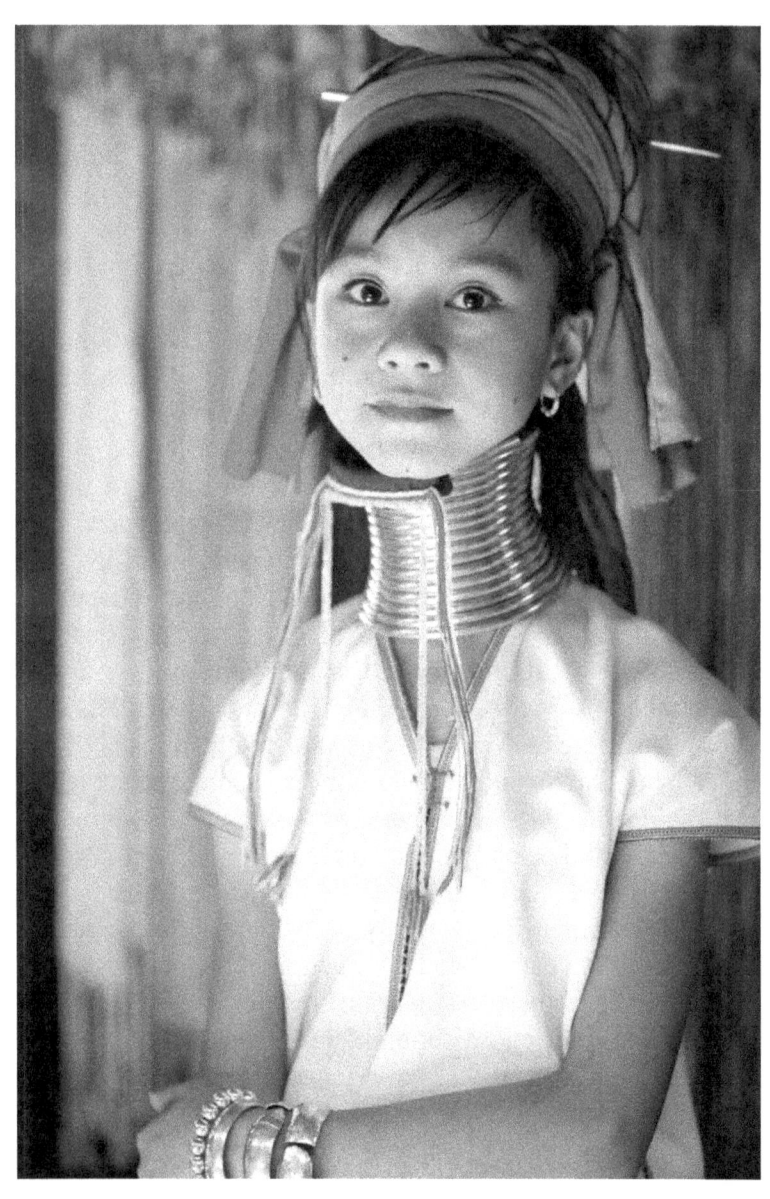

Eddie Chang, *Unsplash* (Sensenay, 2019).

Burton (2001) offers another perspective, which may be considered a facet of the above-stated view. He mentions how when he was in the southern Sudan in the 1970s, he befriended many people of whom a "vast majority… had never, and would never, travel more than twenty miles from where they were born" (p. 33). These people knew one another from birth and almost all had "some degree of kinship" with one another. "Apart from a modest public covering for adult women," Burton continues, "and a string of beads or an ivory armband for men, the public body was subject only to informal control" which led the author to conclude that "[t]he more people share in common, the less they feel compelled to protect themselves from others" (p. 33). Although the author does not develop this reasoning further, it may be argued that a less-dressed body (or even an entirely naked one) is subject to "raw mediation" and unvarnished body-experience, whereas clothes hide us and enable us to disguise certain of our features in communication with others, usually in order to achieve a particular effect. Thus, the body image becomes a vehicle for a message and also the means to an end.

Historically, this has always been the case. However, just as with interpretation of the body image and formation of body-experience, clothes shape who we are – first physically, by forming the shape of the body, and, by the same token, psychologically. "Fashion is a shape, a changing shape," Weston-Thomas (2018) says, a shape that "affects part of the body's natural outline" and subjects it to the dictate of trends, often mandated by the media and advertising agencies (par. 3). In the past, when there were no advertising agencies, people would look at the models of beauty in visual arts, painting, and sculpting. There was also much less shame present for looking "natural" – nudity was common in ancient Greece, especially among athletes, and it might surprise some readers that women used to wear bikini when the Roman Empire was at its height (Laver, 2020, p. 42).

Today, the world is preoccupied with cosmetic surgery, diets, and body-building. Modern "sculptors" re-create and re-shape the natural physical self. Yet, it is always the "other" (often unrealistic) "body image" that the sculpting strives to model. One may wonder who is the artist and how real the canvas or clay are. Such thoughts and ensuing disillusionment have deeply permeated our post-post-modern culture. Lyotard, Baudrillard, and Foucault have all spoken of a "crisis of representation." Foucault did so in the context of language (being overtaken by the world of "pictures"), Lyotard deplored the loss of credibility in representation (because the latter is composed only of fragments and "catchphrases"), and Baudrillard noted that the crisis of representation had erased the meanings from the symbols, creating mere "simulacra" of reality, "empty signs," and "codes without referents" (Baudrillard, 1976, 1981, 1991; Lyotard, 1979 ; Marcus, 1997; Scheerer, et al., 1992).

Our historical excursion into the human preoccupation with the body image began with the phantom limb phenomenon and has, it seems, progressed to today's assumption of "phantom potentiality" or even "phantom reality" not just of the body image but the whole world and all "images" in it. The crisis of representation has turned into the crisis of a referent because the thing re-presented is a void, or can be voided, left empty, or refilled at a whim.

Consequently, the human body is devoid of meaning unless imbued with a meaning; the body schema is a neurolinguistic construct which is subject to fluctuating interpretation; the body experience is the experience of flux and change; and gender is a fluid spectrum, unless filled with gender-ness. In the absence of the original, every image has to be interpreted, and each such act of interpretation re-interpreted *ad infinitum.* Heidegger uses the term

Bewandtnis for a "totality of involvement" with the world, which is to say the totality of all human interpretations.[16] Arguably, however, no such involvement can exist where no "presentation" of reality prior to re-presentation and re-interpretation exists.

In conclusion, if the *body* is a void, the *image* can literally be anything and mean anything. For such an image, the body is no more than a vehicle of communication, a means of mediation, a tool to accomplish a goal.

---

[16] The following notions can also be found in Heidegger, signifying *Bewandtnis*: assignment; indication; reference (Wheeler, 2020). The term is not easily translatable and can be equated to a "large-scale holistic network of interconnected relational significance" that makes the thing what it is, e.g., a hammer ready to hammer, to build a house, to shelter, to drive in a nail, but also to take it out where needed (Wheeler, 2020, Sec. 2.2.3., par. 3). Needless to say, the *Bewandtnis* of the body defies definition, save by concrete examples in specific environments.

The Body

Fashion, Costume, and the Mask

In 1944, Bernard Rudofsky, Director of Apparel Research at the Museum of Modern Art in New York, organized an exhibition called "Are Clothes Modern?" In it, he displayed silhouette figures alongside clothing grouped chronologically, in different periods of human history, showing how differently idealized and transformed by fashion the human body has been.[17] Interestingly, Rudofsky used the word "clothing," and not "costume." The difference is pertinent to the subject of body image in the following respect: "clothing" means various articles of fabric used to cover the human body, while "costume" refers to the period style not only of dress but also accessories and hairstyle characteristic of a particular country, period or people (Chrisman, 2013). Therefore, Rudofsky opted for the word "clothing," in order to show that clothing is not "modern" but, rather, has shaped *the body* for millennia.

On the other hand, modernity is reflected in the *costume.* The French word *costume* was formerly used interchangeably with clothing (or in lieu of *clothing*) in Victorian England, which states more about the Victorian times than that there existed linguistic influences from the Continent: when *costume* is *clothing,* the clothes that alter the body become interchangeable with the cultural normative influence of the *costume.* Disguise and cultural-normative pressures increase in direct proportion with the

---

[17] Bernard Rudofsky (Austrian-American, 1905–1988) was an "architect, curator, critic, exhibition designer, and fashion designer whose entire *oeuvre* was influenced by his lifelong interest in concepts about the body and the use of our senses"(Getty, 2008). He is best known for his controversial exhibitions: Are Clothes Modern? (Museum of Modern Art [MoMA], 1944), Architecture without Architects (MoMA, 1964), and Now I Lay Me Down to Eat (Cooper-Hewitt Museum, 1980).

presence of the interpretation and assumption of dress as a *costume* (which often happens subconsciously). Conversely, *clothes* are utilitarian, keep us warm, and have to be comfortable. The message one sends to others via *clothing* is secondary. People with few body image problems will rarely think of themselves as putting on a "costume" in the morning. On the other hand, those who are extremely socially and body image conscious will do so every time they dress, change, put on make-up, and prepare to meet other human beings.

Weston-Thomas (2018) notes that clothes have been used not only to shape and form, but also to cover, in combination with perfumes, paint, and fashion accessories. To cover what? "The women of Georgian high society" says Weston-Thomas (par. 4), "looked beautiful in their satins and silks," but they rarely bathed, instead "dousing their bodies and clothes in toilet waters and perfumes" (Id.). They wore "scented pomanders and carried small scent bottles… had false teeth, false hair, false bosoms, false calves and induced large eyes which they made to falsely dilate by using Belladonna[18] extracted from the Deadly Nightshade plant" (par. 4). In fact, Thomas concludes, they were "a walking deception" (Ibid.).

There is an underlying shift in body philosophy (the concept of the body image and its relation to the world) that ought to be outlined in this context. Ferguson (2000) points out that in the medieval world, the body "was generally conceived and experienced as a fallen and corrupted being"

---

[18] The "belladonna" (It. "beautiful lady") berry juice used to be used by women to enlarge the pupils of the eye. It is a poisonous agent which numbs nerves, prevents salivation, sweating, urination, disables pupil distention/contraction, as well as digestive functions. Serious side effects include seizures, breathing problems, tiredness, constipation, difficulty urinating, and agitation. It is still used as herbal remedy for bronchial spasms in asthma, whooping cough, hay fever, Parkinson's disease, colic, inflammatory bowel disease, motion sickness, and as a painkiller (in the form of ointment, for the sciatica and joint pain).

which, through its association with mortality, death, putrefaction and decay, was the symbolic extension of the macrocosm of the universe (p. 29). The allegorical symbolic schema in portraying the body as a kin-hierarchical structure was familiar to everyone in the medieval times, and certain elements of this schema can still be found in our modern society: the President as the Head of the Nation, three Arms of the Government, the industrial Heartland, the Soul of the Nation, the Body of Citizenry... The schema begs the following question: If the human body was made in the image of God, what is that image? Surely, it is neither that of Adonis nor that of Athena but, rather, a mediated and co-created *idea* which is as real (or unreal) as its creator's body-selves. Such body-selves assume certain forms in certain times, remain fluid, and often even overlap or absorb one another.

In studying the history of fashion, one soon discovers that there have always been two trends present, not as much based on sex (i.e., trousers *versus* skirts – since men, during different times in history, also wore various gowns, tunics, and skirts), as on form: that between "fitted" and "draped" clothes (Laver, 2020, p. 9). Such distinction appears to follow two paths: social-normative, and natural-free (loose). These are further subdivided into body-concepts according to how the "owner" of the body utilizes it: as a tool (worker), receptacle of knowledge (philosopher), weapon (soldier), or womb of new life and harbor of nurture and love (mother, wife).

Anthropologists distinguish between the "tropical" and the "arctic" dress, but this distinction appears secondary to the influences of wars, conquests, and external pressures throughout history, often caused by various political upheavals or religious indoctrination. For example, the seventeenth century Dutch can be clearly distinguished from the French, on account of their Protestantism and simplicity in dress, influenced by the years of Spanish conquest. Or, one may ask, why did women in Europe in the 1850s wear ten times more clothes than in the 1800s? Napoleon's expedition to Egypt brought to Europe turbans, puffed sleeves, long silky garments, and renewed competition between the British and French clothes manufacturers. Heavy cashmere shawls, imported from India, were now manufactured in Paisley, Scotland. Top hats grew wider, and dandyism developed into a fad not infrequently caricatured by the papers, bestowing men with the pride of narrow waists, puffy pants and stuffed shoulders, sometimes to absurd exaggeration. Skirts grew wider as well, and were weighted at the bottom by a "flounce, frills and other decorations, sometimes even by a band of fur" (p. 157). Such fashion changes have little to do with the anthropological view of fashion, but everything to do with politics, social classification, and normative dictate imposed on the body image.

What can be viewed as an anthropological effect is the overall change in the human body and structure. The average height of a male has increased by four inches in the last 100 years, with a proportionate increase in weight and size (Blaszczak-Boxe, 2014). Changes in the size and reproductive capacities of the female body have been commensurately significant: the age of menarche has decreased from 17 in the 1850s to 12.8 in the 2000s (par. 4). Obesity is the main factor in this decrease, surpassing other environmental and cultural influences, even race. Better nutrition, health, and economic conditions directly influence the natural growth of the human body. Thus, we can still (a generation after the fall of the Berlin Wall) mark a difference in average height between the East and West German males, and similar differences can be shown to exist between the North and South Korean populations.[19]

---

[19] For socioeconomic reasons, pre-school children raised in the developing country of North Korea are up to 13 cm shorter and up to 7 kg lighter than children who were brought up in South Korea. North

Such a comparison can also be made historically. The ribboned breeches, high heels, tight stockings, flaring skirts, turned up, lace-trimmed sleeves, cocked feathery hats, ribbons and starched up lacy collars worn by the 17th century knight or beau would hardly fit a 21st century businessman. This means that the vagaries of fashion follow not just the dictates of society at any given age but, necessarily, also the demands of the ever-changing human body. Or is it the body which is being subjugated?

Burton (2001) argued that the body "has been subjected to culturally contrived rules of body control" (p. 27). Notably, in tandem with fashion, nutritional restrictions constitute the most common form of such contrived subjection. What instantly comes to mind are dietary prohibitions which exist in all religions around the world. These are intended to remind the believer that he is mortal and altogether frail, but also that the body is a mere material shell for the Soul. They also indicate that symbolism permeates all such rules, whether religious or secular. When the police officer dons the uniform, he or she instantly becomes constrained in what actions the body may execute, how the body is allowed to behave, and what interactions are permissible. In such situations, the body is the slave and servant of the social good. When the police officer stuffs his uniform with shoulder pads and enlarges the size of his chest, it is done in order to impress the weight of authority on the passer-by. The reasons why a competitive bodybuilder injects steroids into the same body parts are similar, that is, to conform to certain social stereotypes and unwritten rules, to impress these rules and his own membership in the certain class representing them upon the passer-by, audience, social onlooker.

Korean women were also found to weigh up to 9 kg less than their southern counterparts (Schwekendiek, 2009).

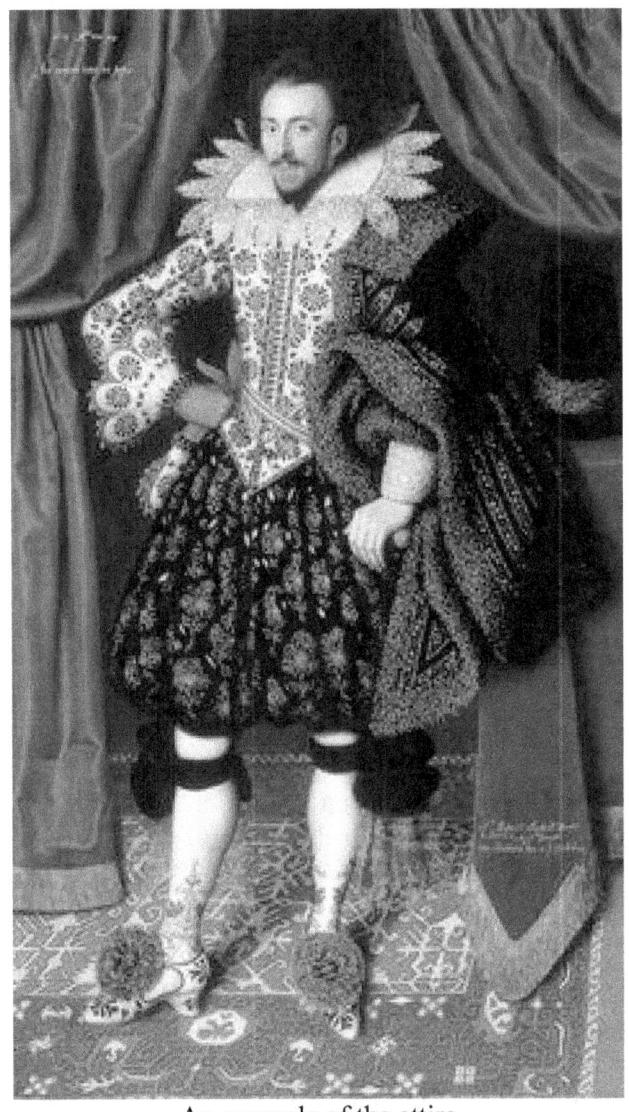

An example of the attire
of a 17th century beau mentioned in the text.

In his sociological study of suicide, Émile Durkheim (1897/1979) suggested that perhaps the human being does not even have a choice in these matters, but does whatever it takes to be accepted and socially secure because such are the dictates of survival. One of the leading causes of suicide, Durkheim noted, is *anomie,* which is a sense of disconnectedness with, and lack of belonging to, the society. While Protestants who are highly educated also have higher rates of suicides than Catholics (who are less educated, says Durkheim), the same is not true of the highly educated Jews, whose education leads to better integration and sense of belonging with their community – whereas, says Durkheim, highly educated Protestants tend to be self-reliant individualists. While whether Catholics or Protestants are more "highly educated" and why is open to debate, such a debate is wholly immaterial to Durkheim's finding that social integration is a key motivator in survival, leading to *conformity.* The fact that this drive is expressed in the way we dress is merely a logical extension of such findings. No-one expects the President of the United States to give the State of the Union Address in his pajamas, no-one appreciates a sloppily dressed attorney in the courtroom, and it is the uniform that we respect and honor, be it that of the police officer or a soldier, because the uniform represents the state, and individual ranking.

The uniform is an interesting example of symbolic dress because it stands for the sum-total of all the heroic deeds of all the professionals in the field. The award is given to the uniform, attached to it, literally and allegorically. Clothes are the man and the man is the clothes he wears. Still, it would border on a fallacy if we assumed that the desire to conform is the sole goal of the individual. Conformity brings about the recognition of a certain place, a certain status in society; but it is also through normative subjugation that the individual acquires a mediated body experience which completes his mental body image, thereby, arguably, achieving a balanced self-image which also corresponds to how others see him.

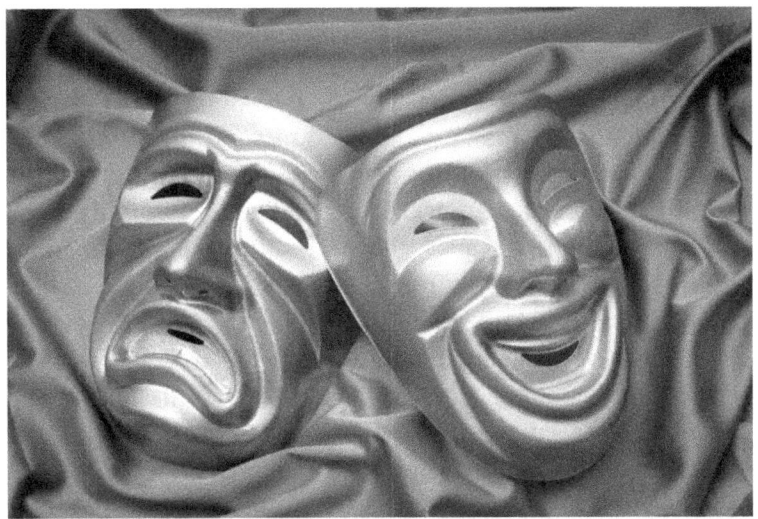

Theatrical Masks-Representations with orifices open just enough to express emotion without communicating the self beneath.

Oravec (2019) discusses dress codes in the academic context. She notes that such dress codes have traditionally been concealing of and limiting to the individuals' expression, such as covering certain body parts (midriff and arms in females) or prescribing what they should look like (absence of beard, short haircut in males). By contrast, the current trend in academia is to allow for "representational choices" (p. 3). They include selfies (Liu, 2018), holography and augmented reality (Díaz et al., 2018), and manipulated or doctored photographs, videos, and avatars (Messinger et al., 2019; Oravec, 2012a, 2012b; Zheng et al., 2016), all of which are used to conceal and control reality in the process of body image mediation. While less stigmatizing with respect to the gender and economic status, race and ethnicity of the "wearer," more often than not, such representations and re-representations tend to be normatively conforming to the "stereotypes of 'desirable' qualities," creating images and "constructions" that make their creators look thinner, younger, and otherwise more desirable and marketable (Messinger et al. 2019; Oravec 2012a; Oravec, 2019, p. 8).

Oravec (Id.) notes that such disguises are akin to theatrical masks which are intended to conceal. By the same token, however, masks reveal. One cannot conceal without revealing. Theatrical masks are used both to amplify the character, and to conceal the real self beneath the mask (Belting, 2017).[20] The mask becomes a persona which completes the costume. The self turns into an image which is "personated" or "sounded through" (*per-sonare*) the mask. If there is a sound, then it accompanies the mask and completes the image. The mask becomes the *imago* or "falsified reality" (p. 52), and this takes place regardless of the intent of the wearer because the wearer's self is concealed, in order for the image to acquire social currency.

In the post-Covid pandemic world, under the mask mandate, it should be emphasized that the mask is not a piece of clothing which would in some way positively contribute to a balanced body image. The primary purpose of this mask *as a mask* is to conceal the face from view because the concealed face appears to be less dangerous than the revealed face, apparently to both the concealer and the onlooker. Our typical understanding of the classical mask is that it conceals the self, in order to portray something or someone else. Once again, however, there is a paradox present even to the most well-intentioned wearer, for the mask creates a new presence which is outside of the wearer's province to wield or master (Belting, 2017). This attempt to

---

[20] This has not always been the case. In the ancient Greek theatre, the orifices in the masks were large enough for the person's mouth and eyes to be visible, conveying a live impression. Modern word mask is etymologically derived from Arabic *mashara*, Italian *maschera*, akin to English "mascara" (Belting, 2017, p. 54). It corresponds to the Latin *larve*, which appears in German *enlarven*, to reveal, unmask. The modern mask is invariably concealing and deceptive, providing little, if any, unity of the self and the image.

master the mask is shown by the individuality some people ascribe to the mask, altering the mask's shape, color, and pattern, matching the mask to the attire of the wearer, and otherwise adapting it to the environment (selecting a dark mask for somber occasions, a bright and flowery one for an informal visit with friends, etc.).

Still, the original self is concealed and substituted, in order for the symbolic or literal message to be conveyed. In the case of Covid masks, the message was "Danger!" resulting in fear, subjugation, and conformity. The latter is what in the Roman world was known as *vultus,* a changeable role which covers the *fascie,* the face.[21] This modern mask betrays the face and manipulates the body image with it. Its impact is similar to some body image distorting advertising which tries to motivate women to lose weight.

What is more, while the thespian mask[22] exists to interact with other faces/masks, the Covid mask is there to hinder interaction, the message being: "The less interaction, the more distance, the safer I am." It is therefore akin to the death masks of the ancient Egyptians, the ritualized "mummy portraits" which preserved the dead as if in a trance, giving them the weight of a cult *imago*, a cultural construct of ritualized, collective value. Thereby, the Covid mask also represents solidarity and unity. It covers the real self in its multi-varied and multifaceted individuality, thus concealing not only the underlying societal division but also stultifying the body-image projection and mediation, as well as potentially critical body-image dissonances.

An argument could be advanced, that the mask (a cover of the face) also weakens the message that the costume

---

[21] *Cf.* to mask or to cover with a mask [Lat.] *vultum alterius larva obtegere*; Masker [Lat.] *Larva* (Riddle, 1838).

[22] *Thespian* literally means "inspired by the gods" but is modernly used as a euphemistic eponym for tragedy or dramatic acting. The word is derived from Greek Thespis, a 6th century B.C. poet of Icaria in Attica, often called the Father of Greek Tragedy.

(dress, attire) is supposed to send about the body image. The clothes one wears always provide context for the face. When the face is concealed, even costume may become irrelevant – because the "whole" cannot be accurately interpreted. The face and the body form this whole, and stand for the whole. The attire completes a symbolic unity with the culture, as well as the unity between nature and the culture.

The theatrical mask (be it an actual mask or the actor's grimace) completes the unity in representing to the outside world the person's character or disposition in the play, but it always requires a willing suspension of disbelief – in order to fully enjoy the act, the audience must forget that they are watching an actor on the stage, in front of the camera, not the real person in real life. In the case of the concealing (Covid) mask, no such suspension of disbelief is possible because the act is absent – the self is concealed without being represented, save for its re-presentation as an expressionless form. Thus both the unity with the Self, as well as the connection to the Other (humans, culture, nature), is broken.

Belting (2017) observes that, from a distance, "the face appears as part of a whole body" while up close, the same face is "separated from that totality and monopolizes the body," thereby "conveying the impression of a whole body," even when it is only the face the observer is looking at (p. 21). Experimental psychologists describe this as a *gaze-distance effect.* Consequently, in close contact, a person wearing a mask which intentionally conceals the face and prevents perception and interpretation, is thereby also deprived of the body. The fashion, costume, clothes do not matter because there is no body image to interpret and no body-experience to convey.[23]

---

[23] Yet another facet of the gaze-distance effect which complicates face-to-face communication and vitiates it when masking is in force is the fact that eye-to-eye contact increases with distance and is more likely to be

How do we accept the body without the face? Either as an immutable, ineffable torso, or as an object-matter with attributions. Both such perceptions cause non-human connotations (lack of free expression makes a person less human) and prejudicial conclusions (conclusions not founded on individuated expression). Therefore, every (concealing) mask not only negates the body-experience, but also leads to prejudice and bigotry. Prejudice results from uniformity and assaults the idea expressed by the voice behind the veil/mask. Bigotry is prejudice by association, i.e., against a body-thing without a face.

Belting (Id.) makes a further observation, namely that a classic theatrical mask does not stand in opposition to the face. The face is a form of a mask, and the mask substitutes for the face. Thus, there ought to be unity between the face and the body even when the person wears the mask, as is the case in theater: the character is happy, sad, crooked, straight, romantic... as the script prescribes. This unity does not exist where the mask lies expressionless over the face, i.e., medical/Covid mask.[24]

Even where the mask carries expression, such expression is stable and immutable, arguably barring multiple representations which would function as a mirror to the body image, thus creating body-experience. Consequently, it may be argued that any form of masking fulfills the function of the cover, which implies the imposition of a representation. For example, burqa is the most stringent form of a mask which covers the entire body, including the eyes, leaving only a fishnet for view (Mubarak, 2009). The cover is employed, in order to thwart males'

---

interrupted and averted when the subjects move closer together (Argyle & Dean, 1965; Knight et al., 1973).

[24] Medical mask, such as the one worn by a surgeon, should properly be distinguished here, as it is also symbolic of the status of the doctor, akin to the white coat of a particular length and designation. Covid mask has the opposite effect, as it is applied uniformly and indiscriminately.

attention to female sexuality (Id.). Sullivan (2021) further notes the cover is used as an imposition of conformity upon women and is inextricably tied to social practices, such as barring women from higher education and higher income-yielding occupations that might bring about their independence. Other Islamic "masks" are less stringent: niqab permits the eyes to be seen, while hijab, al-amira, and shayla cover only the hair and décolleté, and (unlike the burqa) may vary in fashion, style, even color (BBC, 2018). Save for the most orthodox branches of religious practices, fashion prevails and the mask allows for a degree of self-expression, thus also body-mediation.

The contrast of the face versus the mask was starkly presented by the "conflict photographer" Santiago Lyon – literally the photographer of conflict in a conflict. Probably his most well-known photograph is that of a young girl peering out from a group of burqa-clad Afghan women at a Red Cross distribution center in Kabul on November 13, 1996 (Brooke, 2021). The photograph is shown here to illustrate the stark conflict between the nameless, faceless, featureless mask, and the human face, filled with expression. The old saying that a picture is worth a thousand words is doubly relevant and true here, where the photo depicts the contrast within (face vs. mask) and the contrast without: the audience perceiving the photo as a commentary on the situation in Afghanistan. In the case of the latter interpretation, the face represents the other women in the photograph – their anguish, fear, and surprise. In the case of the former, the face emerges as if apart and separate from all the other masked faces, faces which are represented by burqas, whose function may be as much protective as constrictive. That is a matter of interpretation.

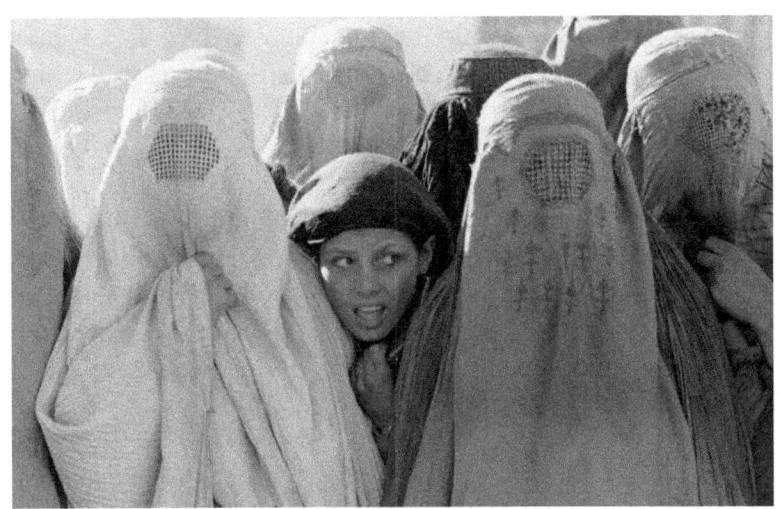
The Message of the Face vs. The Message of the Mask

Nonetheless, protection (safety) always clashes with constriction (freedom). The mask restrains the freedom of the face and, by extension, the freedom of the body. Even if the bodies were visible and the burqas covered only the women's faces, the bodies would stand there like nameless, headless mannequins of different sizes, deprived of individuality. When placed in contrast with a naked face, even the adjacent and surrounding "headless" bodies take on a new social currency and their images are being mediated through the face, which stands centrally in the photo, speaking for them.

The body image is stable (in that the picture is permanent and may be interpreted), but it is also confined to the picture. Even years later, we may interpret the picture as a commentary on the dire situation in Afghanistan, and we may read into the face what emotions we feel mirrored in ourselves: fear, questioning stare, half-open, apprehensive, hungry mouth of the woman; but as to the interpretation of the "masked" women, what can one conclude? For all intents and purposes of a body-experience discussion, they were then, and remain now, indecipherable mute statues. The adjective "mute" should be underscored because even a statue speaks to us – these do not, save for the one face which stands in their midst.

Arguably, the mass of masks does make an existential statement, but the differences in color of the identical costumes are not sufficient to make any individualized statements about the person behind the veil. One is easily incited to prejudice as well as bigotry against the gathering of "headless," faceless bodies. Clearly, by covering the face, the burqa depersonalizes and deindividuates the human being. There is no visual difference between a burqa-clad human and an Egyptian mummy. Should we attempt to trace one, we might conclude that the mummy, with its trance-like death mask and artistic adornments of filigree and scrollwork, is more expressive than a living, breathing person clad in a bland, expressionless, uniform burqa.

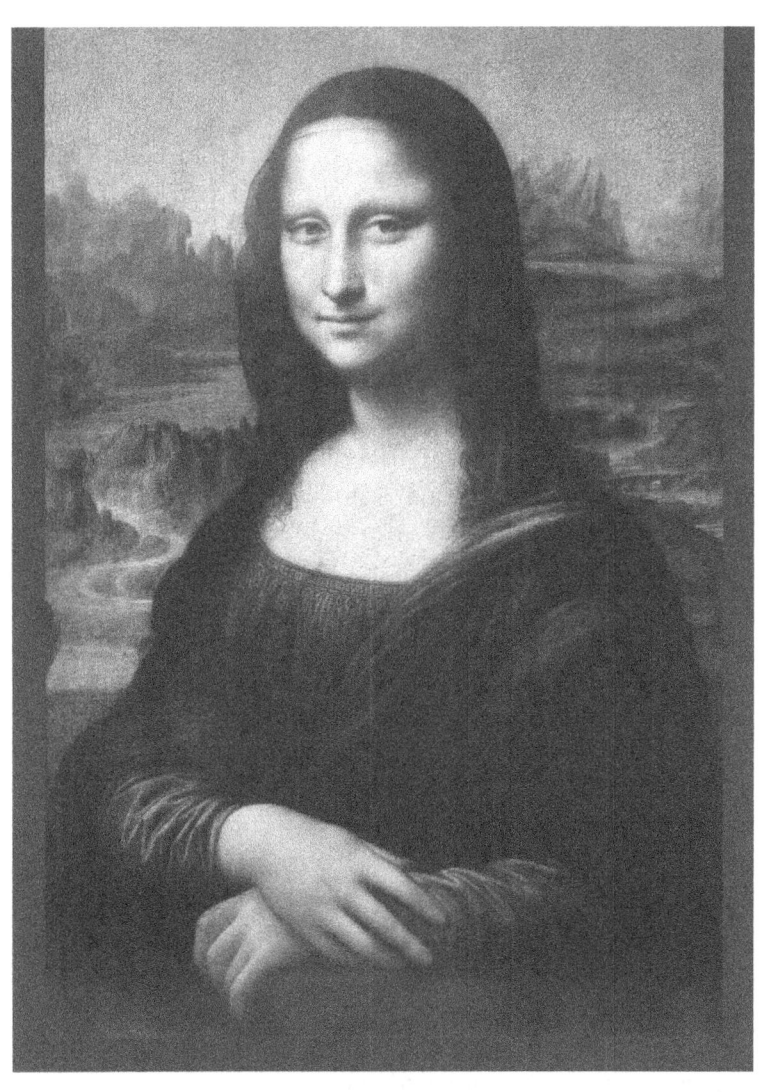

Mona Lisa (1503-1517)

Disrobing the Body[25]

The preceding analysis leads to the question to what extent can we communicate, convey, and reflect the body image without the image of the face being present. Consider a photographic *image* of the painting of Mona Lisa. This public domain image is a common, bland, and generic image of an image of (allegedly) Lisa del Giocondo, the wife of the Florentine merchant Francesco del Giocondo (Heidelberg, 2011). This imputation dates back to the account of Giorgio Vasari (1511-74), but many have noted the resemblance to Madonna, Virgin Mary, and there have been a dozen other "candidates" for the original "model" – Isabella of Aragon, Cecilia Gallerani, Costanza d'Avalos, Duchess of Francavilla, Isabella d'Este, Pacifica Brandano or Brandino, Isabela Gualanda, Caterina Sforza, Bianca Giovanna Sforza (Wilson, 2000). Since so many women may have sat as models to Leonardo, and as Mona Lisa is often compared to Madonna, and because the image itself became a standard paragon of portrait paintings for the next several hundred years, the mediation between the body image of the *image* of the original image and the viewer contains more of the viewer's projection than a mediation of some authentic, particularized body. No matter how concrete in the original, this rendition is an abstract of a beauty, that is to say an image in time, one of many body images the original had possessed.

It has been noted that Mona Lisa projects a "cosmic link connecting humanity and nature" (Britannica, 2021, par. 3). In the half-body image correspondence created by the pleated undulation of the clothes, hair, and Mona Lisa's smile, all set in the background of nature, water, mountains,

---

[25] This chapter deals with the body and its image in symbolic, artistic, and philosophical sense; for nudity, exhibitionism, and related paraphiliac disorders, see p. 339.

and the embankment, we may find an allegorical parallel, to the symbolism of da Vinci's Vitruvian figure, the human inscribed within the cosmological circle which portrays the link between the human body and the totality of the universe (Ferguson, 2000).

While the apparent symbolism connects Mona Lisa to Virgin Mary, the actual expression and communication of the body through the smiling, almost smirking, slightly skewed lips, and sharply pointed eyes staring at the observer, clearly indicate the desire to express the individual beyond the symbol, the persona behind the portrait-mask.

The drawing of the Vitruvian man by Leonardo (viz. below) is comparable but also distinguishable. It depicts the harmony between Man and Nature to the same degree, holding out the human body as a link to the cosmos, and also as a symbol of the totality of the universe. Rather than being "penetrated and fragmented by superior powers," the body was "brought into focus by universal forces immanent in nature" (p. 35). The body is the center-symmetry supporting the frame. It moves as if to fly, yet remains firmly planted in the circle. It stretches, but cannot stretch outside the limits of the circle. The circle is the body and vice-versa. The body attempts to move but can only rotate, and in each rotation remains the same. While there is a similar unity with the universe in Mona Lisa, the woman stands in the foreground – the frame cannot contain her gaze and smile, through which the body image exits and enters the onlooker.

Considering that Marcus Vitruvius Pollio[26] preceded Leonardo by some 1500 years, the idea of bodily harmony can hardly be said to have originated with Leonardo and the Renaissance. The harmony of the body with the environment has been the postulated precondition to the harmony of the body as such (mind-body harmony) for millennia. Sumerian

---

[26] Marcus Vitruvius Pollio (c. 80 BC – c. 15 BC) was a Roman architect and engineer, known for the unity of *firmitas, utilitas*, and *venustas* ("strength, utility, and beauty") in architecture (Macroni, 1966).

cuneiform and the Vedas both reveal a "dynamic and cyclic universe with the harmonic musical ratios" that operate as mediators between the self (observer) and the environment.

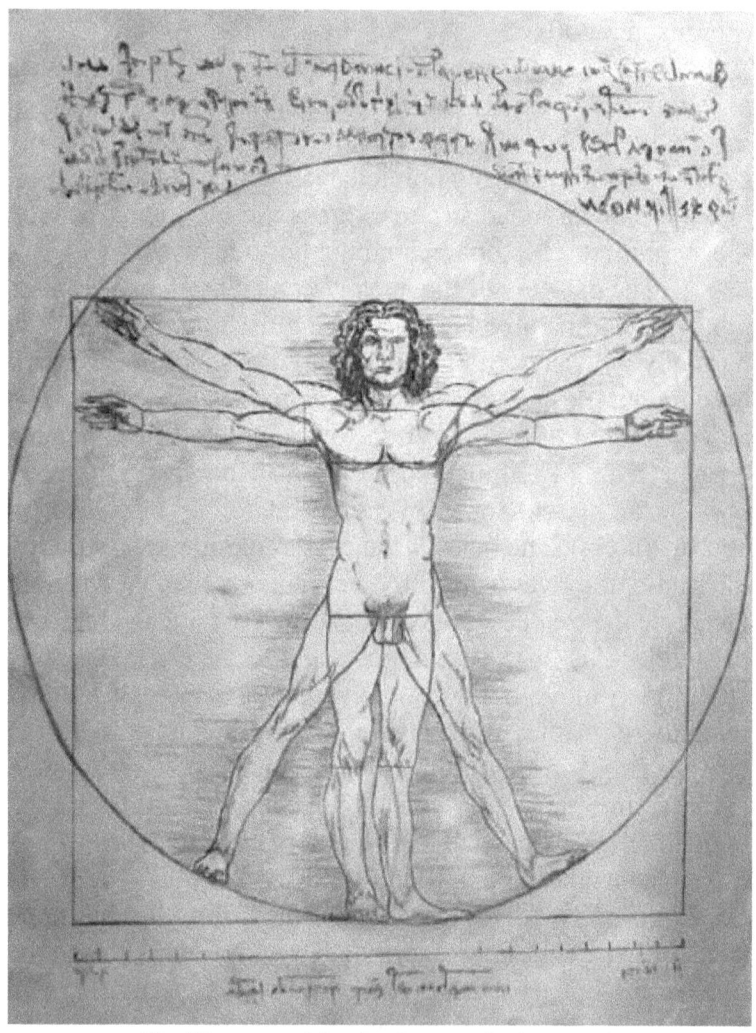

The Vitruvian Man by Leonardo (c. 1487).

The phrase "harmony of the spheres" dates to Pythagoras[27] who discovered that the pitch of a musical note directly relates to the length of the string which produces it (Riedweg, 2005).

The medieval body reflects the universe and represents a universal plane. The costume (fashion) adorns this plane and should contribute to *the harmony of the spheres.*[28] A modern-day reader may ask how is this different from phenomenological *thrownness* of the being-in-the-world and our understanding of this harmony? Our understanding is that the *thrower* is also *thrown* with the object – we are both the body and the projection. The body is not a mere plane, subject, or pragmatic instrument of higher forces upon which (and with which) the ends of the Universe are enacted.

Thereby, the image is co-created by the interpreter. The permanence of the *Mona Lisa* rests not only in the unity with the world (environment) which is an artistic accomplishment, but its significance is also furthered through the multiplicity of interpretations and reflective judgments in the questioning eyes of the modern observer.

What is more, we should not dismiss, with a smirk of superiority, either the notion that Mona Lisa is Leonardo's self-portrait (Watt & Kannampilly, 2010), or that it is the portrait of his transgender lover Salai (Waugh, 2015).

---

[27] Pythagoras of Samos (c. 570 – c. 495 BC), known chiefly for his discoveries in mathematics, astronomy, and music.

[28] This theory was first proposed by Pythagoras, who argued that the Sun, Moon, and planets all emit their own unique hum based on their orbital revolution. Aristotle argued that the reason why humans cannot hear this sound was because it is omnipresent and interminable. Plato also described astronomy and music as twin studies of sensual recognition: astronomy for the eyes, music for the ears, and both requiring knowledge of numerical proportions, based on Pythagoras. In 1619, Johannes Kepler published *Harmonices Mundi* ("Harmony of the Worlds"), positing that musical intervals and harmonies describe the motions of the six known planets of the time.

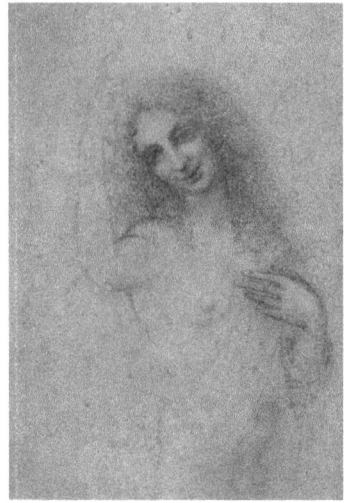 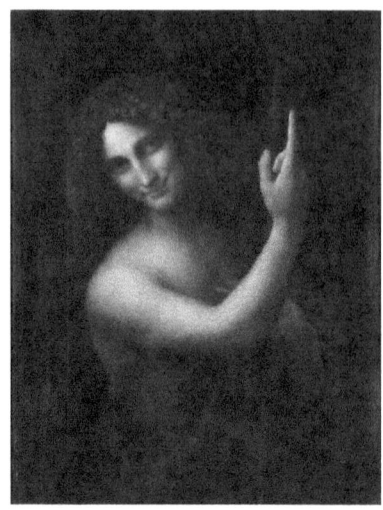

Study of Salai   St. John the Baptist

Above, side by side, are presented for comparison the portrait of Leonardo's lover Salai (left) and his *St. John The Baptist*, for which Salai obviously stood as model. The length of the nose, position of the eyes, and the curvature of the smile are strikingly similar to those of Mona Lisa (Cascone, 2016). Compared to *Mona Lisa,* the difference lies clearly in the immediately apparent fact that the latter two portraits are unclothed – there is no costume which would contribute to the body image mediation. The one expresses the sexual desire of the body, the other stands for the soul, pointing toward the heavens, indicating purity and God, the final arbiter of what is moral, ethical, and good. As such, arguably, they stand in opposition, which is expressed only by the gestures of the body.

Given our understanding of the body image as a "living form" which is constantly being (re)interpreted and mediated, the two may, indeed, also be referred to as two stages ("levels," in the words of John Hughlings Jackson) of the same body image, or (speaking neuro-psychologically) two facets of the same persona. That is not to mention that

Salai's phallus, after all, is (in particular here, in the angle, direction, and size) strikingly similar to St. John's raised finger.[29]

The traditional interpretation of the "raised finger" is that of pointing away from the impermanent, transitory world which is only a shadow (image) of a higher, truer, eternal reality wherein the real truth, beauty, and justice reside. This becomes pellucid in Raphael's School of Athens, where Plato is contrasted with Aristotle.[30]

In Christianity, as well as in Islam, the raised index finger indicates unity with God. In everyday communication, it may mean a threat ("Don't do this!" "Stop!"), request for attention, a command, or even a request to be excused (Mikkelson, 2010). Such meanings differ widely and are not always coherently or logically connected, but they are cross-culturally united in pointing upward, to God. This is sharply contrasted with pointing to oneself, or the proverbial "accusatory finger" pointing at another. Raphael's Plato (see below) raises his finger to God while, at the same time, attracting attention to himself, in contrast to Aristotle's gesture of unity with the earth, which symbolizes a call for tranquility, as if to say: "Harken to the Harmony of the Spheres!"

---

[29] Cf. depiction on the next page. The gesture of giving somebody "the finger" uses the middle finger in the same way. The analogy to the raised phallus is all too obvious. The reason why the one (index finger) as opposed to the other (middle finger) should be different, especially when the fingers are turned face out in the same fashion, is grounded in usage and social custom perhaps originating in the fact that the middle finger is between the index and the ring finger, akin to the lower limbs of the human male. Otherwise, the two gestures are much like two words of opposite meanings with the same root and etymology.

[30] Raphael, Raffaello Sanzio da Urbino (1483–1520). Michelangelo, Leonardo da Vinci, and Raphael form the genial trinity of the High Renaissance (Honour & Fleming, 1982).

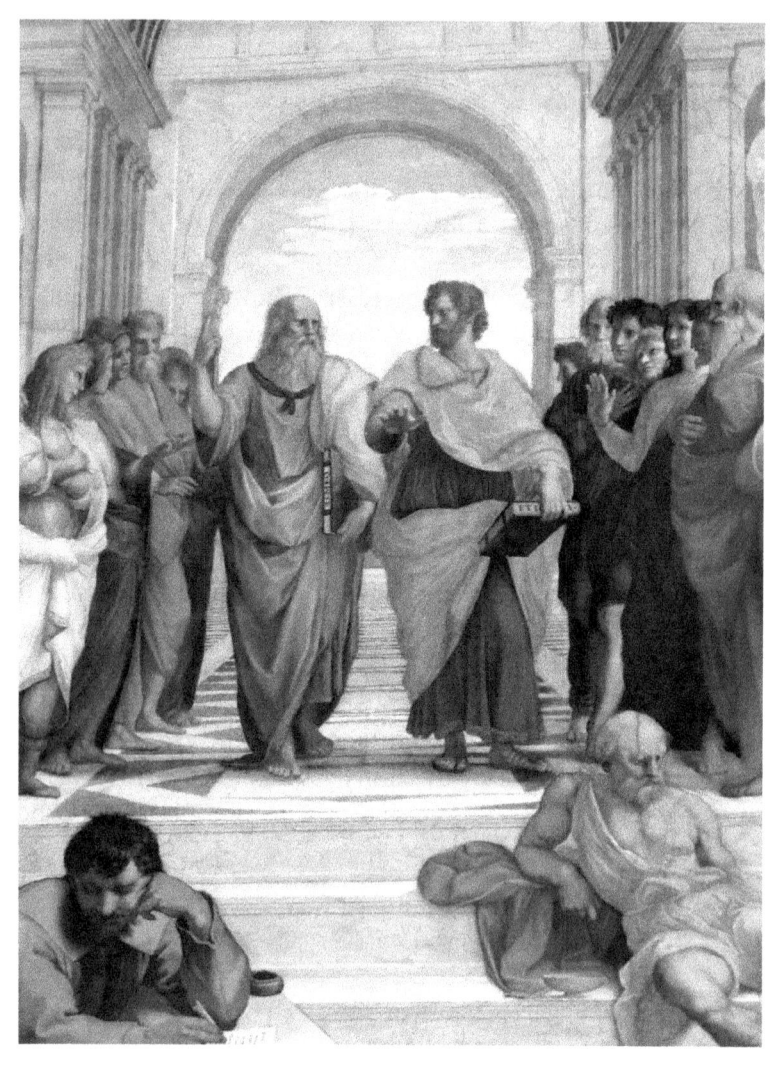

Raphael, the detail of Plato and Aristotle, *School of Athens*, 1509-1511, fresco (Stanza della Segnatura, Palazzi Pontifici, Vatican).

However, Aristotle's outstretched hand also imports a firm command of the forum, power, and primacy of ideas, as well as a disagreement with his fellow philosopher. The two gestures can be contrasted but they do not necessarily stand in opposition. Plato is pointing up to the Heavens, holding his *Timaeus*, a well-known tome which explains the Universe (*Kosmos*) as a creation of some rational, purposive agency, the divine "Demiurgos" (Craftsman). Nothing in the world is haphazard or accidental – all is a product of the higher Intellect (*Nous*). As shall be elucidated further below, this pointing upwards is also symbolic of the separation of the body from its image (psyche).

By contrast, Aristotle holds his hand with the palm down, indicating that the Earth and all that is experienced by our senses is the true reality. The gesture is symbolic of peace, but also motion forward, signifying human progress. Aristotle stands in firm grasp of his *Ethics*, in which the human relationships, justice, friendship, and good government are emphatically the products of the human, not supernatural, intellect (Zeyl & Sattler, 2019).

Arguably, a similar contrast can be seen between Salai and St. John the Baptist. Whereas Salai's right hand is virtually invisible (certainly suppressed and indistinct), his left hand touches the heart, thus becoming symbolic of self-centeredness and mortality, literally emphasizing the body, pointing his "accusatory" phallus at God. Even if we accounted for aging and attributed the lack of emphasis on the raised hand to the wear of the artwork, the hand pointing to the self is undeniably in the center and emphatically overpowering in its symbolism. Meanwhile, St. John's raised hand is clear and sharp, distinct and in full view, pointing toward the Heavens in the same way Plato's hand in Raphael's painting does.

Focusing on their period *costumes,* both Plato and Aristotle are wearing the traditional *chiton,* a loose tunic worn on ceremonial occasions or at festivities, with an *exomis,* a large piece of cloth (six by nine feet) "swathed around the body without fixed fastenings" (Boucher, 1987, p. 109). Both were standards of high fashion, which makes these men normatively representative of their age and society. While Plato is dressed in purple and red, reflecting air and fire, weightless and intangible elements, Aristotle is portrayed in brown and blue, the colors of earth and water. Again, Plato stands for the world of the divine, ethereal (and also "perfect") images; Aristotle for the tangible and substantial ones. By analogy, Aristotle stands for the body, Plato for the image-soul. A similar dichotomy can be found in Salai *versus* St. John, with Salai representing the body, St. John the image-soul.

Perusing the Mona Lisa, the observer instantly notices the interplay between the background and her hair, the surrounding environment and her dark, simple dress with a pleated bodice, embroidered in gold but otherwise without jewelry or adornment, all of which sensibly mediate the veiled body image. This image is transferred to the viewer through the face, rather than the body, which is largely concealed. Thus, the dichotomy arises within the painting itself, between the face and the body, the face representing the *image* through its nakedness, purity, expressivity, revealing no more than a notion of the body, and yet, conveying the entire body image as a purported identity of someone not really identified. The two are reconciled in the process of foreground–background mediation as well as the viewer–image mediation.

Is a similar reconciliation present between Salai and St. John the Baptist? The former uses the body as a primary symbol (instrument), the towering "accusatory" phallus indicating its mortal-physical function; while St. John points away from the body, into the spiritual world, which seems to stand in opposition to the mortal world of the body.

Nevertheless, it may also be proposed that these images do not divide and separate the body (material world) and the mind (spiritual world) but, rather, that they unite them: the sexual function in Salai is that of procreation (arguably the only way a mortal can surpass his death, thus achieving eternity) and it is the body which points to the Spirit in *St. John* – without the mortal body, there would be no immortal "pointing." The Sprit, after all, may not reside "out there" but, rather, "in here," which is to say within the body. One is reminded of the Emersonian *ne te quaesiveris extra* ("do not seek yourself outside yourself") which can be traced, via Persius, to Plato's *First Alcibiades*.[31]

At first blush, this may seem a step too far, given the fact that Salai (allegedly) was Leonardo's male lover (Squires, 2016), and that the symbolic value of all art lies in its ability to remove the material world and place it on a "higher" plane of existence. Nonetheless, this "higher plane" would lie fallow and remain wholly ineffectual without the canvas. What is more, Salai is reported to have been a hermaphrodite, as is apparent from the drawing of his chest/breasts in the portrait, which suggests yet another level of unity. Finally, the observer may wonder: is not pointing up really tantamount to pointing within? When we seek God, do we not find Him within as much as (if not *more than*) without? And is not the materialist pragmatism of self-reliance not directly connected to our bodily autonomy, hence also the ephemerality and mortality of our existence? After all, does not *know thyself* impart an overwhelming sense of *memento mori* of the body?

How different would these two images be if the depicted bodies were dressed in typical 16th century clothes, representing their society and social milieux! Salai's image

---

[31] While Ralph Waldo Emerson (1803–1882) popularized this phrase in his essay on *Self-Reliance* (1841), it is originally attributed to Aulus Persius Flaccus (34–62 AD). The statement is virtually identical to the Ancient Greek aphorism "know thyself" (γνῶθι σεαυτόν), which was one of the famous maxims of the Seven Sages inscribed on the frontispiece of the Temple of Apollo at Delphi.

could convey anything from a wooing knight to a cunning merchant, and St. John the Baptist could easily appear as a philosopher, priest, or even a king. The way the observer would perceive them would then depend on the background in combination with their costume, whether they clash or work in synergy. They are the same person, the same body, which *embodies* different messages.

A synergistically mediating background, as is the case with the Mona Lisa, makes the body image–self-image harmony more likely than a discordant or clashing background, which is why Mona Lisa exudes equanimity and inner peace, while Salai entices the viewer with his lustful phallus, and St. John the Baptist challenges and reprimands the viewer with his raised hand. Notably, in neither of the latter two is there any background present to mediate the image. Thus, the chief mediator of the image is the artist.

An entire branch of criticism has been built around separating the work of art from the artist and inserting the reader-audience (background) into the text via close observation/reading. Such New Criticism tainted views have led to deconstructivist and structuralist philosophies, body image destruction and re-construction while, at the same time, returning us to the pre-New Criticism world in which art was a re-creation of the world of the artist, thereby projecting the artist himself.[32]

---

[32] New Criticism is a 20th-century literary movement which holds that the work of art must be evaluated separately from its context because the context may cause either the *Affective Fallacy*, a confusion or substitution of the work of art for the emotional and psychological responses of the audience; or the *Intentional Fallacy*, which conflates impact of the work with the intentions of the artist. The main representatives of New Criticism are: I. A. Richards, William Empson, T. S. Eliot., John Crowe Ransom, Cleanth Brooks, Allen Tate, Robert Penn Warren, Reni Wellek, and William Wimsatt.

The body image and its perception will no doubt alter the self-representation of the represented (the painter's model), but also that of the artist who represents it – akin to the exposure to criticism and its impact on the author. One may pause to ask who is the medium, and who is the mediator, and what is being mediated? Is such questioning relevant to our aesthetic perception? Whether one is revolted by or attracted to Salai, the desire mediated by his body image and, conversely, the painter's mirror-desire reflected in him, remain the same. A strange merger takes place here, on the canvas between the body image and the self-image, which must have been the real body-experience of the painter. The self-projection and appurtenant self-exposure are, no doubt, forms of self-integration which takes place both within and without the originator of the image. In modern context, one may think of taking "selfies" as a method of presenting one's body image for mediation and integration of body-experience. The clothes a person wears in such "selfies" further underscore the author's normative positioning and sense of belongingness (e.g., association with a political group, artistic feelings, or even sexual preferences), often doing this in a way much more subtle, but no less suggestive, than Leonardo's Salai.

Arguably, those with a more secure self-image will accept criticism with more understanding (complacency, even) and much less rancor than authors who are not certain of the subject matter, style, and impact their work may or should convey. There exists a clear parallel here to the real-life body image. What is more, Petrucelli (2015) shows that the affect[33] flowing from how a person is perceived, and how his or her body image is mediated, shapes the development of neural pathways. His analysis goes back almost two

---

[33] As opposed to "effect" (meaning "result"), the word "affect" implies how the person is influenced by something. Here, the word "affect" means the influence wielded upon the individual from outside, as well as also the resulting effect on the neural pathways and image mediation.

centuries, to Hughlings and Wernicke.[34] The latter spoke of *somatopsyche*, and distinguished two other world-self "orientations:" *allopsyche*, the orientation to the outside world; and *autopsyche*, the orientation toward the self. Expression and impression are two sides of the same coin, the coin which is the currency of the human body structure – not only its self-definition, but its self-expression and its very formation. By "clothing" the one (covering, fashioning, designing), the individual "orients" to the outside, in order to alter the perception of the self by the other – but the same act also involves the orientation toward the self, because the intention is to satisfy one's sense of belongingness and acceptance.

Thus, the human body becomes each individual's "currency" in communication with the world. This has always been the case, but is even more so the case today, in the age of body-shape advertising and commercialization of the image (Ferguson, 2000). If one observed the image of Salai unaware that the great Leonardo painted it, one would probably characterize it as vulgar tripe, an inept personification of the closeted Freudian angst in the painter's psyche. However, as Salai is, after all, Leonardo's, the drawing represents the human body image, and it has a significant commercial value – not just the sketch itself, but the very body acquired the character of a commodity. Today, the owner would easily be able to sell this sketch and purchase a house.

This body-currency is present with us in whatever we do, wherever we go – when one applies for a job, one "dresses up;" when one goes fishing, one "dresses down." The individual dresses to impress, in order to sell his or her self. Women who are single and seeking a partner will invariably dress better than women who are married and

---

[34] Carl Wernicke (1848–1905), German physician, anatomist, psychiatrist and neuropathologist known primarily for his research of encephalopathy (a generic term for a brain dysfunction), and aphasia.

settled. Men who are looking for work or promotion will dress better than men who are tired of their jobs and contemplate retirement. The body image can not only purchase a position or salary, but also respect and admiration. Fungible clothes become unique once they clad the figure of an individual who, like the painter, has a purpose to fulfill.

The obverse aspect is cast by body which is unclothed, unbounded and unconstrained by social norms and moral restraints. Salai's image constitutes a window into Leonardo's heart. If Salai were to be clothed, the "costume" would constrain his (and thus the Painter's) self-expression but it would also necessarily subject the body to normative interpretation and criticism, akin to the one encountered among the critics and audiences whose eyes are endlessly perusing, and minds needlessly analyzing, the *Mona Lisa*. The tradition of bodily self-control and self-disguise is vitiated in Salai, and greatly suppressed in St. John.

The disrobing of the body inevitably opens both the subject (the work of art, here not just the painting but also the model who has been painted), and the author-painter, to humiliation, gossip, and questionable critical condemnation. If the body image is the object and center of perception, as Ferguson (2000, p. 59) argues, constantly undergoing a "largely unconscious and continuous process of construction and transformation," then, one may ask, would not such a process be so much the more "anchored" in space and time if the body was naked? No, because the nature of the body is mutable, and it is by the creation of the "space equilibrium around itself" that the body-self finds its meaning, thereby also becoming "anchored" as (social) currency (Schilder, 1942, p. 234).

Indeed, what happens to the body-self when it is disrobed is shown by one of the most influential avant-garde movements in painting, sculpture, architecture, and literature in the 20th century – Cubism (*The Met*, 2014). Cubists erased the form – or, rather, multiplied the planes of form, so as to provide for spatial ambiguity and literal effacement of the subject. The painting below, by Pablo Picasso, is entitled *Figure dans un Fauteuil* or "Seated Nude" (*Femme nue assise*, oil on canvas, 92.1 × 73 cm, housed at the Tate Gallery of Modern Art, London).

This body image has no head, has no eyes, and the viewer can barely discern her arms. Her nudity is concealed in a multiplicity of planes, and the very body image is dissolved in a strange pastiche of patterns that seem to reflect the viewer's own perception, as if they were a maze of mirrors. Most of all, the key media of communication and body image mediation, the face with the eyes, are absent here. Although we notice eyes strikingly portrayed in other Picasso paintings (viz.), such eyes are unequal, a-symmetrical, reflecting rather than projecting, wanting to be seen, rather than seeing – and yet, once seen, they shatter the body image which forms their surroundings. What is more, the costume is shattered along with the body image, thereby also destroying all social conventions. The eyes offer a mirror to the self, but the self no more than a disintegrated pastiche of incongruous parts.

While social conventions have always prevailed in espousing the *costume*-clad body as a servant-vehicle, fashion *per se* in the modern sense of the word, understood as a specialized industry, had not begun until the dressmaker attached his label to the clothing – which happened in 1858 with the House of Worth. Charles Frederick Worth (1825-1895) was the first to create *haute couture,* a quality, tailor-made fashion design (Milbank, 1997). This design followed the dictates of the rich and powerful, usually the Kings and Queens, displaying their whims and "personality" (Ashelford, 1996).

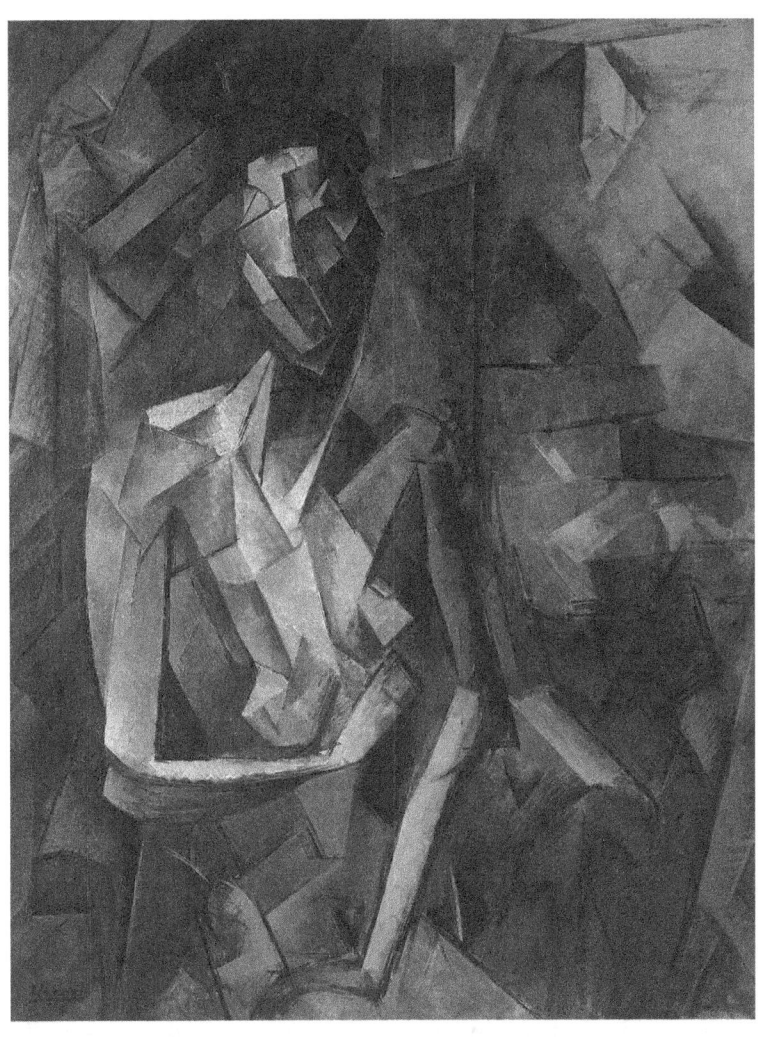

Pablo Picasso (1881–1973) *Figure dans un Fauteuil*
Femme Nue Assise, "Seated Nude"
(Oil on canvas, Tate Gallery, London.)

By the same token, however, having a label attached
to one's *costume* creates a *de facto* normative mask which
associates the wearer with a certain style, brand, culture, or

sub-culture. The mask hides the individuality which is unique, and substitutes it with an image which conforms. The mask serves the *autopsyche* by hiding and protecting the individual, and the *allopsyche* by signaling conformity to the herd.

Consider, for example, one of the pioneers in European fashion, Marie Antoinette. Her dressmaker, Rose Bertin, complied with all her wishes and whims, in turn influencing the contemporary European costume and fashion. Bertin was dubbed "Minister of Fashion," the title which implies a governmental dictate in what is generally perceived as a product of imagination and personal choice. Nonetheless, the fashion whims of the Queen were adopted as symbols of individualism because she, Marie Antoinette, was *the* individualist wearing them. Even today, such widespread fashion features as pastel hair, flower crowns, floral prints, wearing "underwear as outerwear" (e.g., showing a slip lace), and the mottos "more is better" and "the bigger, the better" – all of which had originated with Marie Antoinette – find their place among designers and in the fashion industry, which urges seeming individuality, only just to achieve ultimate conformity (Davies, 2021).[35]

While it is the function of the costume to mask, there can be no masking without conformity because the mask always conceals the uniqueness of the individual self. By the same token, however, the shield of conformity provides not only protection but also the means for self-expression. The naked body is true and unique but society has repeatedly found it inapt and inadequate to portray and accurately mediate the self which it entails. If it is used at all, then it is used primarily in religious context, and for social protest (Jirasek, 2009). Notably, pornography, depicting "hyper

---

[35] For example, consider the "floral crowns" of the 1970s "flower children," the crowns that were worn to symbolize individuality and non-conformity, free spirit and, quite certainly, revulsion against *haute couture* – became unwitting symbols of conformity.

reality of anatomic details," turns the body into a depersonalized commodity (Baudrillard 1996).

Sport has also traditionally extolled the naked body, mainly as the humanistic ideal of beauty and perfection. In sport, however, the body functions as a means to a goal, not as an object of art for its own sake or for the sake of representation. One may argue that the athlete represents a country or team, thereby becoming a token or symbol, akin to a work of art. To the extent to which the athlete dons the uniform and plays the game, he or she is a representative token, wearing a "mask" that symbolizes allegiance. However, once the medal is won, it is the medal which conveys the symbolic value, not the athlete's body image. If the athlete loses, the loss may be borne by the country, but it is not imprinted in the individual's body image.

Even where the athlete becomes an icon, a celebrity, he or she does not cease in individual existence and if the athlete displays the ego with ostentation, for others to idolize and emulate, the athlete runs the risk of losing their individuality (akin to Marie Antoinette losing the uniqueness of her floral prints and flower crowns) because each instance of such emulation creates a copy, a copy which dilutes the original. Eventually, because the image is taken over, depersonalized, and even altered by the crowd, it is the crowd which has the right to terminate it (something which has been done with Marie Antoinette both figuratively and literally).

The Bigger, the Better

The sundry sizes of skirts, wigs, shoulder pads, and other costume accoutrements in fashion that gave rise to fashion design as a profession have traditionally been considered as means of self-expression. However, as discussed in the previous chapter, they can easily be turned into means of preserving the social norm in service of conformity. It has been suggested that the naked body, the body itself is inapt and inadequately equipped to mediate the self of its "wearer." Nonetheless, despite the traditional limitations in body expression to the religious context, social protest, and to a limited degree sports, the focus today increasingly rests on the *body* itself. Focusing on the *image* is often viewed in a Platonic fashion, as obfuscating the real self, even living a hypocritical life (a life of pretense). Almost dogmatically, one wants to *be* what one *feels*, not *seem* what one *should* be or *should* feel. At the same time, this desire is closely linked to the desire to excel, to "be *somebody*," which is created both by peer pressure and mass media but is really a part and parcel of the human condition.[36] To "be somebody" means to be recognized and appreciated for who one is. When this desire is not satisfied and met, the subject often turns inward, consumed with self-doubt. Such self-doubt questions the body as well as its image and may lead to body dysmorphia and disintegration of the self.

Petrucelli (2015) notes that body dysmorphia associated with eating disorders is symptomatic of dissociative processes that represent a "profound detachment" with the body (p. 42). It may not be amiss to state that all human beings suffer from some degree of body

---

[36] This is why the character of Terry in *On the Waterfront* (1954), spoken by Marlon Brando, has such impact on every viewer: "You don't understand. I coulda had class. I coulda been a contender. I coulda been somebody, instead of a bum, which is what I am, let's face it."

detachment. It may even be argued that such detachment is healthy, because only an altogether self-centered egoist or a psychopath would not care a whit about how they are seen by others. Detachment offers a healthy distance and room for growth stimulated by constructive criticism.

The obverse side of such criticism lies in becoming overly self-critical and body-oriented. This psychological impact takes place in human beings regardless of sex and gender. Studies in both Europe and the United States have consistently showed "marked dissatisfaction with body image in men" in both seemingly opposite groups: those with bulimia and anorexia nervosa bent on becoming thinner, and those obsessed with gaining weight and muscle mass (Mangweth, Pope, Kemmler et al., 2001). Indeed, Mangweth et al. concluded that all the bodybuilders who were subject to their research (competitive bodybuilders in gyms across Austria) "revealed a preoccupation with food, body image, and exercise similar to anorexic and bulimic students" (p. 41).[37] Mangweth also concluded that both *anorexic* and *reverse anorexic* men suffered from frequent depressions and were "far mor likely to report 'no sexual desire' than control men" (p. 41).

Two well-known technical terms have been established for muscle-image obsessed men: *reverse anorexia nervosa*, and *muscle dysmorphia* (Pope, Gruber, Choi et al., 1997). While Pope et al. noted that biological and genetic factors may be the root cause here (a predisposition to obsessive compulsive symptomatology, a history of depression in the family, etc.), the origins may lie in societal pressures which trigger such behavior.

---

[37] As explained further below, a "fixation on righteous eating" has been defined as an eating disorder, termed orthorexia (Maine & Kelly 2005, p. 86).

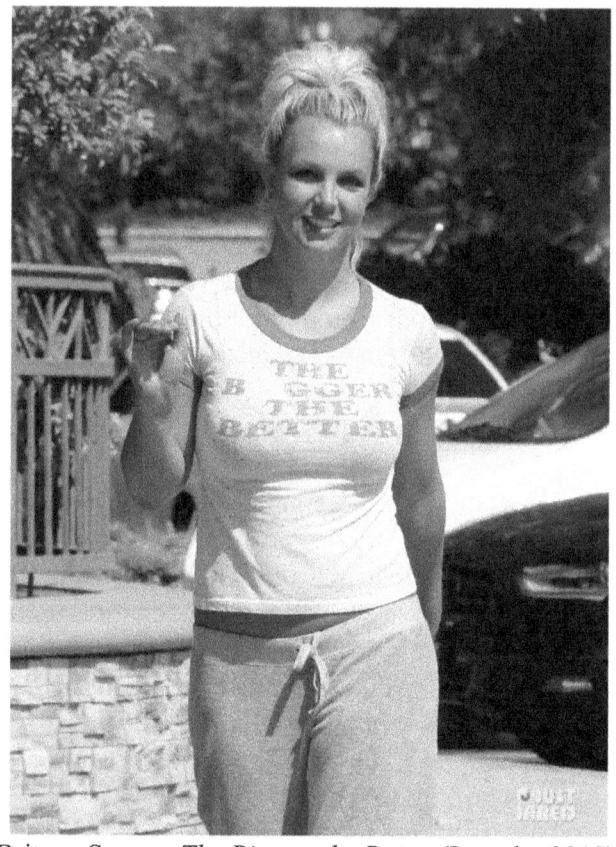

Britney Spears: *The Bigger, the Better* (Lucado, 2013).

What is more, several researchers found that bodybuilders' "fat-phobia" overlaps with the term introduced by Klein (1993), *femiphobia* or fear of becoming "less of a man." Perhaps in female bodybuilding the same is true, only stated slightly differently: the fear of becoming "more of a woman," as female bodybuilders often take umbrage at an outsider's compliment which is usually a variation of: "You lift heavy – for a woman." As the masculinizing effects of heavy lifting are obvious, somewhat different yet akin psychological vectors are in force in female versus male bodybuilding.[38]

In online reviews, Klein has been criticized for bias and a degree of ignorance in attacking a subculture.[39] While such criticisms may be found justifiable and valid by some, bodybuilding is more than a psychological vehicle tending to conceal obsessive-compulsive tendencies, child abuse, and inner (gender, sexual, and other) insecurities. Bodybuilding is, above all, body-sculpting – turning the human body into a work of art – Art built on Nature. It is unique in extolling the naked human body and form (albeit some might object that bodybuilding bodies are not natural but artificial).

The critics of bodybuilding often argue that this sport is "all about drugs." Nevertheless, it is not the drugs (steroids) that make a champion but, rather, determination, indomitable spirit, and the ability to persevere through adverse circumstances (injuries, grief, stress, depression). No-one who relied only on drugs as the key to carrying them over the finish line, or placing them on the podium, has ever become a real champion. They know it, and those who watch them know it.

Still, bodybuilding is outside the norm. Big bodybuilders (not all of them great bodybuilders) are looked upon with awe, often as freaks, often by freak-fans forming

---

[38] Female bodybuilding has become increasingly marginalized in recent years, to the point at which this category was entirely discontinued by the International Federation of Bodybuilding (IFBB), forcing female bodybuilders to either cease competing or to "move down" to the physique category where "masculine" muscle mass is supposed to be downgraded. What is more, prize money comparisons show that muscular women are the least favored category in this sport. Natural, drug tested bodybuilding associations, such as the International Natural Bodybuilding Association (INBA), continue to provide forum to female bodybuilders, although, even there, they remain the least financially rewarded competitors.

[39] *See* the reviews of his book on Amazon.com.

their own subculture or even counter-culture – whereas all main cultures of the human race have always striven to adapt the body to certain socially normative requirements, often in order to conform to sexual or dietary taboos. Circumcision and clitoridectomy are the most common examples. Various forms of body mutilation have been listed in the previous chapter. Bodybuilding.com (2019) goes so far as to suggest that "Men dressing up like women, acting like women and looking like women is big business" but "not the other way around" (Email no. 2, answer). Why is one form of androgyny accepted, the other discriminated against?

When the word "feminization" occurred in the 1990s, describing what some critics termed a "dangerous trend" in our society, it was immediately attacked by powerful politicians (such as Hillary Clinton) as vague, demeaning, and "unfortunate" (Caldwell, 1996). If it were the purpose of making the feminine stand out, these attacks were grossly amiss, underscoring the negative interpretation of the word "feminine" as weak and subservient. By the same token, the term "toxic masculinity" has been advanced, in order to combat the social and political pressures attacking so-called social *feminization.*

What Bodybuilding.com (2019) describes might be referred to as "conformist androgyny" because those who espouse it are, in fact, bent on following the postulated social order so well depicted by Lévi-Strauss (1963). All societies adhere to structural principles which "govern social organization and religious belief" (p. 133). This organization has been referred to as *dual,* because it consists of opposites: sky-earth, heaven-hell, man-woman, sacred-profane, east-west, up-down, raw-cooked, etc. However, as Lévi-Strauss (1963) pointed out, this dualism contains further subdivisions, which are organized concentrically and bear relationship to linguistics and communication. Anthropology is concerned with the search for function (of the individual) in the system, which depends on many exogenous factors. Thus, there are always not only shades of meaning within the pattern, but also separate identities within the same family or class. This deprives the statement "the bigger, the better" of the implication that contrary opposites must clash and be always set apart (big *versus* small), and allows for a graded, comparative scale of meanings.

In discussing the individual within social structure, the parallel that Lévi-Strauss drew was taken from Saussure's (1959) *Course in General Linguistics.* Saussure made a distinction between *langue* (language) and *parole* (speech). A similar distinction can be made between various symbolic identities of each individual within the structure of human society and, by extension, between the body and its various images.

Parole is conveyed without the speaker's *conscious* understanding of the deep grammar or awareness of detailed similarities and oppositions within the given segment of speech or context (social-linguistic structure). Similarly, one lives in the body without necessarily comprehending all the processes that take place in it or the projections of it to the outside. The body-experience is the product of a synthesis of many oppositions, not all of which are recognized and consciously accepted.

The effort to understand the world as a fully consciously projected universe of opposites also collides with the subconscious awareness that this is not the case – in other words, that nothing is black-and-white. As C. G. Jung noted, anima and animus both exist within the same individual body. Their full underlying relationships and interactions are multifaceted, and largely remain in the unconscious sphere.

With regard to androgyny, many different societies and traditions have not only accepted it as natural but have actually imputed healing properties to androgynization (Eliade, 1965; Heilbrun, 1973), mainly because it is said that

79

in the amalgam of the opposites, the individual returns to the original "unbroken totality" (Ross, 1975). Myths of divine androgyny, androgyny in Plato's *Symposium*, the androgyny of the "Golden Age" when the human being was "round with two sexes" are deeply ingrained in the collective subconscious (Fina, 2022). Androgyny has been enacted in agricultural ceremonies, various carnivals, Saturnalia[40], ritual orgies, even in puberty rites and marriage customs (Frazer, 1920; Ross, 1975). The amalgamation of masculine (assertiveness, independence, dominance) and feminine traits (empathy, sensitivity, kindness) has been deemed socially desirable and preferable to a strict separation of these qualities (Kark, 2022).

Consequently, although *conformist androgyny* may be a conscious desire, its root causes lie in the unconscious domain which is both individual and collective. According to C. G. Jung (1959/1990), these domains overlap, because the individual's self-concept contains both conscious and unconscious notions and phenomena. What is more, since the "unconscious psychic processes" are not components of the conscious ego, yet contribute to the formation of *the whole* (persona), they are often inwardly denied, even though they are almost always outwardly manifested by conduct (pp. 275-276). Thus, the "simple" *body* versus *image* division, drawn the by parallel to *body* versus *mind* dichotomy, is in fact the division between the conscious and unconscious self. This suggests that any "mask" the individual puts on (including costume, make up, and accessories) is not merely a cover of the body but, by the same token, an expression of the unconscious self of the person.

---

[40] Every December 17th a sacrifice was offered to Saturn (the God of Agriculture). The holiday originally lasted for two weeks. It included drinking, dressing up in "loud" clothes of bright colors, and changing the assigned social roles (slaves became masters, men could wear women's clothes, etc.). (Parker, 2011).

This conclusion affirms both conformist and non-conformist androgyny. Carroll, Gilroy, and Ryan (2002) conducted research into and survey of various non-conforming gender-identity persons, and found that up to ten percent of the individuals in general population finds themselves gender non-conforming, a datum which far exceeds previous assessments (which had often been founded only on the limited information about those who desire surgical sex-reassignment). However, as the latter (much like other cosmetic surgery procedures) has become more widely accessible and medically safer in recent years, its popularity has increased correspondingly.

While presenting us with an extreme of body image transformation, such treatment merely represents a variation on the scale of self-expression and desire for body image mediation present in all human beings. It also exemplifies a singular embodiment of "the bigger, the better" fashion statement in the title of this chapter: the greater the extreme, the more discernible the body image expression.

Nevertheless, one might pause to ask: Is catering to the extreme conformist or non-conformist? Does a person whose pursuit of plastic surgery or size in bodybuilding never ends attend to the conformist or individualistic social strains? To what extent does the presumption of conformity matter? In the portrait of Salai, the observer notes clear erosion of the conformist dichotomy, not its affirmation. It is this erosion and the appurtenant emphasis on the individuality of the body image which attracts audiences – not just because it is something new or an expression of a secret-cum-open taboo, but also because the artist shows how the body connects to and embodies the inner self. The body is the tool for the expression of the Soul.

Consequently, the meaning of *the Bigger, the Better* imports the depth and breadth of the Self. This conclusion defies the traditional meaning of *the Bigger, the Better* as affirmative of gender and sexual stereotypes. Indeed, both interpretations – the one which says that the pursuit of size is an expression of individual uniqueness, and the one which argues that it is an expression of conformist tendencies and social subjugation – are equally valid and not at all inconsistent. It would be psychologically, socially, and, above all, artistically narrow-minded to focus only on one of the two modes of expression. There are many shades of gray between the black and white of body imagery.

Burton (2001) notes that transforming "or attempting to control" the human body has developed from merely a form of "vanity" into "consumer culture" (p. 61). This consumer "cosmetic culture" is an expression of the "individual's desire for status and power," to achieve a greater social value and esteem (p. 62). While undoubtedly true, such a view encompasses only part of the reasoning. The body is the extension of the Ego, which cannot find fulfilment in a solipsistic existence devoid of body-mediation. First, not always is a cosmetic alteration used to advance social value (Allen, 2020). There are forms of body transformation which actually diminish the individual's social standing and power, such as the gender reassignment surgery, whose sole purpose is to align the mind and the body and place them in unity. This unity is influenced by the environment and upbringing, and conforms to social convention. Second, the cosmetic alteration Burton (2001) speaks of is often used to assert one's unconscious needs of self-affirmation, such as the need for affection and approval, personal admiration and achievement, perfection, and unassailability (Drapela, 1995). It was Horney (1942, 1950) who first pointed out that the lack of fulfilment of these needs leads to neuroticism and compulsiveness.

It appears that the connotative undertones and allegorical implications of "the bigger, the better" lead to the conclusion that the more emphatically the *image* is expressed, the more accurate the *body* will be in its correspondence to the individual's self-perception; should this not be the case, then the expression of "the bigger, the better" will, in turn, shape the Self, so as to make the *body* correspond to the *image* and, ultimately, merge in one.

Size is the most immediately perceptible and palpable dimension. Yet, it is important symbolically, not actually. After all, self-perception is not only "synaesthetic" (Schilder, 1950, p. 39) but also synthetic. In other words, each individual human being perceives the Self through all the faculties, and then synthesizes the inputs into a real-life image. The same is the case with the individual perception of other human beings. The extent to which the perceptions cannot be processed syneasthetically corresponds to the extent to which one's self-affirmation remains subverted, resulting in a correspondingly subverted Self vis-à-vis body image perception. The notion[41] of size helps prevent such a subversion.

---

[41] *Notion*, defined as: belief and understanding about, perception of, awareness and cognizance of. Traditionally, philosophers and cognitive scientists considered the mind to be divided into "input units (perception), central processing (cognition), and output units (action)" (Tillas & Vosgerau, 2015, p. 1). The word *notion* unites this tripartite division. Modern artificial intelligence (AI) research also uses the term *grounding,* asserting that "cognition is grounded in bodily states" (p. 2). As size improves perception, it facilitates cognition and grounding. Body image (body images or body image states) create the synesthetic awareness of the Self, as argued in the text, and thus contribute to *grounding* and cognition. In this regard, there can be no AI unless there is a body image perception.

Body Dissociation, Distortion, Dysmorphia

Each and every time the body image is mediated, it is necessarily also being distorted because such mediation consists of the transfer and translation of the meaning, and imposition of new and added meanings. Indeed, the more precisely one tries to define the self, the more ground for distortion there will be – much like an apparently clear and sharp picture on the modern HDTV screen which, upon closer inspection, will prove to be but a pixelated and fragmented amalgam of millions of seemingly independent pieces. At the same time, the image changes so fast and so smoothly that the minute changes and alterations often remain unnoticed. Yet, one's lifestyle, mental and physical development, environmental factors, willpower, and inner and outer persuasion about what one should look like are constantly impacting the formation and transformation of one's body image.

Each individual absorbs and perceives the world, and immediately reacts to it, trying to contribute to it, to mean and symbolize something. Arthur Schopenhauer stated that there is no Being without Will because the Will is the consciousness of the world – the world which cannot be perceived without "willing something" (Schopenhauer, 1818, p. 23). What does one will the most? To mean something in the world, to be somebody (see note 36, above). But since there can be no being somebody without being interpreted as somebody, and no objective interpretation without symbolization, the identity of Being is formed on the symbolic plane. The body continually "symbolizes a particular identity" (Schöen, 2015, p. 61). Self-identification follows the symbolic representation of the body.

It is the viewer who interprets – and symbolizes – the body, whether it be one's self in the mirror or a stranger one meets in the street. Ogden (2015) called this process *mentalizing* and defined it as "identifying, distinguishing, and predicting" another person's actions and responding to them in "movement, expression, gesture, posture, and so on" (p. 94).

Conversely, individuals may refuse to face and interpret reality. If one encounters something too gruesome to believe, a suspension of belief or outright disbelief and disassociation takes place, aimed at preventing foreseeable consequences one does not want to face and deal with. One refuses to *mentalize* the image. Take, for example, the well-known case of Kitty Genovese. Rosenthal (1964) noted that out of the 38 witnesses that saw this prolonged stabbing and murder of a sweet neighborhood lady returning home from work, "only one called the police, nearly half-an-hour after the murder had occurred" (Condor-Fisher, 2021, p. 169). Not one person from among the thirty-eight tried to help her. Yet, all of them were watching the murder take place, looking on in silent complicity.

"*Depersonalization*" and "fear of getting involved" were cited among most frequent "excuses" (Rosenthal, 1964, p. 75). The word "excuses" is rightfully stated in quote marks because depersonalization is characterized as a dissociative disorder caused by (witnessing) extremely stressful events. When such overwhelming fear occurs, the consequent depersonalization may become a chronic disease (Psychologytoday, 2022).

"Public apathy," Rosenthal (1964) concluded, "is itself a manifestation of aggressiveness" (p. 81).[42] This leads

---

[42] Dissociation may also cause passive-aggressive behavior that occurs in bullying. Consider, for example, the case of Dawn-Marie Wesley (May 5, 1986–November 10, 2000), who was a Canadian student who committed suicide, after a cycle of psychological torture and verbal threats from three female peers at her high school (Knopp, 2006). Her suicide note read: "If I try to get help, it will get worse. They are always looking for a new person to beat up and these are the toughest girls. If I ratted, they would get expelled from school and there would be no stopping them. I love you all so much." (Alphonso, 2000, par. 2) She

to one possible conclusion, namely that people who do not want to be perpetrators (because they are fearful, for various reasons) "vicariously enjoy the act…because our civilization has primed them for such experience" (Condor-Fisher, 2021, p. 170). This *priming* takes place every day, on television, through computer games, mass media – eventually effectuating a "a sort of posthypnotic suggestion" (Rosenthal, 1964, p. 83).

Another possible explanation for the apathy lies in disbelief and reinterpretation of the stressful event in some willfully positive light, such as a "lover's argument" or a "domestic situation" (p. 81). National audiences critical of the apathetic attitude of the actual witnesses were quoted to have used the abstracting and disassociating "they" and the collectivizing, guilt-dissolving "we" in their comments, such as: "What have we come to!" And: "This could never happen in my neighborhood!" (p. 82). Such distancing may be a sign of collective guilt,[43] but it may also be symptomatic of *exospheric apathy*.

Exosphere is thin air in which molecules are so sparse that they do not collide. The term exospheric apathy captures the environment in which body images do not meet, collide, and do not become interpreted and mediated.[44] Whatever the cause, the consequences may be dire, resulting in insomnia, neuroses, family disputes and victimization of

---

killed herself at the age of 14. Her parents found her hanging on a dog leash in her bedroom (Condor-Fisher, 2021, p. 473).

[43] As Karl Jaspers (1883-1969) had proposed in *Die Schuldfrage* (1946; transl. *The Question of German Guilt*, 1947).

[44] The stigma associated with social "invisibility" is well known in psychology as well as literature. Writers as diverse as Ralph Ellison (*Invisible Man*), Herman Melville (*Bartleby, the Scrivener*), H. G. Wells (*Invisible Man*), Alexander Dumas (*The Man in the Iron Mask*), and Franz Kafka (*Metamorphosis*) have used the inexpressibility, inability of mediation and accurate perception of the body-image as symbolic of oppression. Associated ostracism and opprobrium usually lead to personal destruction.

the self, leading to suicide or suicidal ideation. Apathy is invariably present in long-term bullying victims, but not in bullies – unless they are also victims of bullying (Condor-Fisher, 2021; Rivara & Le Menestrel, 2016). The latter can be explained by the fact that bullies are interested in another's body image, in order to escape one's own.

Depersonalization, distancing, and disassociation are all interconnected. Bessel et al. (2022) conducted research into "correlations between PTSD, dissociation, somatization and affect dysregulation" and found not only that there is a "significant" connection but also that the different diagnostic classifications (DSM III and DSM IV) of these dissociative disorders do a disservice to practitioners because they separate what are otherwise interconnected psychological states.

Petrucelli (2016) noted that "parental mis-attunements" in childrearing are causally related to the later "dysregulation of affect, impairment of attachment, impaired cognitive processing, and a greater reliance on external stimulators" such as food (anorexia, bulimia, overeating), drugs, alcohol, and other "soothing mechanisms" (p. 37). The "misattunements" Petrucelli refers to are the inappropriate or inadequate parental responses to the child's (through conduct and gesticulation implied) demands for body image mediation – in essence affirmation of one's self. Parents may either try to project their "idea" of what a child should be (often unrealistic and idealized expectations),[45] or they will insufficiently empathize with the child's emotions, and thus prevent a natural and full body image development in the child.

---

[45] Needless to say, in such instances, the parental expectations are often driven by the adults' very own frustrations and disappointments in body image mediation stemming from *their* childhood and formative years. Body image disassociation or distortion may thus become not only a cyclical, but a generational (if not genetically ingrained) problem.

In such instances, the child develops a distorted or insecure body image and will continue to crave for self-affirmation later in life. Such cravings will be accompanied by emotional dysregulation and misplaced bursts of emotion, amplified, and accompanied by self-anger, self-hate, and the resulting detriment to interpersonal relationships. The fact that even experts in the field cannot agree on how to approach these conditions – suggesting "dynamic therapies" to increase trust and intimacy, on the one hand, and suppression or treatment of the somatic symptoms of these states by medication, on the other – bears testimony to their utmost complexity (Bessel, 2022, pp. 15-16).

It is imperative that we realize that what lies at the core of such a-social or even anti-social conduct is the frustration from the lack of adequate body image mediation, thus body/self-satisfaction which, in turn, leads to the inability of self-fulfillment and self-realization. The affected person then either does everything in their power to create a new body image (be it to adapt to the pressures of the environment, such as childhood bullying, or to accommodate the requirements of parental idealizations), or continues through cyclical disassociation with whatever extant body image they may have, perceiving the body as a burden to the soul, a prison for one's sins – the sins of not satisfactorily reflecting and responding to the needs of society.

Since body image mirrors, integrates, and re-integrates body-self experience, it may be argued that when this process is stultified or hampered, the individual's personal development is also hindered. Conversely, Halsted (2015) notes, that the difficulties with self-regulation and emotional dysfunction projected in (for example) eating disorders, "can be understood as evidence of a poor capacity for reflexive integration" (p. 81). This is seen by the Self as a failure and, naturally, the affected person seeks answers.

Finding none, he feels diminished, weakened, inferior to others. Feelings of fear and insecurity follow. Thus, the misunderstood and misinterpreted body image undermines the psychic structure of the individual, which may result in emotional instability, self-harm, even suicide.

It is also possible that where the microecological (family, school) misattunements are present and the developing child does not come up to the body image expectations of her immediate environment, she succumbs to the pressure and, in order to avoid the feelings of guilt and succumb to potential self-destruction, she will merge or integrate the self-image with the image of another, literally taking on the skin of the perceived oppressor, be it the dominant parent or the bullying peer in school or at the workplace. A naturally insecure and weaker individual may perceive such social pressures as forms of psychological abuse.

This self-destructive detrimental cycle can, however, be broken when the individual (through self-learning process, experience, or contact with a caring and like-minded friend) realize that this process is not uncommon, and that some of the apparently healthy and self-assured individual with seemingly unshakeable body images are in fact carrying those images as shields, carefully constructed to cover their inner insecurities.

Can such a shield become a second skin and grow so deep that the first skin disappears entirely? After all, dissociation may be created consciously, as a self-induced defensive mechanism, necessary to protect the integrity of the Self. Understanding how dissociation works may also lead to reframing one's bodily experience, leading to the comprehension and acceptance of one's body image. The latter was described by Orbach (2006) in the example of a transformation German soldiers had to undergo, in order to become worthy of their Übermensch status, the de-construction then a re-construction of their bodies so that "they developed, through repetitive brutal physical and mental pedagogy, a body armature" which turned them into "impervious fighting machines: solid, impenetrable, steely structures fit to kill" (p. 89). Such pragmatic approach is not unique to the German army in World War II. It is common in parenting and schooling all around the world. Indeed, even in self-improvement and physical education fields. Many "average" people go to the gym precisely with this aim – to deconstruct and rebuild their bodies, in order to become better, stronger, capable of self-defense, endurance under stress, but perhaps also self-abnegation in times of abuse. Likewise, many professionals are trained with the goal to become virtually impervious fighting machines in their respective professions, learning how to cover up their own insecurities and doubts, or even turn them into assets.[46]

However, we would be amiss to characterize their efforts as merely constructing a shield or building second skin. Indeed, we may argue that if there exists dissociation or dysmorphia at the start of the "body deconstruction," it will be there at the end. Depression and disassociation will only become more pronounced because the body image has been reconstructed pursuant to the requirements of society or a certain normative pattern, and not as a true reflection of one's self. Many examples have been provided to confirm such findings (Carroll et al., 2002; Orbach, 2006; Yochai, 2019). Would it therefore not be appropriate to conclude that body image mediation is not a cure-all for body image disassociation and dysmorphia?

---

[46] Lawyers and real estate brokers stand out in this regard. Upon closer inspection of a respected litigator, one may find an intimidated schoolboy bully whose inner needs for belongingness and love have never been met. His entire persona has been frozen and stultified in the eighth grade when he found out that "bullying works." All he has, all he ever will have, is his image. Even his tie, suit, and briefcase are symbolic armor hiding and protecting his real self, deflecting, and shielding him from being recognized for what he really is.

The process described above consisted not of interpretation and mediation of the image but, rather, of the outside forces imposing their "image" regardless of the wants and needs of the individual. Chirisa (2017) noted that body image dissociation originates in disconnectedness of "thoughts, memories, surroundings, actions and or identity" (par. 1). To date, there has been no research showing that one is born with a dissociative disorder in one's head, so to speak. Dissociative disorders are "typically and originally caused by trauma" (par. 2). The problem is that the trauma may be so deeply seated, or so forcefully suppressed, or so distant in the past and defying definition that no conscious memory exists to bring it into the open, deconstruct and reconstruct within the framework of the existing body-experience. Dissociative disorders most often form "in children subjected to long-term physical, sexual or emotional abuse" (par. 3). Post-traumatic stress disorder (PTSD) and various traumatic events may also trigger dissociative disorders. Chirisa (2006) listed the following dissociative disorders:

- **Dissociative amnesia** (which is not caused by a physical but a psychological trauma): dissociative amnesia may be localized, selective, generalized, systemized (related to a category of information, such as all information about the abuser).
- **Dissociative amnesia with fugue**: *fugue state* is a state of memory loss, loss of awareness of one's identity.
- **Dissociative identity disorder** (multiple personality disorder): which consists of the person's loss of one's own identity and association with that of another, which may include a different name, gender, age, identity, even the accent, and (family) history. "One personality state may not be aware of any others" (par. 10).

- **Depersonalization disorder**: when the person perceives surrounding objects and people in different shapes and forms.
- **Derealization**: which consists of detachment from one's own life, when the individual is literally watching one's life as a movie.

Ogden et al. (2006) described a case of a patient suffering from the dissociative identity disorder. When asked about her body-experience (what she was experiencing in her body), she "started rubbing her arms and legs aggressively" while calling her body "dirty" (p. 212). The therapist then inquired about the last time she felt comfortable in her body. She recalled being pushed on a swing by her grandfather. The therapist then asked her to let the sensations "hang out" and report what she felt at that time. The feelings of being "dirty" disappeared and were instantly substituted by the expansion of the lungs, improved posture, muscle tautness and other positive sensations from the swing.

Therefore, body image can be consciously manipulated. The human body is the means and primal tool for regaining a positive self-image. Unfortunately, the path to positive body image is the same as the path to dissociation, only in the opposite direction. Since trauma comes in all shapes and forms, not all of which are conscious to the individual (and when it occurs, it may reverse the positive flow of body image mediation), guided mediation is practicable and useful in cases of body image dysmorphia.

Perhaps the most frequent form of trauma is grief. Grief makes one feel miserable, detached from others, from life itself. It is a common misconception that grief "gets better with time." The only way grief can be overcome is by rationalization and taking a conscious path to positive perception of the world. Otherwise, grief can kill as much as any bullet, only the dying is slower and more painful.

Survivors, those who consciously accepted the positive path, "come to understand and accept that loss is inevitable part of trauma, and that it is ultimately a lifelong task to assimilate the ebb and flow of re-experienced grief with equanimity" (Van der Hart et al., 1993, p. 175).

The positive path to the perception of the world and oneself is the path toward body association. The sensations suffered during grief – extreme anguish, fear, palpitations of the heart, tears, and trepidation – may force the person to disassociate the self from the body image, in order to survive. The image of a curled up, weak, and helpless bundle of pain is a miserable sight. How can a strong, healthy human accept it? One becomes "two bodies in the same body, doing different things" (Ogden et al, 2006, p. 264). The body that gets drunk on alcohol, the body that injects heroin, the body that goes out and has sex with a random stranger... is not the body of one's "real self" – or is it?

The *dissociative split* caused by trauma is associated with cognitive distortions and compartmentalization which, properly directed, may lead to a guided resolution. If one is able to compartmentalize the trauma and then review it under more dispassionate lens, one may find the cause not within but, where it properly lies, without.[47] The acceptance of a positive image is possible because rationalization leads to self-analysis and self-reflection. These processes require reinterpretation of one's body image in context of the trauma. The reframing[48] of the context leads to

---

[47] This applies to trauma-associated body-image disorders only, not BDD caused by other factors, which may be both endogenous, and exogenous.

[48] "Cognitive reframing" is a more sophisticated way of saying "changing the way you look at events." It may require: writing down experiences; researching and brainstorming for the causes (e.g., of trauma); minimizing (avoiding) the stressors; understanding cognitive distortions, and reformulating them in a more positive light; seeking positive social connections; and finding purpose in life.

reformulating the body experience and, ultimately, to a more positive body image.

Phillips (2021) noted that up to 3% of the general population is affected by Body Dysmorphic Disorder, which means that "nearly 10 million people in the United States alone have BDD" (par. 1). Phillips further conceded that the number may be much higher, because "people with this disorder are often reluctant to reveal their BDD symptoms to others" (Ibid.). BDD appears to be more common than obsessive-compulsive disorder (OCD) and more common than anorexia nervosa and schizophrenia. This fact has been noted by professionals in diverse health care settings, from psychiatry to cosmetic surgery (Sarwer et al., 2006). Even social anxiety disorder (social phobia) and obsessive-compulsive disorder were found to be less frequent than BDD.

Body Dysmorphic Disorder consists of a perception of some perceived defect in one's body image or an excessive concern with one's body image (Greenberg, 2021). Three important findings need to be noted on this account: first, the defect is perceived and this perception is the result of comparisons of one's own body to some ideal body image propagated among peers, in commercials, and on social media; second, as stated earlier, the disassociated body image may also stem from emotional dysregulation (which means that BDD and disorders listed in the preceding paragraph may overlap and coincide); third, the defect, although perceived as to the "image," has actual physical and neuropsychological consequences which are so significant and detrimental to normal life that they should be professionally addressed and corrected (Lai et al., 2021).

As to the third finding, Deckersbach et al. (2000) concluded that BDD may cause memory deficiencies, especially in the reproduction of images, excessive attention to detail, causing detail imbalance, and a diminished capacity at information processing. Dunai et al. (2010) and

Hanes (1998) attributed this diminished capacity to inhibition in planning and organization. However, their studies show a mere correlation, not causation. In fact, as Lai et al. (2021) pointed out, while symptoms of BDD have been described sufficiently well, its causes largely remain a mystery.

Neurochemical studies found "decreased serotonin binding densities" in individuals suffering from BDD, compared to healthy cohorts (Lai et al., 2021, par. 7). When treated with serotonin reuptake inhibitors, BDD patients showed an overall decrease in BDD symptoms, relief from emotional distress, and reduced suicidal ideation (Phillips et al., 2008). Several genetic studies into BDD found that a significant number of individuals with BDD is more likely than non-BDD population to have a family member who has also been diagnosed with BDD. This proportion is up to eight times higher than in is the case in general population (Bienvenu et al., 2000, as cited in Lai et al., 2021, par. 8). Genetic information accounts for nearly one half (44%) of the propensity for BDD, and researchers even determined which genes are affected (Richter et al., 2004). MRI studies of the brains of BDD cohorts showed that BDD individuals engage in more detailed processing systems (generally left-sided) compared with non-BDD diagnosed subjects (Feusner et al., 2010, 2011). These studies suggest that body image perceptions may be distorted not only due to environmental factors, but that there exist genetic propensities to image distortion which, arguably, cannot be sufficiently addressed by body-experience mediation alone. Specific distortions in perception may also be symptomatic of a cerebral hemorrhage or spinal lesions, as borne out and documented by the studies of Schilder (1950), Kawamura et al. (1987), and others.

It should be noted that BDD individuals are capable of better perception of detail and can discern detail in complex representations faster than non-BDD individuals

(Feusner et al., 2010, 2011; Monzani et al., 2013). What is more, the way one perceives one's body image reflects and is related to the way one perceives everything else in the world. The preoccupation with one's body image is thus not just a personal narcissistic concern or obsession with one's self but, rather, an indicator of the world-view as well as certain abilities and sensibilities the individual may learn to use to his or her benefit.

In view of the fact that body dysmorphic and dissociated individuals perceive the world differently, and that their perceptions may, in some ways, be more insightful because seeing parts in more detail is beneficial to many fields of human endeavor (as varied as literary arts and engineering) one may reasonably pose the question: Why is BDD deemed to be detrimental to the human being?

Baker-Pitts (2015) described how "psychological splitting of affects" causes dissociated body-states and inner fragmentation, and how the affected subjects view their bodies as "part objects," that is to say a body composed of body parts,[49] not the body as a whole (p. 110). Interestingly, this view is nowhere more prevalent than in the areas of cosmetic surgery and bodybuilding. Bodybuilders invariably speak of "body-parts" with respect to exercise, and measure, assess, and watch their body-parts for the increase in mass, definition, and vascularity.

Similarly, in cosmetic surgery, the client-patient approaches the physician with a request to enlarge, diminish, or alter the shape of a particular part of the body, be it the

---

[49] Body parts (or "body-parts" – hyphenation is acceptable when emphasizing that the body part is not a separate and independent part, but a part of a system) are divided into: regional parts (encompassing a region of the body, such as: head and neck, or the back); internal parts; and external (visible) parts. This "body partitioning" is often used in non-medical context, such as by trainers and personal coaches, but finds its application mainly in the communication between MDs and laypersons about body and body image. The term *bodytomy* has been artificially invented, describing the "anatomy" of body parts.

breasts, stomach, nose, or even the entire face. Cosmetic surgeons charge their patients depending on the complexity of the procedure, whether it involves a single body part, or a body area.

The applicant for a cosmetic procedure may be properly referred to as a patient when she suffers from BDD and overall psychological fragmentation. Yet, rarely are these applicants referred to as patients. Rather, they are called "clients," akin to a customer purchasing a new gadget. The difference ought to be clear, however: when there has been an official medical diagnosis established, the individual should be properly referred to as a patient; when the procedure is wholly elective, not medically necessary, he or she should be referred to as a client. Since there is no medical diagnosis of a crooked nose, sagging breasts, or fat haunches, many cosmetic surgeons do refer to their patients properly as clients.

One may pause to wonder whether it would not behoove all cosmetic surgeons to conduct a psychiatric examination of their "clients" first, in order to determine whether they suffer from a condition treatable by other means (be it medication, meditation, or body image mediation) or what possible other causes are bringing them to the operating room (such as a recent divorce, sex abuse, or trauma). It appears that body dysmorphic disorder can be a profitable business and industry for many: from the mass media magnates, to commercial advertisers, pharmaceutical industry, to body-oriented products to cosmetic surgery, and even underground trade in injectables, steroids, growth hormone and other "beauty enhancing" drugs and procedures.

Every bodybuilder[50] will no doubt object to being associated with cosmetic surgery, at least in the sense of

---

[50] Bodybuilder is used broadly here, including categories such as physique, fitness, sports model, as well as individuals who do not

enhancing particular body-parts (which is officially prohibited in bodybuilding). Yet, Bodybuilding.com (2022) states that there are many cosmetic procedures "popular among bodybuilders, male and female, amateur or pro," such as: "calf implants, pectoral/breast implants, bicep implants, triceps implants, butt implants/lifting, liposuction, abdominal etching and even facial surgeries" (par. 2). Breast implants for women, and facelifts are permitted. Arguably, tummy tucks and certain other "enhancements" are not readily discoverable, for no doping tests are available here. The scope of permitted or even encouraged procedures corresponds to the dominant cultural narrative and the gendered positions assumed and represented in the general population where, as Baker-Pitts (2015) notes, it is usually the man suggesting the "enhancement" for the woman, often in collaboration with the surgeon, who is likewise a man (p. 108).

What adds to the surgeon's dilemma is the fact that the main objective of cosmetic surgery is increase in personal happiness and beauty which, unlike in other surgical specialties, cannot be readily measured in terms of "the reduction or elimination of symptoms or improved function" (Goldwyn, 2006). Yet, improvements in social adaptation and personal life, as well as work performance and professional advancement can be significant. Cosmetic surgery should certainly not be dismissed and rejected where BDD and body image disorders are at issue. However, it must be considered in conjunction with other methods, such as positive psychology, exercise, and guided body image mediation.

---

compete but hire trainers, follow "routines," and "do" bodybuilding after a fashion.

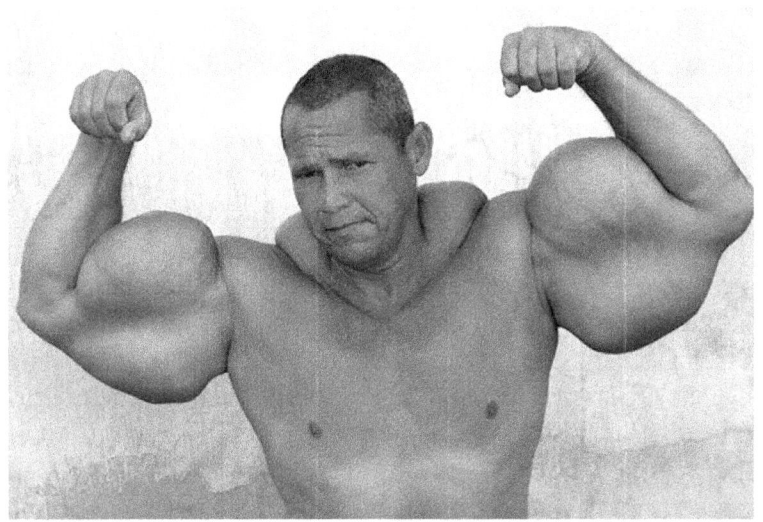
Synthol arms of a self-proclaimed "bodybuilder."

A layperson may wonder why anabolic steroids and substances such as synthol (a mixture of oil, lidocaine, and alcohol) are not considered the same as the use of Botox in cosmetic procedures. Efficiency ought to correspond to the degree to which the use of such substances and procedures enhances the aesthetic sensibility of an average human being. But such criteria are largely subjective, are they not? A man who seeks the utter extremes of human form (primarily in order to please the freak-obsessed fans and judges) no doubt also possesses aesthetic sensibilities that he finds pleasing, although they may be characterized as a distorted perception of reality by someone not familiar with the sport. After all, who is to say what is and is not distorted? As all bodybuilding fans live in the world of bodybuilding distortions, their perception is not that of an average human being. Some seek sensationally freakish bodies to admire, others to emulate, still others watch them from a distance, in order to extol their own "normalcy." The "norm" is shifted here, and it is not until the observer emerges from the distorted environment and looks back on it from a rational distance of an unbiased, "reasonable person" that one begins to perceive various "enhancements" as distortions.

Pope et al. (1997) documented a higher incidence of obsessive-compulsive disorders among bodybuilders, a finding which coincides with the incidence of eating disorders (Mangweth, 2001). Psychopathology may also be similar, as Barth and Starkman (2016) pointed out. Body-shaming is a key trigger for eating disorders, and it may be one of the reasons for overeating-to-dieting-to-overeating cycles. Obsessive eating of healthy foods and constant focus on eating healthy have affected such a significant portion of the population that clinicians were compelled to invent a new term for it – *orthorexia.* Maine and Kelly (2005) define orthorexia simply as "a fixation on righteous eating" (p. 86).

People suffering from orthorexia tend to see deficiencies not only in their own bodies, but often in the bodies of everyone they meet. They are only a step away from body-self shaming. But what is the opposite of body-shaming? Body positivity? Body indifference? Body extolling? Each of these terms carries a significant baggage of connotations and the meaning of each is likewise a matter of interpretation: Is it healthy to be indifferent to one's body? What does "positive" mean in this context? What do we mean by "extolling:" stripping naked, like Leonardo? Showing in public without shame? Revering above the Soul? Panegyrizing and lauding in the Whitmanesque sense?

The primary goal, it would seem, should be to preserve the body as healthy as possible and in harmony with the Soul. There was no word for the Soul in the ancient Hebrew: "And the Lord God formed man of the dust of the ground, and breathed into his nostrils the breath of life; and man became a living soul" states Genesis 2:7. However, the word "nephesh" in Hebrew is better translated as "breath," not a "soul" (Kioulachoglou, 2022, par. 3). Thus, God breathed life into the body. Arguably, this act posits the body above the Soul, because the body preceded the Soul. Therefore, body-awareness and body-pride are not *per se* negative sensations. However, they may become negative by association – with body-shaming, body-blaming, and body-naming – which requires body image interpretation.

It has been stated above that those who suffer from BDD focus on individual body parts, not the body as a whole. However, the focus they attribute to a part of the body is invariably in the perceived proportion to the *image* of the whole. Even among the most at-risk groups, such as fashion models, dancers, and bodybuilders, the overall emphasis is on symmetry and aesthetic perception which, granted, may be skewed by the bias of the profession (e.g., skinny models, puffed-up men, masculine looking women) but the expression of the body image in a sub-culture is primarily a matter of survival, characterized by the need to belong to the group with which the individual shares its peculiar aesthetic sensibilities, and in which the individual feels protected.

Schilder (1964) observed that parts of the whole always remain "psychologically separated" because there is a "distinct space" between them (p. 86). When one pauses to observe the dried up skin on her aging hands, watches her fingers type, or carefully observes the nails and knuckles during various manicuring procedures, she is actively perceiving the skin, the hand, the fingers, the knuckles, and the nails as separate objects that are used as tools or upon which she performs various beautifying procedures, such as applying moisturizer or clipping the nails. In character and type of human endeavor, such procedures are not different from when a surgeon is performing a "nose job" or "tummy tuck." Indeed, this psychological separation of the body into individual parts is so natural to the human being that most everyday activities from very early childhood are learned through focus on body-parts, their coordination, smooth transfer of energy from one body-part to another, and accurate perception, necessary to obtain the desired effect, be it a simple walk, run, pull, strike, squeeze, etc.

Arguably the most well-known expert on body image, Paul Schilder, created a *postural model* based on body parts, parts that are always also parts of some larger whole – be it the body, society, or the world at large (Ferguson, 2000, p. 63). What Schilder (1964) introduced into the body image discussion is a body which goes far beyond its material form, spreading its image, as it were, "into space" (p. 213). Schilder's postural model is helpful in dealing with BDD issues because body image related ailments (such as eating disorders, depression, drug addiction) occur when one starts craving for a complete control over the body image – the control which, needless to say, one can never wield because: for one, there are always multiple images at play (the way I see you may not correspond to the way you see yourself or the way someone else sees you); for the other, the images of various body-parts may appear as discontinuous or even discordant, defying coordination and mastery; and, the body image is never a stable "given" but, rather, a constantly mediated *idea*.

Therefore, some degree of dissociation with the body is always present in our lives, and it can even be concluded that it is healthy for human development and individual growth. Perhaps the only full body-to-image alignment is possible in death, as has been documented in various studies of death masks.[51]

---

[51] The death mask is the mask which refers to "nothing more than itself" (Belting, 2017, p. 80). It is the mask of a mask, the body which ultimately equals the image. Yet, the mask-image which remained is only an empty mask – because the real image was buried or incinerated with the body. This leads to the question what is the Image, and how it differs from the Soul, if that is the case.

The Image

The Ever Changing Ideal

While the body is relatively stable, its image changes with the environment, ambiance, attire, even the individual's mood, not to mention various enterprises and functions. At first blush, Schilder's (1964) *special image* of the body entails personal freedom – one can literally be anything and manipulate one's body image, in order to fit the desired ideal. With such freedom, however, comes not only responsibility but also a potential trade-off. As is commonly known, the more free, the less secure the individual is, simply because being oneself, not a part of "the herd," has its inherent risks and dangers.

An etymological excursion is in order here. The word *ideal* is derived from Latin ideālis, which means "existing in (an) idea." The word *idea* traces its origin to the Ancient Greek ἰδέα, which means a "notion" or "pattern,' from εἴδω, i.e., "I see." On the other hand, the word *image*, stems from the Middle English ymage, via Old French, originally from Latin imāgō, which means "a copy" or "likeness." Thus, a *body idea* purports to say a "notion," while a *body image* implies a likeness, a copy of the real thing.

Each copy may be copied *ad infinitum*, and with each copy the doubt about its faithfulness to the original increases, and its value diminishes (the more there is of something, the cheaper it becomes, not to mention the dubitability of its provenance). That is what expensive fashion industry brands rely on in marketing – the increase in supply cheapens the product value and, conversely, scarcity makes things expensive. Meanwhile, the *idea* remains – or should remain – set in stone (similar to the original of some great Old Master's painting). One may contend that the body idea is therefore more valuable, more unique, and more real than the body image.

The argument that body's image can be transformed, so as to more accurately conform to the idea (whether conceived of by the individual or imposed upon them by the society), requires the freedom to transform the body. The body becomes boundary-less and invaded by this "idealization." The pressure of the environment (family, friends, mass media) may prevail, forcing the individual to compare, assess, transform, and confirm the body to the idea which is not that of the individual, moving it away from the original. This invasion of the body happens so imperceptibly and seemingly innocuously – starting with a change in costume to a change in expression, to a surgery performed on a particular body part – that the individual may one day find themselves standing in front of the mirror, not recognizing what they see, or else looking at their body abstractedly and critically, as if observing a foreign object (Baker-Pitts, 2015, p. 111; Eichenbaum, 2012; Krueger, 2001). This "foreign object" may evoke the original, transforming "time into an image" in a futile attempt to "ground" and anchor the image (Belting, 2011, p. 45). The image is displaced and one's memory creates a story behind it, the story of transformation and development.

Regardless of originality, it is the story behind the image – embodied in the image – that gives it value and currency in the world. Indeed, it might be argued that while no absolute originality is possible, what gives value to body image is the individual's story, the story of the image (which, as stated above, remains a copy by definition). This is equally true of the human body image as it is of any other image or work of art. For example, in primitive psyche and cultures, the inanimate object and its image acquire value only if they are (re)animated, injected with life, given a story: In the mountains and hills of Ireland, there lives a small creature with charcoal eyes, a little trickster called Pooka that can prophesy one's future... Easter Bunny is related to this devilish spirit, especially in his judgmental quality of good vs. bad (naughty-or-nice judgment passed on children at Easter, similar to Christmas). A child touches the bunny, looks into his eyes, perceiving a connection to the unknown which, through the image – its perception, story, cultural meaning – becomes familiar. At the same time, the image becomes the spirit, which is (re)animated in cultural usage, and in the hands of the child. Casey (2021) notes that the spirit-image entails a judgment of mythical qualities, judgment upon the persona of the child.

Judgment is always inexorably connected with the image. Belting (2011) points out that there exists an inevitable tension between the personal "vision of the image" and the normative power of "official pictures" that are embodied in the "collective imagination of the people" (p. 50). As the body is the locus of clashing images, it may be difficult to control. Both the individual's self-conscious perception and the normative collective perception of the image have been affected by this phenomenon: it is the locus (place) of the image which gives it the identity. The birth certificate or the passport betrays the individual's birthplace and age, compelling the customs officer (or any normative official in the vast bureaucracy of image classifications) to pass judgment on the individual. The country, the locale, other people from the region… all provide associations and connotative meanings to the image in the passport, which then superimposes the officer's judgment on the body image of the person standing in front of him.

While customs inspection may be a fitting case in point, image-processing takes place in everyday contact among all individuals all the time. Although it has received a significant media backlash recently (as various forms of "profiling") it would be inaccurate to characterize it as altogether deplorable or unhealthy: with respect to the body image, on the positive side, it forces upon the individual a self-correction of misperceived body image; on the negative side, it may destabilize and even fragment the person's self-image, in particular when the individual is young, teeming with uncertainty about her body image, or when the individual suffers from some form of the body dysmorphic disorder.

FBI provides its agents with multiple tips in profiling training which, among others, include (Bariso, 2022):

1. Create a baseline of personal "mannerisms," i.e., what conduct is "normal" for a given individual (par. 1).
2. Look for deviations, inconsistencies in words and gestures.
3. Notice clusters of gestures (clumps of behavioral aberrations).
4. Compare and contrast the person's behavior in interaction with others versus how they behave in interacting with you.
5. Look into the mirror: Does the person reciprocate your gestures and behavior?
6. Identify the strong voice: Look for posture and gestures to ascertain dominance or submission.
7. Observe how the person walks or holds posture. Shuffle, lack of fluid motions, keeping one's head down, avoiding eye contact, etc. may indicate lack of self-confidence, but also untruthfulness.
8. Pinpoint action words; in particular, various verbs and verbal phrases may provide insight into the individual's thought processes.
9. Look for personality clues, such as: introversion–extroversion; uncertainty–risk-taking; stress–relaxed demeanor, etc.

Virtually all of these points focus on conduct and behavior because body image is never static but, rather, is constantly being formed, molded, and altered by gestures, speech, stance, walk, even a most momentary expression of attitude. It is very well known that photographers for famous model magazines, such as the *Vogue* or *Playboy* and the like set their subjects in precise angles and positions, with exactly timed and directed lighting, all in order to best portray the *image* of the body. In this photoshoot, the photographs are then re-arranged in a specific sequence, in order to show the body image in multiple dimensions, projecting photographic motion and intended focus (e.g., on the advertised product).

Belting (2011) notes that the body is "performing" the image(s) and thus becomes "both the locus and the medium" of the image (p. 49). In psychology of the body image, just as in geography and other spheres of human endeavor, it is the culture that creates place-names and defines the various *loci*. There is a difference in the body image portrayed in the *Vogue*, the *Playboy*, the *New York Times*, or in a CNN commercial. The difference is both, top-down (normative) and bottom-up, based on the demand of the readership/viewership. Linguistically and sociologically speaking, the opposite of "normative" meaning is a meaning "posited" (i.e., imposed) upon the image. Posited is derived from Latin *positus*, which means stood or planted in place. *Posited* does not mean posit*ive,* because the image may be false – although the two words share the root *to posit,* in the first instance, it means placed; in the latter, it purports settled (such as a dispute). Thus, neither normative nor posited are statements of value or veracity (unless the meaning be expanded to embrace positive psychology, mathematics, or phenomenology). One may also argue that a positive answer/statement is not the same as a true answer/statement. A statement such as: "The public wants to see more full-sized models" is not necessarily true, but it is *posited* with normative implications on the *image* of the body. If implicated at all, truth is then a matter of pragmatic interpretation.

However, what the normative implications are remains as vague and ambiguous as the term that defines them. The adjective "full-sized" was chosen because it is a courteous and deferential synonym for the more outspoken "fat" – a word which (not just in body image context) bears invariably negative implications. However, the adjective "fat" has multiple meanings, the primary one listed by Merriam Webster (2022a) being "plump" in the sense of a "cute, fat little baby" or (of a woman) a "little plump but not fat." Interestingly, other denotations are also more positive than negative, such as "full in tone and quality" (a "gorgeous fat bass voice"), and "prosperous" or "wealthy" (e.g., he "grew fat on the war"), and "substantial and impressive" (a "fat bank account"), as well as "richly rewarding or profitable, as in "a fat part in the movie" (par. 1-10). "Fat" may also mean "productive" or "fertile" (a "fat year for crops") but also the very opposite, such as in the phrase "There's a fat chance of" something. An "easy hit" in baseball is also sometimes characterized as "fat" (MerriamWebster, 2022a, Id.).

Perhaps the word "full-sized" has been chosen in order to avoid normative implications of the word *fat*? But is "full-sized" not less ambiguous and more descriptive thus, arguably, more offensive? Is it necessarily more positive than "fat?" Rhymezone.com (2022) lists forty synonyms for "fat" but only twelve for "full-sized." The same is the case with other dictionaries, such as Collins and Merriam Webster. Looking up the word "fat" in the online Merriam Webster thesaurus, one discovers that the very first definition, and a host of synonyms, pertain to the cultural sphere where "fat" refers to "individuals carefully selected as being the best of a class," such as (the) "a-list, aristocracy, best, choice, corps d'elite, cream, crème de la crème, elect, elite, flower, illuminati, pick, pink, pride, priesthood, prime, royalty, upper crust" (MerriamWebster, 2022b). The second listed meaning is that of a "state or an instance of going beyond what is usual, proper, or needed" (par. 2), and only the third definition provides the synonyms of fat as "adipose," "corpulent," or "pudgy." Whether used in the literal sense or not, each word and phrase using this adjective is evocative of an image which triggers the idea implied in the appertaining connotative and denotative meanings.

Linguistic usage and phraseology applied to the body itself and its image (i.e., how it appears to others) can thus be as abstracted and far removed from them (the body, and its image) as masks, makeup, and costumes are from the players who use them to impersonate fictional characters or portray imaginary acts. Belting (2011) noted that the image of the body is created and duplicated in the mask, which is no doubt true. The parallel to the like duplication in language is impossible to overlook here.

Roland Barthes in *Camera Lucida* described how he began to "rediscover" his mother for the first time only when perusing her photographs as a five-year-old girl (cited in Bonomo, 2016):

> The distinctness of her face, the naïve attitude of her hands, the place she had docilely taken without either showing or hiding herself, and finally her expression, which distinguished her, like Good from Evil, from the hysterical little girl, the simpering doll who plays at being a grownup - all this constituted the figure of a *sovereign innocence* (par. 1) [italics added].

It was this image which brought him back to his mother and embodied the truth. Barthes' search for a "just image" (a true image, faithful to reality) as opposed to "just an image" is what Husserl in the phenomenological method termed *eidetic reduction* – reduction to the essence of the image: the object is not formed or co-created by mediation in its environment but, rather, by stripping the object-image of all "secondary" interpretations. Barthes expressed an "ontological desire" to absorb the essence of the object, which would distinguish it from the surrounding "community of images" (par. 7).

What Barthes intended and performed lies on a non-linguistic plane (defined by him as a *stadium* – meaning an "interpretation" – as opposed to *punctum* – absorption of the essence). Whether one says "fat" or "corpulent" or "pudgy" or "full-bodied," one will never capture the essence of the object-image/body image because, in each instance, the observer is interpreting and imputing characteristics that each such word, phrase or description necessarily carries, characteristics which are invariably top-down, thus normative. Does the normative structure thereby prevent the observer from ever matching the description to the image?

Bonomo (2016) pointed out that the essence (*punctum*) is subconscious and largely coincidental, such as a passing momentum of Barthes' mother as captured by the photographic image he described. Barthes (1977) suggests the notion of *satori* in Japanese Zen-Buddhism, a sudden sense of enlightenment which almost mystically illuminates the soul, is the only one which can be accurately used to a body-image description.[52] The reader may be familiar with this sensation from various forms of art, such as when the tones of the music or operatic tenor raise the hair on the back of one's neck, or when a memorable, moving scene in a novel or film moistens one's eye and evokes the innermost vibrations of the heart.

In reference to body image, when the image cannot be described (or one is inapt to describe it in words), the

---

[52] *Satori* is the first step toward *Budhahood*, an enlightenment through seeing one's "self-nature." After seeing one's self-nature, one is guided to deepen this experience through repetition and continuous practice (Sheng, 2006). However, as each such repetition also takes the substance away from the form, abstracts the image from the body, the soul from its terrestrial ties, it can perhaps not be described as the best method of capturing the image, unless it is the instance of the image, captured in time. Then again, time is inconceivable without space and matter…

satori sensation appears. It may appear when staring in the mirror, finding one's image inadequate and inaccurate – but without being able to define where the inadequacy and imperfection lies, or when observing the body image of another individual and finding oneself unable to mediate it or adequately reflect upon it. At this moment, the observer subconsciously understands that the image is not the essence and that whatever speaks to him in the image lies in the aura beyond one moment in space and time. The old saying which describes "seeing" as believing states much more than that one has to see, in order to believe. One has to see the way Little Prince saw – the invisible – in order to understand the visible.

Returning for a moment to Barthes' perusal of his mother's photograph, the most interesting observation he made was that what he suddenly saw in her (in the photograph taken when she had been but five years old) was a trait or characteristic which was there all the time, even when he was looking at many other photographs of her and their family in the past, but which remained hidden from his sight while she was alive. It may have been less apparent and less lucid, less prominent, invisible to the non-circumspect eye, perhaps – but it was always there. Was it a feature of the body, or a pure sensation evoked by the image?

Sometimes, a photograph captures a certain look, angle, grimace which surprises even the person depicted in the photograph, who might then exclaim: "That's not what I look like at all!" Bonomo (2016) notes that the temporal *satori* is the essence of photography. However, it is not the essence of body image perception. It cannot be – because life is motion and a living object can truly only be captured in motion. An observer may suddenly notice his friend, a person he knows very well, in an unexpected position, lighting, from a different angle or viewpoint, and the friend will open a new *satori* for him – but, as soon as the friend moves and the light passes, the observer will be able to automatically integrate the new sensation into the body image of the friend which he, as a habitual observer, formed and constructed over many years. Sometimes, however, the very core concept of the individual is altered by some previously unobserved grimace or gesture, lighting or angle of vision. If body image integration is not fully possible, then the observer is removed and alienated from the image. This often happens with incongruous images that may incite negative feelings in the observer, such as revulsion or disgust.

Development and Interpretation of the Image

All human relationships are founded on seeing and interpreting body images. Given this emphasis on body image interpretation, some notable phenomenologists have posed the question if body image is the content, the self could exist outside of and wholly independently from the image (O'Shaughnessy, 1980; Peacocke, 2014, 2017). Bartolomeo et al. (2017) showed that this is not a purely philosophical contention, as confabulations in people with right hemisphere impairments may create and bring into existence an actual body or body-part images.[53]

In his eponymous and foundational volume on *Body Image,* Schilder (1950) described patients suffering from various forms of brain lesions, thereby losing the sense of the self in different body parts, or transferring sensation from the left to the right part of the body and vice versa (alloesthesia). Indeed, these descriptions date much further back in history, as far as Ambroise Paré (1510-1590) and René Descartes (1596-1650). Schilder (1950) suggested that "perception is *synaesthetic*"[54] [italics mine] and synergistically consists of various "units of perception" (p. 39). He noted that there was "no question that the subject 'body' presents itself to all senses," thus creating a body–self reference. Driven to its logical conclusion, Schilder's analysis means no body image is perfect by definition, because perfection would require perfectly accurate perception by all faculties at all times.

---

[53] Confabulations usually refer to "memory distortions, characterized by the production of verbal statements or actions that are inconsistent with the patient's history and present situation" (Bartolomeo et al., 2017, Abstract). However, behavioral patterns "reminiscent of memory confabulations" can also occur in patients with right hemisphere damage, "in relation to their personal, peripersonal or extrapersonal space" (Ibid.).

[54] *Synaesthetic* means concomitant feeling with image, stimulation of a body-part evoking a particular sense or imagery.

This is also the case when an individual perceives one's own body image in the mirror, a perception generated mainly by sight and created upon perception. This is also the reason justifying the phenomenological "independence" of the body image from the body self, noted above. What further supports this notion of independence is the phenomenon considered by Fisher et al. (1984) that each individual's self-image is first described and imprinted upon them by their parents, thereby creating a body-image imprint which is not necessarily concomitant with the accurate self-perception (or, indeed, any perception at all, as it often precedes a full development of the faculties which would enable the individual to perceive the self): "When the parents first meet the infant and ask, 'Is the child normal?' they are really asking whether the physical product of themselves conforms to the image they have created" (p. 14). This questioning never ceases, and is further expanded in adulthood when every individual's body image is compared first to her peers, then to various ideals that society imposes through mass and social media, advertising, and branding.

Interestingly, the word "normal" has etymological connotations not only those of being "typical" or "common" (from Latin *normalis,* meaning "in conformity with a rule"), but it also means "standing at a right angle" – in classical Latin "made according to a carpenter's square," this being the *norma* or "rule" for everyone else (Etymonline, 2021). Thus, a "normal school" is a "training college for teachers" (French *école normale,* 1794) because it serves to set a national standard (a norm, rule) which the teachers are to advance and perpetuate.

With respect to the body, the right side of the body is *normally* "not only stronger" but also "more 'dexterous'," as human beings "generally make more use of the right side of their body" and the motor impulses "go more easily to the right side" (Schilder, 1950, p. 37). This indicates that the orientation to the right is the norm (standard), and that whatever diverges from the right is a deviation, therefore "not normal." Consequently, the "right" body image is the "normal" normative body image, whatever it may be conceived of in a given milieu and culture.

Norms and normativity would be impossible without grounding the rules that make it normal. This grounding limits (or altogether denies) flexibility and latitude to the individual with respect to their own body image, and makes the imposition of some stable, socially acceptable image imperative. However, as Bonomo (2016) elucidated, such stability is undesirable and, indeed, unnatural: first, because the essence of life is motion and only motion can capture life (reflect on the grace of a gazelle escaping a lion – can words ever do justice to the actual or imagined sight?); second, because everyone's body image develops and alters with the growth and evolution of the individual; third, because something which is abstracted from its material substance cannot be captured by it.

Where perception is concerned, motion is naturally superior to a still image. A motionless body appears lifeless. Absorbing a beautiful painting, the viewer is thrilled to find signs of motion in figures, expressions which convey seemingly live and living moods, dimensionality in the countryside, such as flow of a river or waterfall. Similarly, connecting with one's body requires perception of motion vis-à-vis topography of the locus. Snowden and Freeman (2004) showed that brain cells in the middle temporal area (MT) are "directionally sensitive" and that human beings, much like many other animal species, cannot very well perceive an image as still unless it is distinguished against a moving background, and vice versa (p. R829). Even a brick wall is better perceived as still when leaves on the trees above it and roses in front of it flutter in the wind. Optical illusions may be constructed which create a semblance of motion (such as rocks seemingly moving up against a waterfall). Similarly, when one is lying or sitting still on a flat surface, one may achieve a sense of illusion of motion of Self away from one's body or, when being in motion, the illusion of stillness and composure of the self. Interestingly, those who are unable to connect with the body often seek help in various retreats, where they are taught how to "feel" their own bodies by means of sensory imagination, such as imagining a heavy ball dropping from the position of the head down to the lap or center of the torso (Jones, 2016). MT and medial superior temporal (MST) areas in the brain can be manipulated both internally and externally.[55]

There is a "field tension" between the ego and the outside world which may be mitigated through the MT and MST manipulation (Schilder, 1950, p. 51). This seems to suggest that body image fragmentation and dissonance can also be reduced commensurately, such as by meditation during which the body is abstracted from the image. "The knowledge of one's own body is an absolute necessity," stated Schilder (Ibid.). This statement is at once common-sense but also uncommonly difficult to bring about in real world because either the self or the body are constantly in motion.[56]

As Belting (2011) suggested, the body is a locus of the image, wherein all normative images reside, clashing with the individual's Self. Belting also made the point that the individual's "mental images" always stand in opposition to the "artificial, exogenous pictures" (p. 126). These are composed not only of mass media, commercials, and movies, but also of all sundry facets of virtual reality. The I-pads and I-phones contain the localization in their very names: "I" is where the images reside, where the reality is

---

[55] The MT cells distinguish directionality but not optic flow patterns. MST cells are sensitive to "movements that expand, contract, rotate or deform" (Snowden & Freeman, Ibid.).

[56] For instance, when one is lying in bed at night, unable to fall asleep, the body is still, yet the self is all over the place, flying through air, attending to work, relationships, etc. Where is the body image then?

being re-enacted and re-created. The image on these devices moves in time and space and is altogether devoid from the often motionless real world body.

Tovian (2002) noted that psychoanalysts see body image as a "crucial element in ego formation" and that one's personality cannot be fully developed in the absence of a healthy body image (p. 362). A mature body image develops only through motion, through sequences of crises and conflicts that the individual has to overcome on their path to adulthood and in life in general. Much like an artistic masterpiece, the image starts with a sketch and proceeds until all the figures, background and foreground, colors, shades, the play of light and shadow... are completed in every detail. Only then, does the masterpiece fulfil its role.

Developmental psychologist Erik Erikson (1902-1994) outlined eight stages of psychosocial development which he termed "crises" (Woolfolk, 2013, p. 88). It is through these crises that a person "creates their Self-Image and becomes an autonomous human being" (Condor-Fisher, 2021, p. 130). The first stage, that of "basic trust" versus "basic mistrust," corresponds to Piaget's Sensorimotor Stage: here, the child develops awareness of and either trust or distrust (doubt) about her caregiver.

Interestingly, Lewis and Brooks-Gunn (1984) conducted an experiment in which they applied a red dot onto an infant's nose and then held the child up to a mirror. Children who recognized themselves in the mirror would reach for their own noses rather than the reflection of the dot on the nose in the mirror. Lewis et al. (Id.) found that almost no children under one year of age would reach for their own nose rather than the reflection in the mirror. This indicates that the image each individual associates with his or her own body is not innate but, rather, forms and develops as the Self detects and appropriates it.

Swiss developmental psychologist Jean Piaget (1896-1980) called the earliest stage of self-development

Sensorimotor – because it is through coordinating sensory experiences (seeing, hearing) with motor actions (reaching, touching) that infants begin to understand the world and their position in it (McLeod, 2019). The main developmental objective at this stage is to comprehend that objects exist independent of the actions of the self – so called *object permanence*. This requires a concomitant development of the object-image in the mind. Conversely, it is during this period that the initial self-object image is created, as distinguished from the other-object image (i.e., the body image of one's self, as opposed to the body image of another human being).

This finding fully comports to the established description of body schema as a "changeable" blueprint, the creation of which is enabled only through collaboration of all senses and faculties at all times (Schilder, 1950, p. 114). "The development of the body-schema," stated Schilder, "runs to a great extent parallel to the sensory motor development" (p. 105). The mental picture of the self develops as a result of accumulated perception, synthesized in the brain – which is why positive reaction from the environment is paramount to healthy development of every human being. If the response is negative and trust does not develop during the First Stage, then the Second Stage (18 months to 3 years) is characterized by mistrust (Erikson, 1956, 1963). Mistrust is the "founding stone of shame and (self)doubt" (Condor-Fisher, 2021, p. 131). Mistrust undermines autonomy, self-control, and self-confidence, which are all supposed to develop during the Second Stage.

The analogy between the human body image and an artistic masterpiece could, once again, be drawn here: few, if any, artistic masterpieces are begun in doubt and shame, and even fewer of such have withstood the test of time. According to Erikson, shame turns into guilt, which leads to inferiority, confusion of self-identity, stagnation in development, and despair (Woolfolk, 2013):

Erikson's Stages of Development

Stage 1

Infancy:	Trust vs. Mistrust
Virtue:	Hope
Maldevelopment:	Withdrawal
Freudian stage:	Oral stage
Example:	Secure environment provided by the caregiver, with regular access to affection and food

Stage 2

Early Childhood:	Autonomy vs. Shame, doubt
Virtue:	Will
Maldevelopment:	Compulsion
Freudian stage:	Anal stage
Example:	Caregiver promotes self-sufficiency while maintaining a secure environment

Stage 3

Play Age period:	Initiative vs. Guilt
Virtue:	Purpose
Maldevelopment:	Inhibition
Freudian stage:	Genital stage
Example:	Caregiver encourages, supports, and guides the child's own initiatives and interests

Stage 4

School Age period:	Industry vs. Inferiority
Virtue:	Competence
Maldevelopment:	Inertia (passivity)
Freudian stage:	Latency stage
Example:	Reasonable expectations set in school and at home, with praise for accomplishments

Stage 5

Adolescence period:	Identity vs. Identity confusion
Virtue:	Fidelity
Maldevelopment:	Repudiation
Example:	Individual weighs out their previous experiences, societal expectations, and their aspirations in establishing values and finding themselves.

Stage 6

Young Adulthood:	Intimacy vs. Isolation
Virtue:	Love
Maldevelopment:	Distantiation
Example:	Individual forms close friendships or long-term partnerships

Stage 7

Adulthood period:	Generativity v. Stagnation or Self-absorption
Virtue:	Care
Maldevelopment:	Rejectivity
Example:	Engagement with the next generation through parenting, coaching, or teaching

Stage 8

Old Age period:	Integrity vs. Despair
Virtue:	Wisdom
Maldevelopment:	Disdain
Example:	Contemplation and acknowledgment of personal life accomplishments

This "staging" of human development is founded on the so-called *epigenetic principle*[57] which involves the study of the changes of phenotypic traits (individual character traits) and how gene expression can be regulated or impacted by the environment. Note that Stages 1 through 3, Oral, Anal, and Genital respectively, are the ages of self-discovery through perception and self-exploration. Stage 4 may be marked by Latency, and Stage 5 by uncertainty as to one's identity which may go far beyond body image issues, although those are the most marked manifestation of such maladaptation. Other symptoms include self-rejection, abnegation, and distancing from one's body. Since the affirmation-of-self (Stage 1) and environmental security (Stage 2) and support of self-interests (Stage 3) had been lacking or inadequate, individual turns body image inward – it becomes "latent" and "inert," and a stage of inferiority (Stage 4) is followed by repudiation and inability to love (Stages 5 and 6). When one is incapable of loving one's self, one is unable to love anyone else's self either. Purported love may then turn into obsession with material or imagined things outside one's self. Thereby, the distortion of self-image poses severe limitations not only on the body but also on the Soul.

It is this recoil and distancing from the image that has plagued the human race ever since Adam and Eve were repudiated from their divine Image original in Paradise. It was Plato who is said to have given the first impetus "in the direction of enlightenment" when he described images as "empty" and secondary to their originals (Belting, 2011, p.

---

[57] Epigenetics is the study of DNA "marks" (stable, non-alterable parts of the DNA sequence) vis-à-vis parts that mutate, divide, are altered or silenced. Epi- (ἐπι-) is Greek for "over," "outside," or "around") and the word *epigenetics* thus implies the study of features that lie around and outside the inherited DNA.

111).[58] What does "empty" mean? Void, opposite of full, imbued with meaning and life. Belting (Ibid.) referred to the image as an "artifact" which, according to Belting, implies that it is created by the individual for cultural purposes. However, the life-force in the image is not that of the culture but of the individual.

Plato would not disagree. In *Phaedrus* (370 BC), Plato went so far as to state that written word was "no more than an image" of the original form (p. 87). In the very next paragraph, his protagonist Socrates postulated that man "will not seriously incline to 'write' his thoughts 'in water' with pen and ink, sowing words which can neither speak for themselves nor teach the truth adequately to others" (p. 88). Socrates was famous for never writing anything, leaving the bulk of his intellectual heritage to his pupil Plato and Plato's literary endowments and aspirations. Thus, all extant Socratic teachings about the image-original *versus* an image-copy are passed on to the reader as second-hand images, copies of the original. Whether this is to the detriment or benefit of the reader is arguable but seeing Socrates through Plato's eyes is certainly helpful to the modern interpretation of the self (including the selves of the great philosophers in the environments that shaped them).

An image-idol (the third meaning of the image per Plato/Socrates) may be deceptive, stable, even illusory – but it is far from "dead" in the sense expressed by Socrates. For example, take the "image" of a thought expressed "with pen and ink," so as to pass on a seemingly stale idea to posterity. Not only is the writing not dead because it speaks to the reader, perhaps centuries later but, more important, it is revived through the reader and re-injected with life, once again re-interpreted, spoken, and reconveyed, often even re-

---

[58] Plato held that there is a hierarchy of images (Gk. εἶδος, εἰκών, and φάντασμα/εἴδωλον): 1) an image-eidos, or Divine original; 2) an image-icon, a true likeness; 3) an image-idol, a seeming likeness.

written, in a different light. This is how civilizations move forward – on re-interpretation of images.

Akin to the image of the body, the image of a thought-idea in writing takes on the form which is, in part, formed, reformed, and mediated by the environment, and, in part, changes the environment it has been revived in – because nothing can be injected with life force without exerting life force upon its creator, be it its originator in the contemporaneous world or its re-interpreter elsewhere. Therefore, the very opposite may be argued, which is to say that the image is more potent than the original, because it creates something meaningful anew, long after its creator has met his Creator, and it may even prevail over and destroy the original. Consider when a bullied child commits suicide because she is unable to reconcile the original body image (self) with the copy (refashioned and bended by environmental pressures).[59]

The potency of an image becomes even more apparent when we realize that every image represents an idea and may also be interpreted as a sign, or a symbol, apart from conveying the meaning directly. The analogy with semiotic interpretation of an expression can easily be drawn. Kristeva (2002) created the term *semiotic chora* for spaces or environments in which the *I* encounters language, thus *the Other*. Her analogy of an infant in the womb associating with "sounds and rhythms that set up the possibility of

---

[59] Although there has been a strong backlash against the verb "to commit" in this context, proponents of which argue that suicide is neither a crime nor a sin, therefore "to commit" is improper here (Freedenthal, 2017): when a person dies of suicide having succumbed to, for example, bullying or PTSD, then it is the culturally bended image of the self which lends the hand to the Devil. It would be more proper to speak of committing self-homicide, which poses no legal liability because it is excusable or justifiable, depending on the circumstances. In some cases, moral liability lies with third persons, so the verb "to commit" is redeemable and applicable on such narrow grounds, akin to one being "committed" involuntarily to an asylum (note: a linguistic parallel only).

signification before the infant (mis)recognizes itself in the mirror image" indicates the potentiality of two levels of body image perception which may occur in sequence or separately but need not necessarily coexist (p. 24). After all, the parents of the child in the womb already have a preconceived image of the body of their baby which is also *symbolic* of their union (image-icon) and whose *signs* of life react to and intersect with the "possibility of signification" possessed by the child in the womb (image-idol).

How is this analogy helpful to body image analysis? All individuals cohabit in the world of signs and symbols. There is always a signifier and a signified that long to be united. However, it is not always clear which is which because, indeed, they can be one and indivisible, and they can also be interchangeable: there is a concept of the image as signifier, and the body as signified – the image provides a plane of content to the body. Where the image is not real (an imagined body image construct), the body is meaningless.

What is more, just as there is an arbitrary relationship between the sign and its real-world referent, there is an arbitrary relationship between the concept of the body and the mediated image. This is why some body image researchers and experts explore this topic so far as to question the very existence of Self and the extent to which an individual is capable of possessing or owning a Self. On that point, one might argue that the Self is constantly being structured and reconstructed from a multitude of images which are constantly being perceived and reflected by the individual.

Saussure (1959) suggested that the signifier (that which points at something else) does not always exist prior to the signified (p. 65). In other words, they are correlated but not necessarily causally related, which means that either one can be the impetus to the creation of the other, but neither can exist without the other. The body–image analogy is at hand, especially when one realizes the degree to which the body language and facial expression convey one's thoughts and intentions, and to which costume expresses the individual, his or her occupation, social situation and standing in the world. Indeed, the body and its image do not separate – until death.

Whatever does not express literal meaning has symbolic potentiality which, needless to say, is virtually everything, including the body image. Whatever is symbolically understood may become culturally ingrained and may take on culturally stabilizing functions, such as the police uniform, the red cross, the symbol of the body on the sign "men at work." The interesting part is that symbolic representations unify both the material, and non-material world.

Therefore, it is imperative that the image be seen and reflected by the observer as a symbolic interpretation of the body of the subject. What other purpose does the body serve *in society* other than to symbolize and represent? Costume may carry ideological meanings or project conformity of the wearer to his social milieu (isomorphic symbolism). An individual's body image is constantly being compared to other individuals' body images (comparative symbolism). Sometimes subliminally, sometimes ostensibly, the image-symbol points beyond itself, such as when a person wears a rainbow-colored T-shirt. These symbolic messages may be conveyed by the costume as well as the body (e.g., tattooing, earrings, affected gesticulation, use of jargon in speech, etc.). Even conventional symbols (such as the red cross) may be analyzed and found to be pointing beyond the symbol-image, to the body (red for blood, the cross for the body of Jesus on the cross).

Symbolic Character of the Image - Implications

The symbolic character of body image lies at the very core of many body dysmorphic disorders. It has two significant implications which are both interconnected and intertwined: the first is the internalization of affect; the second the internalization of symbolic projection.

First, the degree of affect is causally related and commensurate to the extent of "internalization of socially reflected appraisals" which result from the symbolic function of the body and turn back into it, altering its image (Cash & Pruzinsky, 2004, p. 278). Cash and Pruzinsky (Ibid.) describe a phenomenon called *attributive projection*, which causes all individuals to alter "how they see themselves" based on their "social cognition and behavior" (p. 278). A woman who "feels fat" will project such feelings outwardly and elicit corresponding reaction from the environment. She will interpret compliments as disguised criticisms causing her embarrassment, hence she will try to dress down and avoid social contact.

Cash and Pruzinsky (2004) cited research conducted by Kleck and Strenta in 1980, during which female participants were to wear a "made up" scar on their faces in personal contact. Unbeknownst to the cohorts, the horrid scar was removed shortly before the interaction with the "stranger" who, in fact, was the researchers' confederate trained to act uniformly with all cohorts. The women who believed they had the scar on their faces felt they were viewed as "less attractive," had less frequent eye contact with the stranger, and alleged that they "observed" that the stranger was "uncomfortable" with them (p. 278).

The researchers concluded that health and value of social interactions are directly proportional to healthy self-esteem and self-image of the interacting individuals. What is more, symbolic value of the image directly impacts how the individuals see themselves. Interacting individuals adopt the symbol as their defining characteristic: it is not a far-fetched mental stretch from "I have a scar" to "I am the scar."

Consider the quote from a great French psychiatrist, philosopher, and linguist Phillipe Chaslin (1857-1923):

> Delusional ideas seem to have their source in the emotions of the patient of which they are symbolic representations... One could illustrate the origins of delusions by recollecting the mechanisms of dreaming. Propensities, desires, and feelings from the waking state reappear in dreams in symbolic scenes (1912, p. 178, as cited in Blaney et al., 2015, p. 28).

Clearly, one should be cautious of naming that which defies naming because naming is always defining and *per se* definitive – it may limit and degrade the named; but it may also elevate it, or even free it from the shackles of its context. Calling oneself a "scar" may serve as one example, calling a birthmark a "beauty spot" as another. In social context, the connection between the signifier and its referent impacts individual's feelings more than any logical notion of similarity, likeness, or descriptive representation (Stokke & Selboe, 2009).

Symbolic representation is grounded in belief. The symbol has to be credible, in order to pass the muster of representation – if the birthmark is so ugly that no reasonable person would call it beautiful, it hardly helps the individual to refer to it as a "beauty spot." What is more, one has to have a certain degree of self-esteem and security in one's being – in other words, one has to believe in oneself – in order to project a credible self-image. Whenever such belief is absent, the image cannot carry the symbolic weight necessary to substantiate the body behind it.

Ferguson (2000) stated: "We live through images because they are substantially unreal" (p. 69). He made this statement in connection with images of war to the presence of which we have become numbed and accustomed. However, how have they become "unreal" and to what degree is both psychologically and philosophically arguable. When Matthew Brady published his photographs from Antietam,[60] the horrendous pictures of death caused a great public opprobrium and disenchantment with the war. The bodies devoid of life signified the only thing they could signify – death.

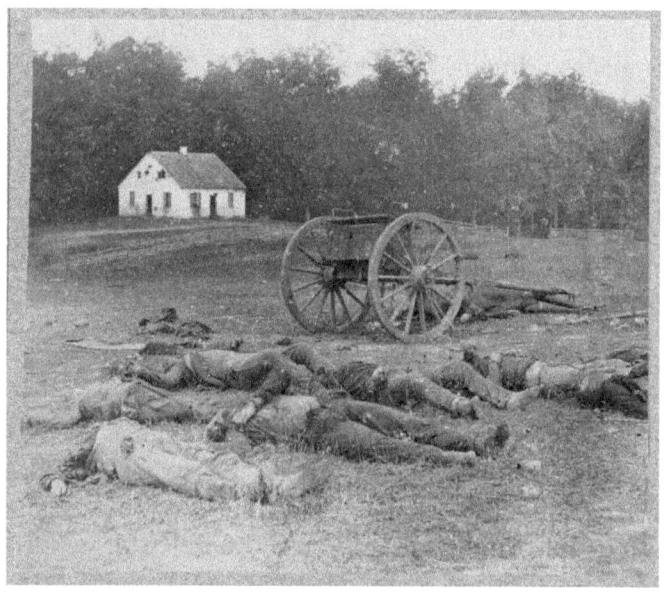

Gardner (1862)

---

[60] These photographs were taken by Alexander Gardner, a Scottish immigrant who was employed by Brady. Brady learned photography from Samuel B. Morse, the inventor of the Morse Code, and daguerreotype.
After victory at the Second Battle of Bull Run on August 30, 1862, General Robert E. Lee led the Confederate Army into Maryland. On September 17, the Union Army attacked Confederate forces at Antietam Creek near Sharpsburg, Maryland. With over 23,000 dead by the end of the day, the Battle of Antietam was "the bloodiest single day of warfare in American history" (Stanford.edu, 2023).

Fergusson's statement about images being "substantially unreal" has more general implications. For example, health-food and diet commercials in the form of: "I have lost 50 pounds on this diet!" and: "Look how slim I am now!" – or those that appeal to physical strength and muscularity purportedly brought about by the secret formulas of diverse "male enhancers" – are so ubiquitous that individuals with BDD, diminished self-esteem, or distorted body image will crave them as means to realize their hidden potential, even as they are thereby going to conform to the prophesy of the unreal images, exacerbating their body image dysmorphic issues. Even in people with a healthy self-image, the impact may be felt, lasting, and not insignificant.

But what then is real? Should an effort to be fitter be considered less real because it is stimulated by some commercial, or peer pressure? The answer is that it should not, provided that the main driving force comes from within and corresponds to the image of the body the individual forms about themselves (without submission to the drive of the norm), as opposed to what someone else says about them.

The optical and the tactile impulses are always initially separated which creates fertile ground for body dysmorphic disorders and what Schilder (1964) referred to as *psychological dismembering*. According to Schilder, psychological dismembering is the result of the optical and tactile differences in perception of various body-parts, creating the notion of interchangeability of body-parts, as well as a psychological delusion in focus on one body-part at a time, which may happen when the individual is obsessed with, for example, the size and shape of her nose, or the size of his biceps.

However, not only can one not reasonably avoid psychological dismembering but it can be argued that this process facilitates acceptance of the body as a "social estate" – thereby anchoring and grounding the self in their environment, be it their family, tribe, nation, or culture (Belting, 2011, p. 62). This symbolic function of the image would not be possible if one focused solely on the body. Belting (Ibid.) notes that the dismembering of the body into representative symbols of the image facilitates human understanding of the genealogy of the body itself. He uses the heraldic symbolism to exemplify this, pointing out that the image fulfils the function of the *medium,* and because the image may be literal, symbolic, or a sign, it may ultimately stand in competition, if not opposition, with itself. The painting on the portrait panel would compete with the coat of arms of the individual's family, which would include genealogy and nationality, combining symbols and signs, and often also faces. For example, consider this heraldic symbolism in the crest of the House of Bourbon (see the next page).

This symbol combines identification via language, two identical mirror-faced human faces, which constitute both images as well as signs here, and symbols representing the empire (chiefly the fleur-de-lis and the royal mantle or ermine).[61] The very name Bourbon is topographical (the surname originated in a village in Allier, site of the now ruined castle of Bourbon) and the phrase "Montjoie Saint Denis!" was the battle-cry and motto of the Kingdom of France. The phrase is akin to the English "Hold the line!" *Montjoie* is said to have referred to the pile of stones where the war counsel was held, possibly with the crucifix affixed (Duggan, 1976).

---

[61] A sign is used to communicate information, usually of a warning or prohibitory nature (e.g., a stop sign). A symbol has a deeper meaning which may differ from culture to culture. For example, the cross is a symbol of Christianity but it may also carry a broader meaning (i.e., death). The heart is a symbol of love. Rainbow may symbolize hope in general, but it may also be a sign (as well as symbol) of "Pride."

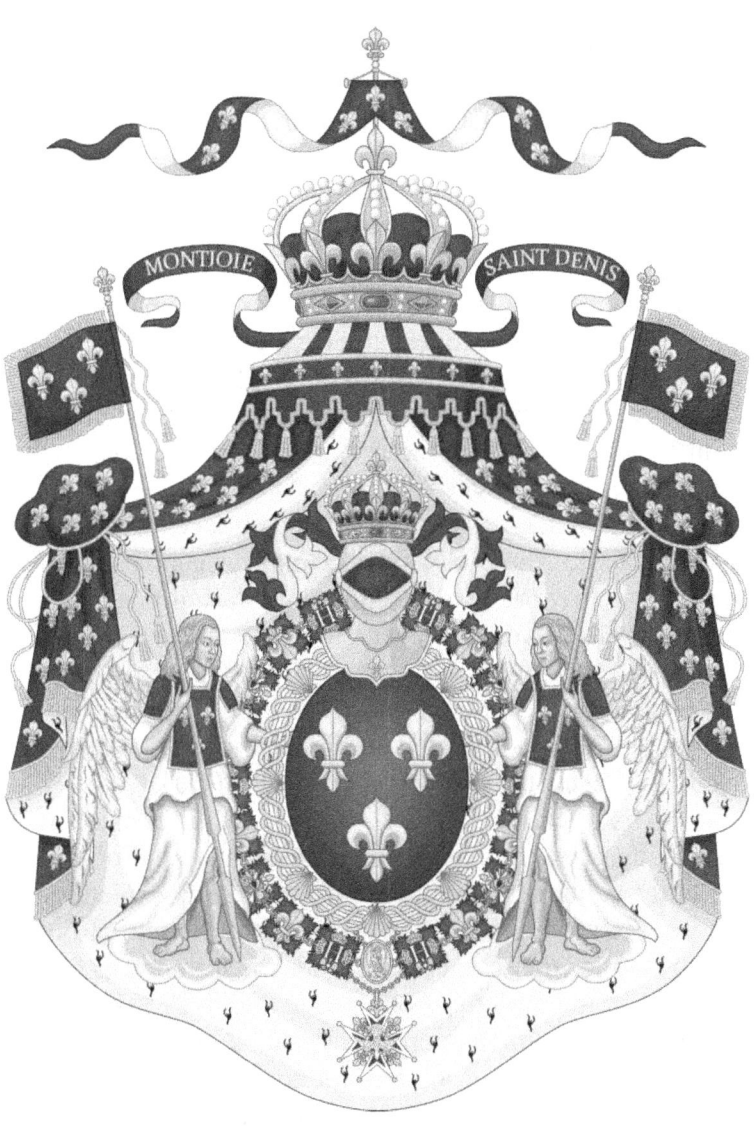

The fleur-de-lis (French for the "flower of lily") is a symbol that depicts a lily or iris, signifying life, light, and perfection. The three fleur-de-lis on the shield here clearly symbolize the Holy Trinity. They are printed in the center of

131

the crest, which depicts a suit of armor of the warrior-king, complete with the helmet and royal crown.

Notably, the faces of the two guardians of the shield are portrayed opposite each other and gaze or point toward the center, thus neither clashing nor coming in conflict with each other nor with the central image. Again, however, they are "dismembered" in that each has a hand cut off or hidden (apparently holding the shield), the faces are separated from their bodies, and the one bare leg of each person-image stands parallel with the spear, firmly planted at their feet. This dismembering reinforces the impact of the heraldic symbol where the images are portrayed as independent mediated as one, in synergy.[62]

This synergy is healthy for body image interpretation in that it unites the body and the image, making them one whole which carries social and cultural significance. It is important to note, however, that no body is directly displayed anywhere but, rather, remains portrayed by representation in the sign and the symbolic import of the image. It is this represented and representative body which becomes the currency of social existence.

Historically, there existed a difference with distinction between the coat of arms and a shield of arms – the latter being more of a portrait or *tableau* depicting the person, the "living bearer of the name in his mortal body" which "carried the social rank;" while the former was further removed from any actual body image (Belting, 2011, p. 66). One may, for example, consider Gainsborough's *Blue Boy*, where the costume and colors are used to emphasize the rank and social standing (see below). The painting remains the

---

[62] The very words "heraldic" and "herald" refer to a "messenger" or "envoy," which means a representative, bearer of the symbolic tradition and custom. The origin lies in the Frankish *hariwald* which means a "commander of an army" (Proto-Germanic *harja* "army" and *waldaz* "to command" (cognate of *wield*). For more information on this topic, *see* Fox-Davies *Guide to Heraldry* (2012).

"epitome of British culture" (Wilson, 2022, par. 1). Wilson (2022) further speculates that the Blue Boy has become a "powerful symbol of non-conformist gender identity and same-sex attraction" during the rise of the homosexual movement and the Gay Rights agenda, thus taking on a new role with the changing social milieu. As such, it would properly be described as a shield of arms.

By the same token, however, we may ask whether such refinement of symbolic representation is not merely a slight of hand performed by some slick post-modernist social scientist familiar with Jacques Derrida.[63] After all, it is the viewer who is interpreting the meaning here, not the painter, and especially not the subject himself who, to all practical intents and purposes, remains mute. What would the Blue Boy himself do or say in the face of such criticism? In the Huntington Gallery, he stands opposite the Pink Lady ("Pinkie") by Thomas Lawrence, not as a contrasting figure but, rather, as her contemporary companion, thus a beau apposite a belle, suitor, and his paramour, or, perhaps, a brother and sister. They are skillfully juxtaposed, not "juxt-opposed" – that even though these two paintings had never been listed in any association or relationship until Henry Huntington purchased them and placed them in the same room, opposite each other (Bernal, 1992). They have been positively contrasted and connected ever since (Wilson, 1984). Such positive correlation stands in stark contrast with the symbolic interpretation of the Blue Boy as a heraldic shield. Clearly, it is not the body itself, but the image which suggests meanings to the viewer, imbuing significance onto the body as a symbolic vehicle.

---

[63] Jacques Derrida (1930–2004), French philosopher, founder of Deconstruction, a movement which distinguishes among symbolic levels of text, and argues that there exist endless levels of meanings and oppositions which may be wholly unrelated to what the author wanted to say.

The body is an immutable given – some people are tall, others short; some overweight, others slim; some are lovable, pudgy endomorphs, others are neuroticism-prone ectomorphs; differences in the shape of the skull, hair or eye color, hand size, etc. are all immutable characteristics. The ultimate body symbol is the hollow skull, *memento mori*, symbol of death. Death is the inevitable end for all bodies. As such, the body can only convey individualized meaning as an image during life.

Body-as-image, on the other hand, may be preserved – in a painting, photograph, statue, or as a heraldic symbol. Its attractiveness lies in its imperishable nature as much as in its malleability. Who is to say what the *Blue Boy* represents? Who is to say what *Me* represents? Arguably, the image can be "processed" altogether without taking into account the existence of the body. Nevertheless, in real life, one has to deal with the realities of the body, be it because of the body's perpetual aches and ailments, or because of its constant physical needs.

Supposing then that the body is the ultimate reality, the image must be a derivative reality. As such, it cannot exist independent of the body. Indeed, the image (such as that of the *Blue Boy*) is a mere shadow of the real boy in blue, allegedly Gainsborough Dupont (Sloman, 2013), who is reproduced here from a certain perspective which, at the same time, disembodies the image and creates a perception which triggers image mediation in the observer, which may include self-comparison or comparison to a known body image, including attire, expression, and background (all of which facilitate recognition and contribute to the interpretation).

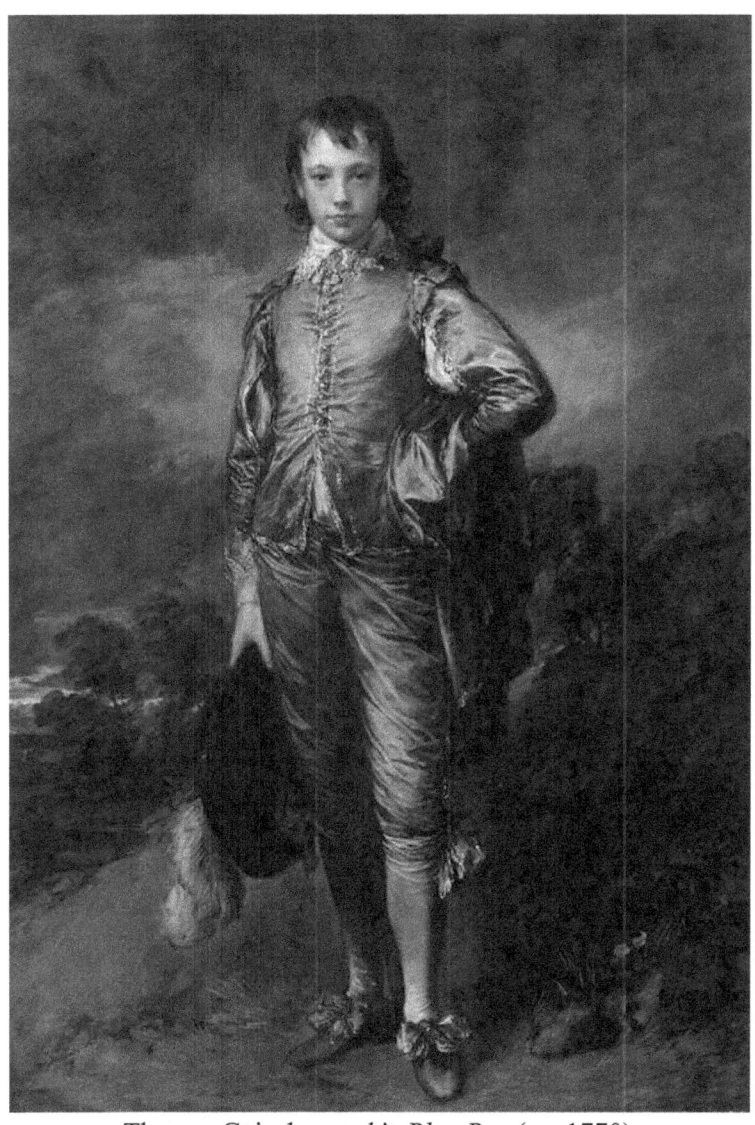

Thomas Gainsborough's *Blue Boy* (ca. 1770).

The interaction between the disembodied image and the observer's sensomotoric system is what "brings into play the dynamics of our consciousness and our inner images," employing "our imagination and our desires" (Belting, 2011,

p. 29). Therefore, the image belongs neither to the painter-mediator, nor to the object himself; rather, its disembodied content is deconstructed by the subject-observer. The word "subject" is necessary, in order to preserve the clarity of construction: the observer is the *agent*, the observed is the *patient*.[64]

Ferguson (2000) notes that, historically, the body's image has been interpreted as its "nonmaterial conception of the soul" or *psyche* (p. 83). Consider the contrast in Raphael's *School of Athens* between Plato and Aristotle (*see* p. 62, above). Plato is pointing up to the Heavens, holding his *Timaeus,* wherein he described the soul as an entity abstracted from the body. According to Plato, each man has "three kinds of soul," the function of each not being dissimilar to Freud's Ego, Id, and Super Ego. Much like the image, the Soul is "plastic," malleable, responsive to the individual's feelings (Ferguson, 2000, pp. 180-183). It is an ever changing image, bound to the *terra firma* through the dumb body.

On the other hand, Aristotle saw the soul as an intermediary between the body and "changeable forms of nature" (p. 84). In Aristotle's view, the soul is neither inferior nor superior to the body – it simply is. Platonic Soul is clearly superior, capable of attaining the ultimate goodness of God. Plato placed the Soul on a pedestal, from which the Soul looks down upon the body. But neither Plato nor Aristotle spoke of a dichotomy between the soul and the body. Indeed, this dichotomy came to the fore only with the rise of Christianity, subsequent suppression of science in the

---

[64] Semantically, the *agent* is the "doer" or instigator of the action denoted by the predicate; and the *patient* is the "undergoer" of the action or event denoted by the predicate. This semantic distinction has been carried over to ethical deontology where the distinction lies between "agent-centered deontological theories," which focus upon agents' duties, and "patient-centered (or victim-centered) deontological theories," which focus upon individual rights (Schroth, 2019).

Dark Ages,[65] and became of particular interest to the philosophers and artists of the Renaissance period.

Why was this so? In mythology, even before Christianity, the concept of the soul has always been likened to *psyche*. Psyche is the *anima* or what animates the body. The body only gains life through the *psyche*. Two social currents underlay the formation of the body-*versus*-soul and body-*versus*-image dichotomy: the medieval "fostering of magical arts," such as alchemy, numerology, and astrology was to liberate the soul from the "controlling authority of feudal institutions" (Ferguson, 2000, p. 87); and the related emphasis on self-reliance, independence and autonomy was to be realized through the liberation of the soul, regardless of the body. Indeed, the body's form and penance became almost irrelevant. Lord Byron's *Prisoner of Chillon* is symptomatic of this condition:[66]

> It was at length the same to me,
> Fetter'd or fetterless to be,
> I learn'd to love despair.
> And thus when they appear'd at last,
> And all my bonds aside were cast,
> These heavy walls to me had grown
> A hermitage—and all my own!

Although the poem is dated 1816, it describes the travails of François Bonivard, a Swiss monk imprisoned

---

[65] Dark Ages refers to the period between the fall of the Roman Empire in the fifth century A.D. and the rise of Renaissance in the fifteenth century A.D. The term was coined by Petrarch (Francesco Petrarca, 1304–1374), whose rediscovery of Cicero's letters revived Antiquity and posed the "dark" ignorance that followed its fall to the preceding "light" of arts and philosophy.

[66] George Gordon Byron (1788–1824), English Romantic poet. The *Prisoner of Chillon* (1816) is a narrative poem which chronicles the imprisonment of a Genevois monk, François Bonivard, from 1532 to 1536.

during the first half of the sixteenth century (the period of High Renaissance) – the century which saw the burning at stake of Girodano Bruno, the clash between the "darkness" of the Church and the "light" of the sciences, and the century which also originated the Copernican Revolution, giving rise to the concept of the universe and our galaxy. This revolutionary schism coincided with the rise of Neoplatonism which emphasized the substantiation of the body as a "vehicle" for the soul, akin to the Platonic concept of stars as vehicles Gods use to "circle the heavens" (Dillon & Gerson, 2004; Plato, 370 BC, 247b; Sorabji, 2005).[67]

Note that Byron uses the word "bonds" as a synonym for "fetters," thus abstracting the idea of imprisonment (boundness) from the physical to the psychical[68] world. In the subsequent, final lines of the poem, he returns to the physical as substantial and binding:

> My very chains and I grew friends,
> So much a long communion tends
> To make us what we are:—even I
> Regain'd my freedom with a sigh.

This sigh is not only a sign of desperation, but also of the realization that the liberation of the Soul from the body is impossible. The image is permanently bound to the body. It would not be until Jean-Paul Sartre rephrased this bond as a "condemnation to be free" that new body image

---

[67] Neoplatonism (300-500 A.D.) Plotinus (c. 204-270 A.D.) is considered to be its key proponent. He countered Plato's (c. 428-347 B.C.) dualistic thought (ideal-*versus*-real) by locating the One in human consciousness, that is in self-reflection: it is in trying to understand oneself that one creates one's ideal (idea/image) self, as opposed to the real (reality/body) self.

[68] Relating to the psyche (from Greek *psyche* – the soul), lying outside physical sphere and material knowledge (not "psychological," which relates to the conative function of the will and mind studied by psychology).

potentiality arose. Still, hidden within it lies the foundational paradox of the human condition, which is that no "body" can become a whole and wholesome Self unless accompanied by an image carved in time and space – an image which, by its symbolic nature, interminably subjected to interpretation, undermines the very body of its creator.

Is the Image the Soul of the Body?

What an intriguing question! Most notably, it was the founder of sociology Émile Durkheim (1858-1917) who noted that "in many societies, the soul has been thought of as an image of the body" (Durkheim, 1995, p. 48). Today, we often hear the term "the Soul of the Nation" which is purported to mean the essence or embodiment of what the nation represents. There is "soul music" and "soul food" as well as "food for the soul." One can "bare one's soul" to someone as well as "put body and soul" into an activity. The soul is both an immaterial, intangible percept, an inner drive, animating principle of existence, but also the totality of the person's self and selfhood. If someone appears soulless, they are in a trance, zombie-like state of abandon, abstracted from other human beings, their feelings, their ethics, their souls. Evil is soulless, so is a stone.

Plato equates the soul and the idea. For Plato, the term "*Idea* represents the absolute, metaphysical reality" (Bugiulescu, 2021, p. 80) [italics added], as opposed to the "idea" used for the generic ideas people may have. Etymologically, the word *idea* is derived from Greek, where it means a "form." This may seem paradoxical to the modern reader who conceives of an idea as something immaterial and abstract, without a definite form. According to Etymonline (2023) notes that the origin of the word stems from *idein* "to see," from Proto-Indo-European *wid-es-ya-*, which is a suffixed form of the root *weid-* "to see" (par. 1). Contrary to the modern reader's common sense concept, Plato held that Idea represents a pure form. A cognate of "idea" is the Greek *ennoia,* meaning a "mental image or picture" produced by the thinking process (para 3). This means that it is a thought product in its ideal *form*. By nature of this paradox, the idea is seen (image) and yet remains impalpable because immaterial, without a "body."

In *Phaedo*, in the dialogue with Simmias,[69] Socrates postulates that human beings have an innate knowledge of ideas such as beauty, truth, virtue, vice, good and evil, and that, therefore, human souls (ideas) preexist human bodies, which means that they are immortal (Plato, n/d): "But when did our souls acquire this knowledge?" asks Socrates, and rhetorically answers himself: "—not since we were born as men?" He concludes that our knowledge of ideas came from recollection, which implies recollection of something previously known.[70] The entire method of so-called Socratic instruction is founded on this concept. "Then, Simmias," Socrates concludes, "our souls must also have existed without bodies before they were in the form of man, and must have had intelligence."

This conclusion not only gives a whole new meaning to intelligence, as something far beyond and above learned knowledge, but it also leads Socrates to the following logical conclusion:

[if,] as we are always repeating, there is an absolute beauty, and goodness, and an absolute essence of all things; and if to this, which is now discovered to have existed in our former state, we refer all our sensations, and with this compare them, finding these ideas to be pre-existent and our inborn possession—then our souls must have had a prior existence, but if not, there would be no force in the argument? There is the same proof that these ideas must have existed before we were born, as that our souls existed before we were born; and if not the ideas, then not the souls.

---

[69] Simmias of Thebes was Socrates' disciple, one of his "inner circle" of followers (as alleged by Xenophon in *Memorabilia*, 1.2.48, 3.10.17). He also appears in *Crito*, *Phaedrus*, and *Epistle XIII*.
[70] From Latin *recollectus*, past participle of *recolligere*, from *re-* "again" and *colligere* "gather." The English meaning is thus a direct translation from Latin: to recover, recall, bring back to the mind.

This is certainly a *déjà vu* to every reader who has, time and again, realized that *nihil sub sōle novum* – nothing is new under the sun; in other words, that all ideas that ever occur to human beings have occurred to others before them, and that, therefore, the best one can hope for is to place old ideas in a new light, and to contribute to the world of ideas with personal perspective and experience. Harold Bloom's term "anxiety of influence" (i.e., that every subsequent writer suffers from anxiety of having to build on preexisting ideas) is not just a literary critical statement – it applies to body image influences in the world of images in general.

Socrates' conclusion that "the soul is immortal, because the idea is immortal" also means (in Plato's interpretation) that ideas are "not simple mental concepts," but "ontologically distinct entities in the World of Ideas" to which, however, we are granted access only through our bodies (Bugiulescu, 2021). In Plato's philosophy, the Soul pre-exists the body and is "configured in three parts: one rational, opposite to the other two, the sensual and the passionate" (p. 81).

Similarly, Persian philosopher Avicenna (980-1037)[71] expounded on the subject, further underscoring the importance of the *form* for the matter:

> To treat now of the definition of the Soul at large, I mean the universal, absolute, generic soul. This will become apparent, according to the tenets I hold, that among truths that are plainly manifest one is that every one of all natural bodies is compounded of "hyle" [sic] I mean matter, and of form. As for hyle, one of its properties is that through it a natural body is affected (or acted upon) in its very self; seeing that the sword, for

---

[71] Avicenna (original Arabic name: Abu-`Aly al-Husayn Ibn `Abdallah Ibn Sina, often abbreviated to Ibn Sina), Persian philosopher and polymath who was familiar with the philosophers of ancient Greece.

instance, does not cut through its iron, but through its sharpness, which is its form; whereas it gets jagged owing to its iron, and not owing to its form. (Avicenna, n/d, Sub-Section B)

Here, Avicenna followed Plato and Socrates in identifying the idea with the form. While the body is but a mass of cells, the image of the body (literally the body-idea) consists of its sharpness (or bluntness, as the case may be), which means of a *form*. One may argue that using "consists of" in this context is inaccurate and misleading because the matter is what makes up the body.

Nevertheless, to *con-sist* literally means to stand-together. As such, the word bears upon the firmness of the matter, which may be said of a material, material thing or matter – but it need not be. Firmness is also a quality or characteristic, similar to sharpness. Sharpness is a property which relates primarily to the function and utility, not the substance of the object. Thus, it is a property not of the body but its image. Conversely, in the same vein, where the image is infirm, it is referred to as a body dysmorphic disorder (BDD) or some similar body-image related condition (pertinent not to the body but to the image).

Having conceded that sharpness is a characteristic necessary for the proper functioning of a knife, then one must concede that firmness is the characteristics necessary for the proper functioning of the body. Where is this firmness located unless in the image of the body? However, while Avicenna could observe that the sword "cuts through its sharpness," one could not claim with the same certitude that the body performs its functions through the image – unless one should also concede that the image is its soul.

Image in itself is a mute picture, but body image is not mute – the very opposite! It is the coin of social currency. It speaks through the gesticulation and imagery which the soul wields. Is it too far-fetched then to say that the image is the soul?

Aristotle[72] considered the soul as something which "arises from the normal functioning" of the body (Ferguson, 2000, p. 85). Psychology, for Aristotle, was a "branch of physics" (Taylor, 2015, p. 2). Neither Aristotle nor Plato thought of the soul/image as standing in opposition to the body but, rather, thought of them as one. For Aristotle, psyche or the soul embraced an entire "process of nutrition and growth and the adaptation of motor responses" to the external world (Ibid.). Consciousness of these processes was said to permeate and live *with* the body, as did the soul (Windberg, 2021). Since consciousness implies awareness of the self, therefore self-reflection, it is a pre-requisite for body image formation. For Plotinus and the Neoplatonists, consciousness *arose from* (literal translation would be "fell out of") the First Matter, and only then did the soul *arise from* Consciousness.[73] Thus, the soul and consciousness were separate entities.

The Greek word *psyche* is translated as "anima" into Latin.[74] In virtually all other languages, it is identical with "soul" (English "soul," German as "Seele," French "âme," and Russian "dusha" all mean the "soul"). Taylor (2015) pointed out a salient fact in Aristotle, namely that the concept of the body is an organic amalgam with the soul: "If," said Aristotle, "the whole body was one vast eye," then "seeing would be its soul." This means that the body is an instrumentality in the service of the soul. Further, the

---

[72] *Cf.* Aristotle's (384–322 BC) essay *Concerning the Psyche* (Greek: "Peri psyches," transl. as *De Anima* in Latin).

[73] The resemblance to Heidegger's *thrownness* as the primary ontological state of Being seems more than coincidental. Such *thrownness* into Being is a manifestation of both motion (in becoming) and image-creation (in self-reflection and realization).

[74] This word is tinted with Jungian psychology, where it is used as the female part of a male personality. It is derived from Latin *animus* which was originally applied to the soul, breath, and the vital principle of life.

144

presence of the soul, *the first entelechy* of the living body, is the first precondition for intelligent life and good character of a human being.[75]

For Aristotle, the soul is neither acting on the body nor acted upon by the body, nor is it a series of body-states. Yet, there is a parallelism which he considered to coexist in unity. Aristotle's concept of the soul is therefore directly opposed to the western Christian notion of the soul as an immortal part of the self, for which the body is but a conch.

In trying to describe somatic events that had no apparent somatic causation, C. J. Jung (1969) arrived at the conclusion that the human psyche interacts with the surrounding matter, creating a *liminal space* (Jung described it as a *zero-point*) between the somatic domain and the psychic sphere, in which both the symbol (idea) and its representations (soma, somatic symptoms) become *embodied metaphors,* metaphors like: a "broken heart" or "cold feet" or "the guts to do something" (Miranda, 2014). For Jung, the image of the metaphor is a situational embodiment of an act of the living, material body, and it must have existed in the body prior to the event which has given rise to it. "Such an image is an a priori type," noted Jung, which is "inborn" in the animal form even "prior to any activity" (Jung, 1960, p. 201).

All human beings share similar inborn instincts or patterns of behavior, such as the motherhood instinct. It is through these archetypal patterns that people can relate to one another, but also to other animal species (e.g., when imputing certain feelings or thoughts to domestic animals). For Jung, the soul is the embodiment of these instincts and patterns of behavior, whereas the *psyche* is a broader, poetic concept of the soul, which "evokes the unconscious, the

---

[75] *Entelechy* is sometimes also translated as the soul, or a biological force. Etymologically, the word came to English via late Latin, from Greek *entelekheia* (coined by Aristotle): *en-* meaning "within," *telos* "end," or "perfection," and *ekhein,* to "be in a certain state."

imaginal, the emotional, the intuitive, the somatic, and perhaps the spiritual" (Erickson, 2022, p. 12). Therefore, putting aside this soul-psyche distinction, Jung's analysis leads to the conclusion that the soul is the intangible image of the body because it represents archetypal patterns embodied in the body and its activities.

This conclusion comports to the materialistic and mechanistic theories which stem from T. Hobbes (1588–1679), J. O. La Mettrie (1709–1751), and others, holding that the psyche is a "function of the brain and nervous system" (Dafermos, 2014, p. 1530). Nevertheless, opposing theories have also been many, starting with G.W. Leibnitz (1646–1716), and C. Wolff (1679–1754), who have traditionally held that the psyche (the soul) has a life of its own, and is able to introspect and rationalize in the abstract. It was the father of modern psychology Wilhelm Maximilian Wundt (1832–1920) who coined the term "discipline of consciousness" (*Bewusstseinswissenschaft*) for the realm of the psyche (Graumann, 1996).[76]

---

[76] Thomas Hobbes, English philosopher and what today would be called a "political scientist." In *Leviathan* (1651), Hobbes argued for a social contract and the rule by an absolute sovereign as the only means of avoiding the war of all against all which, he asserted, was the true natural state of humanity.

Julien Offray de La Mettrie, a French physician and philosopher, known for his *L'homme machine* (Man a Machine), published 1747, which expanded on Descartes' argument that animals are "machines" and denied the existence of the soul as separate from the matter.

Gottfried Wilhelm von Leibnitz, a German mathematician and philosopher, pioneer in calculus and mechanical calculators. In philosophy, he argued for logical deduction as means to knowledge.

Christian Wolff, a German philosopher, represents the apex of the Enlightenment period in Germany. The knowledge of the soul for him was a matter of empirical (rational) deduction, boiling down to the principle of non-contradiction (a thing cannot be and not be at the same time).

Wilhelm Maximilian Wundt, a German physiologist and philosopher, considered the "father of experimental psychology," predecessor to

The reader is well aware that scientists rarely, if ever, use the word "soul." Modern ("new") psychology has replaced the soul with the "mind," "brain," and "psyche," sometimes even "spirit," all conceived of non-spiritually. Spiritual connotations of the term have largely focused on the intellect and cognitive processes. The advent of Marxism and materialism facilitated a new branch of psychology, behaviorism, which eliminated the term "soul" altogether, and, instead, focused almost exclusively on "the study of external, observed, measured stimulus and reactions" (Dafermos, 2014, Ibid.). The very term "psychology" implies a science of the psyche – i.e., the soul – but there is very little of the soul left in it today. Most "psychotherapy" methods focus on the body, treatments of symptoms, and take advantage of various medications that directly affect the brain. Only poets and, sometimes, philosophers venture upon the intricacies of the human soul.

However, the very notion that the modern society suffers from the illness called narcissism (narcissistic personality disorder) and that this "pathology represents a heightened version of normality" (Lasch, 1979, p. 38), is symptomatic of the search for one's self. Who (save, perhaps, for an AI engineer) would deny that there can be a self without a soul? Since the soul is seen as an immaterial image of the self, during one's life, this soul-image is tied to the body, and inseparable from one's body image. That is why the focus is diverted to the body, not to the soul. The body is perceived as material, something the individual can master and shape. This mastery consists in trying to understand and master one's body – only then is one supposed to understand and love the soul.

---

cultural psychology. (Butler-Bowdon, 2013). Wundt was an anti-empiricist, proponent of Leibnitz's "Nihil est in intellectu quod non fuerit in sensu, nisi intellectu ipse." – "Nothing is in the intellect that was not first in the senses, except the intellect itself." (Leibniz, 1765).

A different dichotomy was described by Rousseau, who distinguished between *amour proper*, and *amour du soi même* (Ferguson, 2000, p. 94).[77] The first assumes that self-esteem and self-love are grounded in the approval of others, while the latter focuses on the feelings for oneself alone, without any intervening concerns about how one is seen by society. It can thus be stated that *amour proper* depends on the body, how it is viewed and interpreted by others, while *amour du soi même* is love of the soul, regardless of how the others view it, with or without the body. Therefore, by logical deduction, body image and the soul are different concepts, although the soul inhabits the body.

---

[77] Walt Whitman makes the same differentiation (between the I, and Me myself) in the Leaves of Grass, *Song of Myself*: "Battles, the horrors of fratricidal war, the fever of doubtful news, the fitful events;/ These come to me days and nights and go from me again,/ But they are not the *Me myself*. (Pt. 4) [italics added]

Body vs. Image

Most people grow up with very little abnormal preoccupation with their body image – children eat what they are given, what is available and provided for them, and pursue physical activities as they are taught or as learned by imitation from their peers.. In most people, the body–image dichotomy, although natural and present in all human beings, does not become problematic unless and until a triggering event occurs, affecting (or preventing the affect of) regulation, reflective functioning and coherence of the mind. Such a triggering event may be caused by a sudden trauma (loss, grief, severe harassment and bullying, ostracism, etc.) or by a gradually ripening crisis. Tasca and Balfour (2014) reported these symptoms to be causally related to anorexia nervosa (AN) and bulimic disorder (BD). Singh and Veale (2019) made similar findings of correlation to the body dysmorphic disorder (BDD) in cosmetic surgery patients.

It has been noted that "parental misattunements" in childrearing are causally related to the "dysregulation of affect, impairment of attachment, impaired cognitive processing, and a greater reliance on external stimulators" such as food, drugs, alcohol, and other "soothing mechanisms" (Petrucelli, 2016, p. 37). This indicates that, for example, in cases of obesity and eating disorders (ED), it is not the food-shaping-the-body which triggers body dis-satisfaction or dysmorphia but, rather, the neural impetus from the image to the body which takes food as the means of self-regulation and self-affirmation. Petrucelli (Id.) blamed inappropriate or inadequate parental responses to the child's implied requests for body image mediation, which are fundamental for growth and self-affirmation. Demasio (2010) described the process of image formation in detail, noting that not just the body but everything in the individual's proximate environment is subject to image "mapping" (p. 68).

The "misattunements" that Petrucelli (Ibid.) referred to may occur in any environment and may be triggered by any third persons or even by inanimate experiences (such as encountering posters of models or muscular men, social postings which may evoke anger at one's own weaknesses or perceived inadequacies of one's physique). As Trottier et al. (2022) concluded, PTSD can become such a "trigger" because PTSD and eating disorders "frequently co-occur and can share a functional relationship" (p. 687). By definition, PTSD itself is caused by a preceding traumatic event ("post-traumatic" stress disorder) which means that, in analysis as well as in therapy, the approach must address past trauma.

Developmentally, original parental projections may turn into self-projections later in life, thwarting the integration of body image, and altering self-affirmation into self-disaffirmation. Traumatic events and predispositions to them may thus be passed on to the child by the parents acquired from them. Not unrelated to such image processing is the interest in one's body which has originated in youth from the parents' own preoccupations with their bodies (or directly with the body of the child). Schilder (1950) offered an example of a boy born with some form of "an anomaly in his genitals" whose mother was consequently "very much interested in it" and "touched him frequently in the genital region" (p. 133). This resulted in his own lifelong preoccupation with his body and body image, unspecified physical pains,[78] discomfort, and a "masochistic attitude" to

---

[78] There is evidence of a "high prevalence of psychiatric comorbidities in fibromyalgia syndrome (FMS), in particular: depression, anxiety, borderline personality, obsessive-compulsive personality, and post-traumatic stress disorder; as well as "high levels of negative affect," such as: neuroticism, perfectionism, stress, anger, and alexithymia (Galvez-Sánchez et al., 2019, p. 117). Researches showed that FMS patients "tend to have a negative self-image and body image perception" as well as "low self-esteem and perceived self-efficacy" (Ibid.).

the body (Id.).[79] When he was four-and-a-half years old, his mother gave birth to his sister, the procedure which he witnessed, and to which he would often return in his masturbatory fantasies, imagining that he was the mother in labor and reliving the perceived torture performed on her by the attending physician. His "fear of castration," Schilder (1950) stated, was "connected to this phantasy" (p. 134). What is more, his mother's interest in his "anal region," administration of frequent enemas when he was a child, and his earliest fears that "rats might crawl into his anus" resulted in homosexual and "passive masochistic and anal tendencies" (Ibid.). Nevertheless, his Super Ego enabled him to adapt to reality; internally though, he suffered from the Oedipus complex.

The term "complex" was first mentioned by Breuer and Freud (1895, p. 187; as quoted by Laplanche and Pontalis 1983). Freud himself used the term "Oedipal conflict" (Boothe, 2017, p. 1401). In order to understand this complex, the story of Oedipus must be told. The most succinct version is as follows.

In the original myth, King Laius of Thebes, learns from an oracle that he will be killed by his own recently born son Oedipus. Therefore, he orders his wife Jocasta to kill the baby by throwing him off Mt. Cithaeron. Instead, she gives him to the Theban Royal shepherd, who brings him up for a while, then passes him on to the Corinthian Royal Shepherd, who takes him to the court of the childless King Polybus of Corinth. King Polybus adopts Oedipus and treats him as his very own.

When Oedipus turns 18, someone at a palace feast scornfully remarks that Oedipus is an adopted stranger, and

---

[79] Such and similar events are commonly mentioned in sincere confessions of adult men. One may find them in Rousseau's *Confessions,* Stendhal's *Red and Black,* Dickens' *Great Expectations*, and many other works of both fiction and non-fiction, indubitably rooted in real-life experiences.

not a true Corinthian. Extremely upset, not knowing what to think, Oedipus leaves and travels to consult Apollo at the Oracle of Delphi, where he is told that he is doomed to kill his father and sleep with his mother. Resolved to never return to Corinth, in order to prevent the materialization of this prophecy, he leaves without looking back – but, alas, accidentally encounters his real father at The Three Ways junction on his way to Thebes. Assuming that this man (who, in fact, is his real father) is but a stranger, Oedipus slays him without a second thought. He then conquers the monstrous Sphinx and arrives in Thebes where he is received as a great hero, and is offered the hand of Jocasta, his real mother.

Subsequently, Oedipus and Jocasta have four children, Antigone being one of them. There is a sudden bout of sterility followed by an ensuing plague at Thebes. Oedipus consults the Oracle at Delphi and learns that they must seek the murderer of King Laius and slay or exile him from the city. Shortly thereafter, the King of Corinth dies and Oedipus learns that he is not his blood son, but was born in Thebes. The Royal Theban Shepherd is summoned and reveals the truth to him. Jocasta, having learned that she had married her own son and had four children by him, hangs herself. Ashamed and humiliated, Oedipus blinds himself.

The Oedipus complex is derived from this myth, which Freud interpreted as: 1) the wishful fantasy of the son to be his mother's exclusive object of affection, which 2) results in anxiety and fantasy of being punished for this by castration, which is connected to 3) aggression against the father who is perceived as a rival. The myth extends beyond the section summarized above – a civil war follows and Thebes falls prey to the tyranny of Creon.

The name of the intersection where Oedipus slays his father, "The Three Ways," is symbolic of the decision-making process each man must undertake, as well as being pertinent to the three-way self-image development, the dilemma between the like-mother, like-father, and self-image.[80] There is also the three-way orientation to the body and punishment: the Origin, the Expulsion, and the Punishment; as well as the tripartite divine and social retribution in the form of: 1) sterility/infertility, 2) ostracism/expulsion, and 3) blindness. The latter, in particular, the loss of sight, is symbolically important – the individual is trying to deal with shame and humiliation by not seeing it, not seeing one's own reflection in others. One may also interpret the act of intentional blindness as a forceful expression of belief in the self, i.e., "Now I can see with my Heart, I do not need the eyes." By the same token, such a resolution imports rejection of society, along with the social transcription of body image – the mediation of one's self, based primarily on sight.

Consider the following quote from the reflections of George Bernard Shaw which follows the remark that, as a boy, he often *saw* himself "theatrically," acting "as a good boy" being "in the character," but not really himself:

When Nature completed my countenance in 1880 or thereabouts (I had only the tenderest sprouting of hair on my face until I was 24), I found myself equipped with the upgrowing moustaches and eyebrows, and the sarcastic nostrils of the operatic fiend whose airs (by Gounod[81]) I had sung as a child, and whose attitudes I had affected in my boyhood. Later on, as the generations moved past me, I... began to perceive that imaginative fiction is to life what the sketch is to the picture or the conception to the statue. (Erikson, 1968, p. 148)

---

[80] The parallel to the Holy Trinity is also apparent here, as is that of the Biblical tradition expressed by Milton: God was betrayed by Satan, Son of Light; Satan married his own daughter; and produced a son by this union. This daughter and her child together complete the "third way," a bridge which spans the way to Heaven, and the way to the Earth, at the point where Eden had been.
[81] Charles-François Gounod (1818–1893), French operatic composer.

It was not until Shaw "blinded himself" to what he saw in the mirror that he began to develop his real self. Before one conceives what Erikson (Id.) calls one's "lasting idols and guardians of a final identity," one must face many discontinuous and temporary selves, some of which may be wholly unacceptable to the developing person (p. 128).

Facing an unacceptable image is always challenging. Often, the viewer will refuse to see "things" because it is impossible to "unsee them." Take, for example, Ernest Hemingway's story *The Indian Camp*, where Dr. Adams is summoned to help an American Indian woman who has been in painful labor for two days. Dr. Adams takes his young son Nick with him, as a form of undiscussed and undisclosed initiation (to face life or death, possibly both). He performs the cesarean with a fishing knife, catgut, and no anesthetic, reminding the boy that he must ignore the shrieks of the woman at all costs – even as her husband cuts his own throat because he is unable to face the suffering of his wife.

Love is the ultimate emotion a human being can experience; hence, to feel the suffering of the loved one is the ultimate level of empathy. Yet, it is the body which suffers, not the image of the body. Is the image of the body projected onto the vicarious sufferer, thus the image causes the suffering; or is the suffering caused solely by the body? Is the suffering the husband experiences that of the body or of the image? If it is by the image, then the power the image has over the body is ultimate (death).

No birth or death can ever be "unseen" by a human being. It is self-projected, either accepted or rejected, thus, triggering either affirmation or disaffirmation of the self. The body image which has instigated the initiation must be absorbed, although it can never be fully understood. Can it be interpreted without being fully understood? The ability to live is the ability to cope with and interpret images of crucial transformation, fashioning one's true self. Arguably, therefore, since one cannot experience the body of another, one can only relate to it through the image. Thus, the image becomes both the medium (the interpreter-signifier) and the subject (the interpreted-signified). The image is where the signifier and the signified merge.

There is a degree of self-fascination in all human beings which, arguably, is necessary for human self-development and what Ferguson (2000) calls "self-fashioning" (p. 87). This self-fashioning is emphatically the province of the human soul, and has been identified with and equated to the self-image in the Western Tradition. It is through the interconnectedness of images that the individual relates to the universe. As such, body image is not only the medium for the body but stands above the body in its infinitude of variations. On this plane, body image is a place-holder for the soul in more than just a name.

There is never just one image but a multiplicity of images, a multiverse which lies without (outside of) the soul which, however, reflects the multiverse within. Hence, introspection can never lead to a determinable and well-defined end – because behind every image-signifier appears a new image-signified. On the obverse side, as has been well documented by Christopher Lasch, such self-introspection can lead to vanity, ebullition[82] of self-indulgence, and effluvium of narcissism. Historically, however, it has also led to the development of Protestant ethic and Western civilization, founded on constant advancement, growth, and improvement of the self.

There is an innate paradox in all human beings, present on both social and intimate-personal levels, that comes from human self-awareness, consciousness of one's own mortality, and craving to "leave something behind" that

---

[82] Eruption, outburst, bubbling and boiling. Ebullition and effluvium are emotion-focused terms, placed in stark contrast here with the obverse side of narcissism in the subsequent sentence, juxtaposing Lasch and Weber.

will outlive and surpass the apparently ephemeral self: Does Hamlet see a ghost, the body image of his father, his own body image, or a self-projected future of himself strolling by the wall? Carnal knowledge (knowledge by and through the body) has often been scorned and looked down upon as something altogether animalistic and undignified. It was not until the rise of Empiricism in the Renaissance Italy that it came to the forefront as a formidable opponent of rationalism, then often based on some dogmatic thought or theorem.

However, as Dawes (2017) pointed out, empiricism did not appear as a *creatio e nihilo* and does not exist *e nihilo*, which is to say that no philosophers exist as black-or-white, either clear-cut empiricists or pure rationalists. Epistemology (theory of knowledge) has been the chief preoccupation of philosophy since Confucius and Aristotle. All epistemological investigations overlap – but it is easier to negotiate the overlaps in philosophy than in real life, especially when we speak of personal experiences and creation and knowledge of the self.

Despite themselves, philosophers tend to be absolutist in one direction or another, for example: *Nihil est in intellectu quod non prius fuerit in sensu* (nothing is in the intellect which was not first in the senses) is an absolutist position.[83] If one approached the body image through such lens, it would be equally absolutist to abstract and separate it as an image, perhaps implying that it is no more than an illusory, immaterial, wishful thought. All that is real, must be empirically founded, therefore derived from the body, claim the empiricists – which, as everyone knows, is far from accurate. There is as much, if not more, derived from

---

[83] This being a guiding principle of empiricism, accepted in some form by Aristotle, Aquinas, Locke, Berkeley, and Hume. Leibniz added (with a Cartesian smirk, no doubt): *nisi intellectus ipse* (except the intellect itself), opening the way to the popular concept that reason conditions experience (Blackburn, 2016).

the mind and therefore, arguably, exists wholly apart from the body, such as your favorite painting or the text you are now reading. You may wish to pause and reflect upon the paradox that this very text, in which the author dissects body image dichotomies, comes into being as a material substance from which it is reconverted back into a host of thoughts and images by the reader. These reconstituted images are absorbed by the self: Hemingway's initiation rite can then be interpreted in light of both self-experience (as a reader of the story or its rendition here), and as a mediated position of the author of this text.

So-called *constructive empiricists* hold that science aims at "truth about observable aspects of the world," but that it shuns unobservable aspects, which means that whatever scientists say is "empirically adequate" but not necessarily true (Monton & Mohler, 2021, par. 1). In lay, non-philosophical language, this means that my image of my body is true for me and yours is true for you because of the empirical and epistemological differences in our individual foundations. Further, consider my image of your body image and your image of your own body image, and vice versa. Neither is necessarily true, although both are true from the point of view of each of us. Yet, there are only two material bodies which a physician can study. Therefore, it is the mind (*ratio*) that creates the body, or each instance of it, as perceived by us.[84] This rephrases Schilder's argument that the *image* re-creates the body.

However, if it is the image that creates the body, not the other way round, then the malleability and subjectivity of the image should mean that the dictates of the body are subject to the whims and vagaries of the mind. Both

---

[84] C. I. Lewis, via C. S. Peirce, introduced the term *qualia* into modern philosophy. It originated with Leibnitz who attacked materialism on the grounds that even minutest description of matter does not explain the mind. *Qualia* can be equated to body-states of perception, thus, by analogy, also as body images.

arguments are scientifically supportable. For example, Young and Watson (2006) documented that physical symptoms (e.g., backache) were the main cause of breast reduction surgery in approximately one half of the patients, the other half complained of "heightened self-consciousness, poor self-esteem, decreased self-confidence, and a negative body image" (p. 191). Psychosocial concerns predominate in younger patients. With age, the physical sphere prevails, possibly because of pragmatic issues, such as increase in non-active matter (weight), rise in blood pressure, diabetes, skeletal structural problems, such as arthritis, and others. Although Young and Watson did not state whether the groups of cohorts overlapped or were separate (such as the two halves of women who underwent breast augmentation), other researchers (cited by Sarwer et al., 2006) indicated that psychosocial concerns are always a major consideration in cosmetic surgery patients, and that "the relationships between physical appearance and psychological adjustment are more complex" (p. 65). Nonetheless, psychological adjustment invariably results in a more positive self-concept.[85] The fact that adolescents who were *less* socially isolated reported an increase in dissatisfaction with their body image, and correspondingly a rise in preoccupation with cosmetic surgery (Topolski et al., 2004), merely means that social congeniality and adjustment are two different concepts. It is interesting that Topolski studied adolescents only. One may wonder what would the results be had the pool of cohorts been expanded. Craighead and Nemeroff (2004) noted that the thalamus is the key tactile processing center in the brain. The thalamus relays all information to the somatosensory cortex, which is the primary brain region dealing with sensation.

---

[85] This phenomenon (and its obverse side, i.e., body image fragmentation) was studied by Alfred Binet (1890), Jean-Martin Charcot (1889), Sigmund Freud (1953-74), Morton Prince (1906), and others. It will be discussed in more depth in the following chapter.

Anatomy of the brain

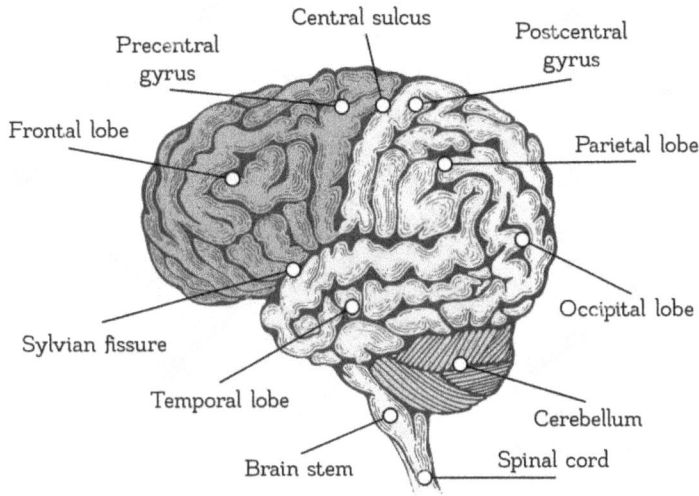

Central sulcus

Precentral
gyrus

Postcentral
gyrus

Frontal lobe

Parietal lobe

Sylvian fissure

Occipital lobe

Temporal lobe

Cerebellum

Brain stem

Spinal cord

The thalamus lies in the parietal lobe, close to the central sulcus, which separates the sensory cortex from the motor cortex (*see* the figure above). The closer to the center of the brain in the sensory anchoring, the closer to the center the mapped parts of the body are: the sensation centers related to the mouth, eyes, and face, are more proximal to the core of the brain than those related to the torso and the legs. Further, each side of the body is mapped in the contralateral (opposite) side of the brain. Physicians have long observed that injuries to the brain regions can be localized from observed impairments in sensory and motor functions of various parts of the body. What is more, the hands, face, and lips take up a disproportionately large part of this chart – they are the most sensitive loci and supply disproportionately greater sensory data and information to the brain.

Stories do more than entertain.
They enter our brain and they remain.

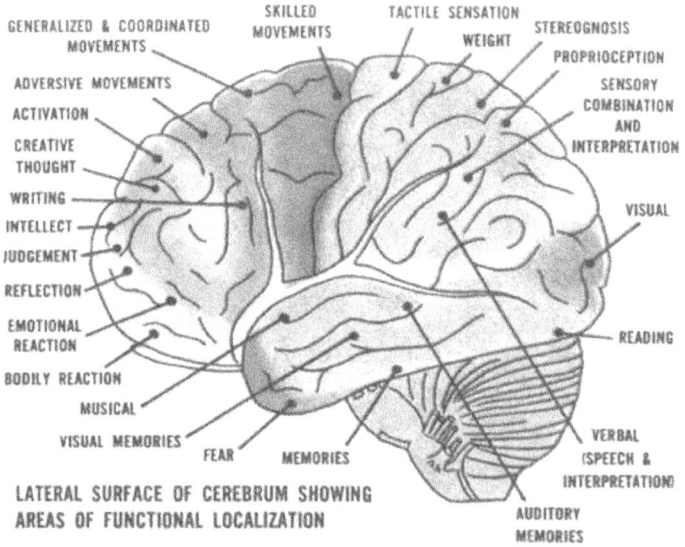

LATERAL SURFACE OF CEREBRUM SHOWING AREAS OF FUNCTIONAL LOCALIZATION

The findings reported by Topolski et al. (2004) – that adolescents who were *less* socially isolated suffered from a greater dissatisfaction with their body image (and correspondingly increased interest in cosmetic surgery) – correspond to the conclusion that since the majority of sensory stimuli enter the brain through the eyes, mouth, and hands, it is these inputs that play key role in the formation of body image, while decreasing the emphasis on the bodily inputs that enter the brain through the secondary sensory system (through the spinal cord and the brain stem). What is more, the primary sensory interaction not only diminishes with age but becomes both less frequent and less prominent,

160

thus leading to the reduced preoccupation with the body *image* in older people.

It may also be argued that the secondary processing mechanisms become more precious to the individual with age because they monitor and relay information about various bodily discomforts, aches and pains which increase with age. Sensory receptors send their information to the spinal cord through peripheral afferent nerves in the arms, legs, body, and head. There are 31 pairs of nerves that enter the spinal cord from the body. Four cranial nerves supply sensory information from the head. This information travels to the brain via two major pathways: the dorsal column–lemniscal system and the spinothalamic system.

The dorsal column–lemniscal system transmits mainly touch and pressure, does so fast (30 to 110 m/s), and provides a high spatial resolution, which means that one can locate the stimulus and its intensity with a high degree of accuracy.

The second system is the spinothalamic system, which is slower (8-40 m/s) because it uses mainly smaller nerves, and provides lower resolution. It also does not adapt quickly, forcing the individual to avoid the pain or any unpleasant sensation thus perceived. Imagine localizing a painful spot on the hip of your body or your leg caused by a sudden rise in temperature. One commonly requires verification by touch that all is well with the affected area. The unpleasant feeling increases, however, when the primary sensory input (e.g., sight) cannot be corroborated by a secondary one (e.g., touch).[86]

One of the five sensory inputs (sight, touch, smell, taste, and hearing) is usually considered as primary by the individual, with others being supportive. Sight and touch are particularly important. Schilder (1950) noted that "optic

---

[86] When one has been bitten by a mosquito in the scapular region, the sensation is doubly unpleasant because its verification defies both the touch and sight inputs.

161

orientation" has an immediate influence on the body schema (p. 112), which has two implications: first, a singular instance of body image can be altered by variation or experimentation with optic impressions; and, second, body image is more accurately portrayed in motion and action: "movement leads to a better orientation in relation to our own body" (Ibid.).

Experiments conducted by Straton, Scholl, and Wooster have shown that the knowledge of one's own body is "to a great extent dependent upon our action" (p. 113). When one is in an elevator or stands on an escalator, the whole body "feels" different. All the faculties contribute to this altered sensation, and although the individual still perceives his or her body as one, this oneness is perceptibly composed of many parts – many separate and distinct perceptions collaborate in the creation of the sequence of body image instances which comprise the one body schema.

Damasio (2010) argued that it is through constant interaction with the environment that the "mapping" of the self is accomplished (p. 67). "The human brain," stated Damasio, "is a born cartographer" (p. 68). This cartography began the moment the individual was conceived and takes place with respect to every sensory input, be it sight, sound, taste, or even a feeling stemming from an inner, apparently non-mechanical, intangible stimulus, such as an upset stomach.[87] What is more, the brain is able to affect the states of the body and, in the course of executing (literally running through) its patterns of mapping, it can evoke and "*stimulate*

---

[87] Note that in language, the intensity of the feeling is linguistically underscored by the use of the present participle: "I am having" is much more intensive than "I have" – and it is also an expression of a passing, momentary state. It can also be used sarcastically, such as in: "She is being facetious." It is not used with states, such as: "He is thirsty." Or: "She is delighted." Language thus captures the difference between body-states and body-images as temporal perceptive functions of the self.

body states that have not yet occurred" (p. 99) [italics original].

On the opposite seat of this mapping seesaw, one may suddenly observe a sudden multiple sensory overload which may result in body image fragmentation, even a complete temporary loss (a sense of being lost in oneself, not finding one's bearings in the world) because the body's topography cannot be detected and analyzed in real time. On the obverse side, such feelings may result in severe depression and suicidal ideation. On the positive side, they may be self-induced – bungee jumping or a rollercoaster ride are good examples. The "high" that daredevils obtain from this temporary bodily confusion is akin to the effects of a psychedelic drug which heightens human perceptions to the point where they also cannot be analyzed and absorbed.

Schilder (1950) concluded that it is primarily and chiefly these actual perceptions, as opposed to imagination and visualization, that create individual body image. This may be the reason why people with body image problems tend to crave such feelings – feelings often self-induced by various daredevil actions, but also through drugs, self-mutilation, cutting, tattooing, or doing pretty much anything which would intensify the perception of one's self and redefine the body image boundaries, thereby enabling the individual to perceive control over their body image.

However, Schilder (Ibid.) did not omit to also note that imagination does influence motor impulses. On that account, Tanaka et al. (2022) conducted experiments into how the feeling of one's body changes with suggestibility of sense-perception. The results of testing with a rubber-hand and heat exposure were assessed both subjectively, via a questionnaire, and objectively, by a proprioceptive drift and electrodermal activity.[88] Their conclusion was that

---

[88] The integration of multisensory input (vision, proprioceptive, and touch) through inference results in the generation of a sense of ownership (SoO) over the object: "When the real and rubber hands are stroked

subjective perception (feeling) was always affected by suggestion (verbal input), but contemporaneous objective measurements (electrodermal activity) were not altered. In a less sophisticated fashion, one may look at time, how it passes subjectively faster with an enjoyable companion in a pleasing environment vis-à-vis the TSA line in the airport. Also, all athletes know that their personal and very subjective feelings affect the outcome of the race, although such feelings are completely invisible and impalpable. Such intangible feelings are wholly unrelated to objective measurements, such as time, distance, or weight. The fact that they do affect results rests in training and preparation. They have been many athletes who have felt "good" about the race – until they saw the time; and vice versa.

Sheerha and Mukta (2016) noted that, regardless of the interaction with (or action within) the environment, it is the top-down factors from within that wield central influence over one's body image. They listed various forms of visualization and their impact on body image, concluding that they all affect and shape self-belief and self-image. They suggested that a sequence of visualization from the current to a future (ideal) body image start with controlled symbolic visualization of one's self in a *"predetermined form"* (p. 473) [italics original], in order to learn to effectively control the image and strengthen it; only then is the subject advised to move on to controlled visualization of symbolic scenes and representations (such as reaching the lighthouse, walking hand-in-hand as a couple, imagining oneself on top of the mountain, etc.).

---

simultaneously, the participant gradually feels as if the rubber hand were a part of their body" (Tanaka et al., 2022, p. 1). Using a virtual arm has been shown to result in similar perceptions (virtual hand illusion: VHI) (Slater et al., 2008). Bottom-up factors (visual, tactile, and proprioception) as well as top-down factors (manipulating the appearance of the rubber hand, e.g., swelling, light alteration) affected the illusion (Matamala-Gomez et al., 2020).

Symbolic visualizations of affective states directly impact one's body image and happiness. It is therefore important to take small steps in positive direction and not to visualize an extreme, unrealizable image as a model. Sheerha and Mukta (2016) concluded that the closer the "ideal image" is to the real image, the more likely it is that the individual will feel internally satisfied and happy. Such happiness is a matter of body esteem, which requires "sexual attractiveness, weight concern, and physical condition" (p. 476).

The problem is that the image often precedes the body, trying to shape it while disregarding its real-life needs and limitations. Maine and Kelly (2005) described this phenomenon as a "body myth" – by which they mean that a persuasion to follow some strict diet, or undergo some radical cosmetic surgery will make the individual happier, is a "myth." By myth they mean falsehood. However, the word "myth" should be understood more in the sense of a popular belief, social practice or phenomenon of symbolic importance, key to social cohesion and constituent of the human culture (Lugli, 2014; MerriamWebster, 2022c). It should therefore not be dismissed lightly.

When King (2001) asked his group of cohorts to write a description of themselves in their best possible future condition for 20 minutes on 4 consecutive days, he noted a "significant immediate increase in positive mood, with an increase in subjective well-being 3 weeks subsequent to the intervention, and with decreased illness 5 months later" (as cited in Sheerha and Mukta, Ibid.). In other words, the more the cohorts thought of themselves in positive light, the more positively attuned they became, and their body image and self-image improved commensurately. This finding leads to the conclusion that an abstract image is superior to the concrete form, thus validating the "body myth" phenomenon in that the actual body alteration (such as having a cosmetic surgical procedure done) is inferior to the impact of a mental, image-motivated action, and may even be futile in the attempt to suppress or overturn it (such as a gender affirming/denying surgery).

It should be noted (just as Topolski et al. (2004) have done), that most researchers have focused on adolescents, simply because most body–image dissonances arise in formative years and frequently take forms that defy concealment. Dacey and Kenny (1994) described physical characteristics as central to adolescents' sense of the self. However, these physical characteristics are not those of the body as much as those of the image, mainly regarding self-consciousness and concerns about peer evaluation (Davison & McCabe, 2006). It is psychological (not physical) functioning that researchers repeatedly address in connection with body–image dissonance: depression, anxiety, bullying and harassment, negative self-esteem, and associated symptoms (Condor-Fisher, 2021). The body is then seen as a physical appendage of the image because its physical attributes (general attractiveness) are mental projections and introjections.[89]

Note that these representations are referred to in plural because each body representation has its own image representation. Kammers et al. (2010) emphasized that different body representations "have been dissociated on multiple levels, including conscious versus unconscious, dynamic versus static, and top–down versus bottom–up" (p. 203). In order to simplify this model for descriptive and research purposes, two general representations of the body have been chosen: its image, and its schema.

---

[89] Introjections implies unconscious internalizations of aspects of the body within the self in such a way that the internalized representation takes over the psychological functions of these aspects (*aspects* implies forms and functions). By losing control over body image, one loses control over the body. In extreme circumstances, the attempt to regain power over one's body may end in suicide.

The image integrates experiences and perceptual judgments; the schema describes the forms and functions of the body. The body schema underlies the action; the body image underlies the perceptual judgments (Id., p. 204). It follows that physicians are primarily interested in the body schema while psychologists are partial to the body image. Body schema is based on the bottom-up proprioceptive information and is less disturbed by the sensory conflicts which affect primarily the body image.

Body Image	Body Schema
Psychological	Physical
Top-down	Bottom-up
Perceptual Judgments	Action
Aesthetic Presentation	Forms and functions
Multiplicity	Unity

Consequently, the body schema is a more objective representation of the body than body image. In fact, the image may not only contradict the body (most blatantly in the cases of sex *versus* gender identity), but it may also defy the body schema – as happens with phantom limb cases, or during rubber hand experiments (described above). The image may embrace and encompass the schema, but it will always add to it and modify it, as our mind always manipulates the sensory and motor inputs to and from the brain.

Further, although the schema captures action, it is actually more static, in that it locates body parts and maps the body in the subconscious (Paillard, 1999). The body schema should be distinguished from the self-schema, defined as "cognitive generalizations about the self, derived from past experiences that organize and guide the processing of self-related information contained in an individual's

167

social experience" (Marcus, 1977, p. 65). Therefore, body schema does not stand in opposition or apart from the body, as body image may; but, by engaging consciousness in proprioception, self-schema corresponds more to the body image than to the body schema.[90]

In conclusion, the opposition is twofold: it consists of the multiplicity of body images, and of the inaccurate and incomplete correspondence of the unified self-schema to the body. How these phenomena interact and correlate shall be dealt with in the following chapter.

---

[90] Proprioception or kinesthesia is the sense of movement and body position, action, and location. It is the ability to detect velocity, load, strength, and resistance via sensory fibers, neurons, and muscles.

Fragmentation of the Body Image

Fragmented self was first described by Jacques Lacan as a natural consequence of the *mirror stage* during the development of the Ego in the process of the formation of human psyche. When a child looks at its own image in the mirror, at about six months of age, the human child will be interested in her image, experiment with it, try to define the self – on the other hand, a chimpanzee will not show any great interest in the image because, Lacan alleged, the ape believes it is an illusion (Lacan, 1953).

Lewis and Brooks-Gunn's (1984) experiments with a red dot on the nose of a toddler (discussed above, p. 117) showed that children under the age of one invariably failed to recognize the mirror image with the dot as their own face. Once recognized, however, the "mapping" of the image begins, and body schema in the brain will reflect the dot. Lacan's point was that the structure of the self (subjectivity) is neither given nor stable, and that the image has to be captured and owned before it is incorporated into one's Ego and given value as one's body image.

However, this identification is fluid, changes with the changes in the body, and thus remains incomplete, unstable, and (needless to say) is never perfect. At the time when this identification first takes place, the little human can barely stand on its own feet, has poor coordination, and feels trapped in a tiny body which is overflowing with physical needs and desires which cannot be reined in or satiated by self-help. The little body causes the little human pain, which seems far from little. The body is lamentably unreliable, imperfect, and weak.

It is the contrast between the fluid image which defies capture, and the body itself which produces fragmentation and tension (Lacan, 1977). Seemingly, the only way to relieve this tension and resolve this fragmentation is to identify with the image. By the same token, this identification with the weak, immature, unreliable body results in a weak, immature, unreliable self – though it be one's true self. This self, compared to the adult self, appears inadequate and misunderstood. Circumstances may arise when, in order to forestall the feelings of immaturity and tension, the child will identify with the *self* of the closest *other* who is much more mature – most often one of the parents, sometimes an elder sibling, or another dominant figure in the child's microsphere. Through such identification, a sense of unity is achieved but – at a great cost: identifying with another causes alienation from the self, especially when the image of the other is dissonant with the image of one's true self. For example, a boy may identify with the seemingly omnipotent mother, a girl with an older male sibling, etc. They then wish to acquire the power of this person, begin to imitate them, and may even completely lose grasp of their original selves. Freud's libidinal theories are at hand in this context. The very popularity of these theories may serve as a testimony to how fast and facile self-reflection and self-identification with the other may become.

Freud's key focus was on repressed desires. Jung underscored repressed memories, both individual and collective. Such repressions are the function of self-projection onto the dominant figure in childhood (akin to what may take place during transference in psychoanalysis). What is more, most individuals will preserve memories of earliest childhood body image fragmentation and carry them throughout their entire lives. These memories may lie dormant, in the subconscious, and may one day be triggered to life by a sudden traumatic event (Yochai, 2019), thus reviving early childhood doubts and insecurities. They may even lead to the fragmentation of the self, causing a plethora of psychological as well as somatic problems (Sapolsky, 2004).

Both memories and desires are interconnected: not only do individuals create memories of their desires at any particular moment in life, but "memories" can also be created by desires – a person's desire to be loved may be so strong that they reconstruct the past and create something which never was. Desires may be so strong that they create memories which will lead to new desires. Whether by the force of the Id or through repressions or desires, the self may be forged into a functioning whole – but it may also be fragmented. Sometimes, the seemingly united self is but a façade, under which the doom of the House of Usher is looming and the cracks reappear in a slightest tremor. Needless to say, the individual is then unable to mediate and respond to mediated body images. The body image, which is *per se* unstable and fluid, takes over the Self.

The best and most frequently practiced way of dealing with this problem is compartmentalization of the body image into body parts. Such compartmentalization is also the product of body image dissociation which originates in trauma. Dissociative responses occur in instances of either hyper- or hypoarousal.[91] Ogden et al. (2006) further argued that they do not occur in non-traumatized individuals. No research has been conducted to-date which would determine whether compartmentalization (thus also fragmentation) is solely causally related to trauma. It would seem natural that the degree of dissociation corresponds to the extent of traumatization and may occur in degrees commensurate to the degrees of traumatization. The problem for researchers is that degrees of traumatization are not clearly measurable and determinable, not to mention comparable, on a scale.

Regulation of affect and tolerance for affect is a complex process developed during early childhood. In

---

[91] Arousal is a state in which the fight, flight, or freeze defense responses are activated. Hyperarousal is caused by an extreme stress which results in the fight-or-flight reaction. When there is no opportunity to escape (such as in chronic stress), the senses may be blunted, the mind freezes and the individual may collapse into hypoarousal (a partial or complete shutdown).

particular, it originates in the interactions between the infant and the mother. Schore (2003) observed that rapid interaction and interchange in the mother-child play creates imprinting of corresponding emotional responses, showing "sympathetic cardiac acceleration and then parasympathetic deceleration" in response to the signals "produced by the autonomic involuntary nervous system in both parties," such as smiles, exclamations, gesticulations (p. 277). It is through these interactions that the infant learns tolerance of affect and self-regulation, and it is through these interactions that the first mirror image of the self is shown to the infant. When the mother's or close caretaker's responses are positive and reinforcing, the infant develops trust, which implies that commensurate trust is being vested in the mirror image of the infant's self. This trust is imperative for acquiring security in one's body and body image during crucial formative years. Where the positive reinforcement is not present, various forms of disassociation and fragmentation arise. These may be projected later in life in various character aberrations (e.g. philandering, hatred for the other sex, child abuse, etc.) or abnormal desires (such as inner insecurity projected in the extreme craving to get married and "be taken care of").

Ainsworth et al. (1978) identified three attachment patterns: secure; insecure-avoidant; secure-ambivalent. Main and Solomon (1990) contributed a fourth attachment pattern: disorganized-disoriented (see also Condor-Fisher, 2021). Ogden et al. (2006) summarized these patterns as follows:

Secure Attachment provides a "healthy bond to the primary caregiver" (p. 46). It creates a defensive mechanism against trauma and distress, with a wide latitude for tolerance and acceptance of the self and others. It also creates a healthy and tolerant behavior toward one's body and body image.

Insecure Avoidant pattern is created by lack of response and affection in the mother when sought by the

172

child, "focusing instead on toys and objects" (p. 49). Avoidance or ignorance of the mother, mother-image and mother's response may lead to the avoidance of one's self or minimization of the importance of one's needs, including disregarding or minimizing or devaluing one's body image. Orientation on toys and objects outside the self and caretaker's mediation valences can be both positive or negative at the time but, if it persists, it will subsequently turn into a preoccupation with outside body images, as portrayed by the media, advertising, etc., with invariably negative results for the self and body image (leading to eventual dissociation and fragmentation).

Insecure Ambivalent attachment develops as a result of inconsistent and unpredictable responses of the mother to the emotional needs of the child. Insecure ambivalent patterns lead to a "difficult temperament" with "tendencies to immense expressiveness and negative mood responses, slow adaptability to change, and irregularity of biological functions" (Schore, 2003, p. 29). Later in life, this insecurity results in ambivalent feelings toward one's body image, marked by, for example, craving for cosmetic surgery, in blind hope of gaining the attention of a love-object, creating a permanent bond which is abnormal (abnormal preoccupation with someone, resulting in extreme jealousy), and outward representation of the self as "belonging" to the self-secure other (or group of others, such as a gang or subculture), while clinging to the naïve belief that such perceived security is real. Social status and wealth are more than incidental to such body image issues – they are indispensable for the sufferer and invariably tied to her desires.

Disorganized/Disoriented Attachment is created where the mother's response to the emotional need of the child creates fear, either by retraction in reaction to the infant, exaggerated response, fearful voice or facial expression (Ogden et al., 2006). Such a caregiver "induces

173

traumatic states of enduring negative affect" (p. 51) which trigger instantaneous defensive mechanisms, such as the fight-or-flight reaction, freezing or extreme hypoarousal (feigned death). This may lead to total abnegation and destruction of the body image, such as may be witnessed in certain cases of drug abuse, or even gender transitioning (alteration of one's body-self to fit the body image imprint of the dominant figure).

The integration of the mirrored reception takes place in the *Dorsal Vagal Complex* which mediates the reflexes and relays autonomic neural responses to stress. The dorsal vagal complex "displays adult neurogenesis, intrinsic neural stem cells and a high brain-derived neurotrophic factor (BDNF) content" which comprise "effectors of plasticity that are modulated by stress in the hippocampus" (Chigr et al., 2009). The dorsal vagal complex reacts to the mother-attachment patterns in the infant and mediates the integration of the body image in the adult.

Siegel et al. (2021) referred to this integration as "relational" and posited that it is indispensable to the formation of one's *identity* (p. 24). The Self can thus be represented as a system of em*bodied* energy whose physical boundaries in no way limit the scope and reach of the Self. Identity is a matter of *consilient integration* of the mind-set and the body-set, flow of mind-states and body-states. This integration is both horizontal (body—image mediation) and vertical (integration of the self), but it is multi-dimensional because it takes place in emotional space and time, governed by the right hemisphere. It is altogether natural, and fluid. Where the self resists, problems arise (Serafino, 2016).[92]

Cash and Pruzinsky (1990) depicted self-integration as a "developmental process" from functional (what the body does or can do to the self/me), to formalistic and

---

[92] Serafino (2016) noted prevalence of eating disorders (ED) connected to body image inflexibility, and the "unwillingness to experience negative appearance-related thoughts and emotions" (p. 28).

conceptual, to symbolic (p. 257). This analysis is founded in part on Piaget's (1946) stages of development, wherein the child first realizes the permanence of the self and, shortly thereafter, the permanence of objects around the self (at 13-18 months of age). Organized self-awareness begins at this time, and it is also at this time that the seeds of fragmentation are sown. Fisher (1986/2014) noted that self-recognition is crucial to self-growth, and that "greater closeness to mother" is positively correlated with increased self-awareness (p. 10). Conversely, distancing from the mother results in decreased self-awareness and self-integration, thereby increasing body image fragmentation.

Where the integration of self-states is either lacking or inadequate, fragmentation of body image occurs. Arguably, the brain can be "embodied" without identifying with the body or "embodying" another human being. The term *embodied brain* is used by Siegel et al. (2021), to describe a brain which is not limited to the skull but can be located all across the synapses of the body. However, the concept of self is "broader than the brain and bigger than the body" (p. 18). It is created through the sensory input to the brain, as well as by the "process of reasoning, decision, and action" that makes images (Demasio, 2012, p. 79). The image of the body can literally be anything created by the embodied brain on any given occasion.

It should be noted that the broader the definition, the more susceptible it is to vagueness. It is the drive to entropy of the image, not the body, that the mind must integrate and contain. In this sense, the Mind preforms the function of Maxwell's Demon, sitting atop the gate between the body and the image, letting in the atoms of its choice, projecting the mirror photons back, to seemingly equalize the vessels.[93]

---

[93] Maxwell's Demon was proposed by James Clerk Maxwell in 1867 as a "finite being" and later called a "demon" by Lord Kelvin (Kelvin, 1879; Maxwell, 1867). The demon controls a small door between two chambers of gas, quickly opening and closing the door to allow only fast-

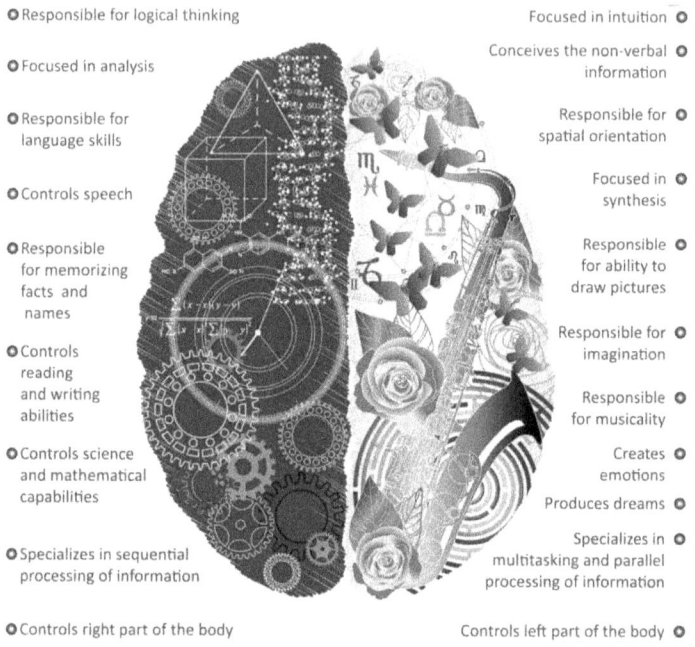

O Responsible for logical thinking

O Focused in analysis

O Responsible for language skills

O Controls speech

O Responsible for memorizing facts and names

O Controls reading and writing abilities

O Controls science and mathematical capabilities

O Specializes in sequential processing of information

O Controls right part of the body

Focused in intuition O

Conceives the non-verbal O information

Responsible for O spatial orientation

Focused in O synthesis

Responsible O for ability to draw pictures

Responsible for O imagination

Responsible O for musicality

Creates O emotions

Produces dreams O

Specializes in O multitasking and parallel processing of information

Controls left part of the body O

Since the limbic-autonomic communications precondition empathy, a person deprived in body image imprint is deprived of the most fundamental human ability to share emotional states and synchronize them with the environment. Such individuals often avoid eye contact, feel inferior, doubt themselves, become easy pray for bullies, and

moving molecules to pass through in one direction, and only slow-moving molecules to pass through in the other, thus increasing the high velocity molecules and temperature in one, and decreasing it in the other. This causes the decrease in the total entropy of the two vessels of gases without applying any work, thereby violating the second law of thermodynamics. The *mirror matter* (sometimes referred to also as *shadow matter* or *Alice matter*) is a hypothetical counterpart to ordinary matter (Zyga, 2010).

suffer from debilitating attachment-related symptomatology. Their right-lateralized interpersonal brain synchronization is defective, and the left brain hemisphere cannot accurately interpret what takes place in the right temporoparietal junction.[94] The affected person finds it difficult to follow a reasoned narrative and transfer it to a spontaneous conversation. Affiliated conditions, associated with the inferiority complex, may also be present.

For all the beautiful divisions of the brain, schematics of information processing, and "executive systems" located in the brain, no-one has yet established where the body image is formed and integrated. Demasio (2012) focused on the cortex, but that is a wide area, and even his division into bi-directional "relay nuclei" (which bring images and sensory inputs from the environment) and "associative nuclei" (in the brain) does not quite elucidate how body image is created in the brain. Space and time, functional abilities, and executive functions overlap and intertwine. It is in where impulses are insulated and localized where body image problems arise – such as focus on a particular body-part with respect to its size or function, or focus on a perceived deficiency (or even pain) localized in a particular body part. Such focus allows researchers to isolate the image-making processes with relative facility in pathological cases by their symptomatology. Where the body operates as it should, in healthy individuals, the mapping process is more complicated to describe in detail.

What is more, body image machinery expands beyond sensory phenomenology of the body. It expresses a unique value of the body for the self, which requires a sense of ownership, what Vignemont (2020) called *myness*. It is

---

[94] The temporoparietal junction (TPJ) is an area of the brain where the temporal and parietal lobes meet, at the posterior end of the lateral sulcus (Sylvian fissure). The TPJ incorporates information from the thalamus and the limbic system as well as from the visual, auditory, and somatosensory systems (Abu-Akel & Shamay-Tsoory, 2011).

necessary for the preservation of the Self: "This body is mine, without it, I would not exist." It is only when one feels such personal possessive attachment, and perceives its unique personal value, that one can satisfy the basic needs of love and belongingness. No matter how narcissistic and egocentric such experience may seem to be, body–image dissonance and dysmorphia may have much more serious consequences than a degree of self-ideation and self-love. That is also why cosmetic surgery is often found to be effective in ameliorating body image fragmentation, and in uniting the body and the image in a more complete self-image. Whether this "myness" of body image can be achieved by non-surgical means (such as diligent exercise, yoga, meditation, psychotherapy, etc.) is a different question. Nonetheless, Sarwer et al. (2006) clearly showed that surgical interventions, from rhinoplasty to gender reassignment surgery, may offer fast and effective resolution here. While science encounters the problem of perception (i.e., perceived self-identification, perceived need for surgery), self-perception is always superior to an objective determination or to whatever "reasonable" perception a third party may provide. After all, the issue is the fragmentation of the self, not the other.

Not all visual-spatial relations are of personal significance. In fact, individuals mostly tend to ignore the world around them until and unless it begins to personally affect them. Such affectation arises from the mediation of one's body image in the environment and from how the individual relates one's self to others. Arising relatedness is similar to the feeling of myness with regard to one's own body. In fact, it is a part of this feeling because it affects the body and self-formation, defines the affective self, and co-creates a sense of ownership in one's self. There is no myness without personal significance – both the image and the body must be given some meaning before they are possessed (owned).

Vignemont (2020) distinguishes between the personal significance of an object (such as a drawing representing one's own body) and the body itself, arguing that "what happens to the drawing does not happen to the body" (p. 120). Actually, a drawing of the body is used in clinical psychiatry and psychology as a representation of the self (in both, projective techniques of assessment and treatment, as well as to detect transference and counter-transference). The affective part of relatedness is always present in the drawing, but also in the interpretation (e.g., Rorschach[95]). Meanwhile, the actual body proceeds to comply with all the biological and evolutionary needs of the individual, thus gaining significance independent of the drawing. This significance is diminished and disowned, as the drawing is possessed (self-appropriated) as a signifier.

Arguably, once the drawing is subjected to interpretation by a third party (friend, viewer, audience), it cannot be said to have still retained the "myness" of the original body. Only to the extent to which it still matters to the drawer, and is adopted by him or her, will it do so. It is in this narrow, affective overlap that there the difference between the body and the image is negotiated to a minimum.

Conversely, the interpreter may mirror his or her own body image in the process of interpreting the "drawn myness" of another individual. For example, Sam (2018)

---

[95] Rorschach was originally developed by a Swiss psychiatrist and psychoanalyst Hermann Rorschach (1884–1922) as a differential diagnostic test for schizophrenia, not as a personality test. It is still widely used as such. For example: Porcelli and Mihura (2010) studied 219 patients and reported a sensitivity of 88%, and a specificity of 94% to alexithymia; Liebman, Porcerelli, and Abell (2005) reported a validity coefficient of 0.71 in 150 adolescents when comparing the Rorschach aggression variables with the Violence Rating Scale; Smith et al. (2010) evaluated the validity of the Rorschach in assessing the effects of trauma, and found that Rorschach may have validity in the assessment of trauma-related cases (Collura, 2020).

notes that the interpretation of a blot figure may indicate either a skin-related, or inner-related condition of the body:

A new interpretation called a "barrier score" has been developed which indicates the sharpness of distinction between the body and its surroundings. Responses like "alligator" and "armadillo" contribute to a high barrier score since the skin of these animals has unusual qualities. These responses have been found among people with symptoms that lie in or near the surface of their bodies, such as dermatitis, rheumatoid arthritis, and conversion reaction. They are not usually given by people who suffer from internal conditions such as stomach disturbances and ulcerative colitis. (par. 1)

Fisher (1986/2014) was the first to conduct a large-scale research and analysis of body image projection surveys among children and adolescents, pointing out the existence of significant "internal discrepancies and negative attributes" (p. 8). While the ability of cohorts to self-identify in shadow photographs, and nude photographs (in briefs, with head and neck covered) taken from various angles was about similar regardless of gender, it significantly increased with age, indicating that body image integration is a process, not a stable "picture" that all humans are born with. As an example, consider the accuracy of self-identification from a photograph taken from the back which improved with age from 52%, 5-9 years to 88%, 9.5 years (p. 4).

However, self-identification was much less accurate when the cohorts were presented with various body-parts, such as when the photographs were cut into strips showing only the head, thorax, abdomen, arms and legs, the torso, and top and bottom half of the body. Fisher (Id.) noted the following findings (p. 5):

The front view of the full body was correctly recognized by 94% of the males and 100% of the females. The respective correct identifications for the rear view were 63% and 92%; and for the side view, 81% and 100%, respectively. The males correctly identified 100% of the pictures of the front view of their bottom half, whereas the females had only 92% success. This sex difference was reversed for the front view of the top half of the body: males, 94% and females, 100% success.

Analysis showed that males have "relative difficulty in perceiving aniseikonic[96] change in the upper body region" and that "females display such difficulty in relation to the lower body region" (Collins et al., 1976, as cited in Fisher, 1986/2014, Ibid.). Collins (1981) found higher accuracy in female self-identification. The accuracy was high in both sexes when the photographs depicted the genital region. Women were 100% accurate "in identifying their own breasts," whereas men correctly identified their chests "in only 88% of their judgments" (Ibid.). Interestingly, both sexes identified their right arm with much more facility than their left arm (81% versus 50% for males, and 67% versus 58% for females). Girls could better identify their hands, and their self-judgment corresponded conversely to their sociability (i.e., more sociable females judged themselves to be smaller; more sociable and self-assured males, bigger).

Enough has been stated about the importance of integration of body image at different levels of perception. Such integration is key to both inner and outer perception of the body. The problem is that the integration of the image through the observer takes place primarily on the level of language, which is invariably deceptive, often resulting in

---

[96] *Anis-* (unequal) + *eikōn* Gk. "image" (cf. *icon*): a defect of binocular vision in which the two retinal images of an object differ in size. The term was invented by American ophthalmologist Walter B. Lancaster (1863-1951).

misinterpretation and maladaptation. Siegel et al. (2021) observed that maladaptive states and body–image misalignments throw the individual back into an "earlier stage" which is generally referred to as *regression* (p. 43). While Jung (1926/1992) portrayed regression in a more positive light (as returning to innocence), majority of experts in the field interpret it negatively, mostly as a state of hopelessness resulting from stress, frustration, neurosis, or traumatization (Freud, 1920/1977).

It should further be noted that the younger the individual, the more susceptible he or she will be to the impact of language interpretation (linguistic mediation) of the body image, be it by one's peers (consider remarks such as: "You have a big nose!" or "You are fat!"), or from the dominant figures in the individual's micro and mesosphere ("You were born white, thus you are a racist!" Or: "How do you know you are a -- ?" playing the strings of youthful insecurity). Unfortunately, it is almost impossible to express how one feels, or what one is, comprehensively enough to satisfy body mediating criticisms and inquiries which, furthermore, are often veiled in seemingly unbiased objective criteria: big/small, fat/skinny, tall/short, etc. The end is often to detract from the speaker's own body image fragmentation or state of disembodied identity which may be characterized by one or more of the frequent defense mechanisms, such as projection, denial, repression, displacement, regression, or sublimation (Freud, 1937). Among children, the conversation will then frequently turn into a physical altercation and name-calling; among adolescents and adults, it will take on the form of more serious bullying and harassment, often on reciprocal grounds (Condor-Fisher, 2021).

Body image fragmentation and regression are correlated. It was the father of British neurology John Hughlings Jackson who pointed out that both hemispheres cooperate in perception, and that there is a certain process of *regression* which takes place in both hemispheres and which is associated with "more primitive methods of expression and representation" (Freud, 1900, 1915, p. 186; et Ibid.) [italics added]. Naturally, such regressive reactive modes of self-perception may not only be uncomfortable, because they suppress the Super Ego and evoke the Ego level of self-image, but also because they tend to be difficult to control and manipulate, not to mention interpreting and understanding them. What is more, regression is often associated with depersonalization and derealization, which also accompany the states of PTSD. In fact, the fifth edition of the Diagnostic and Statistical Manual of Mental Disorders (DSM-5) introduced the dissociative subtype of post-traumatic stress disorder as a specific diagnosis (PTSD-DS).

These diagnoses (regression, depersonalization, derealization, PTSD) overlap, and what really matters is how they are defined in symptomatology. For the purposes of this argument, whether the dissociation and fragmentation are or are not products of PTSD is less relevant than their detection and actual correlation to the fragmented body image. One may ask if there can there be such a thing as body image (image) regression and, if so, whether or not it is somatically detectable, and psychologically reversible.

An example from psycho-oncology provides some ground for optimism here. In the 1970s, the concept of a Type C "cancer-prone" personality was introduced. This was characterized by lack of autonomy, avoidance of conflicts, and emotional recalcitrance, almost as if one was afraid of associating the image with the body because the body was diagnosed with a grave, almost certainly fatal, disease (Temoshok, 1987). The patient may become reactive and fatalistic, or the opposite – proactive and positive. When regression is maladaptive, the patient slumps into a state of chronic stress and dysregulation, leading to a spiral of pathogenic responses (Temoshok, 1990, 2003; Temoshok & Dreher, 1992). On the contrary, *adaptive regression* will lead to control and self-possession. This is the case even where the treatment of the body is ineffective.

Hopwood et al. (2001) developed a Body Image Scale compatible with the quality of life assessments of the European Organization for Research and Treatment of Cancer Quality of Life. Their goal was to assess the extent to which the body disintegrates the image. White (2004) suggested that "investment in appearance and body integrity" are not only worthwhile in diagnosis, but in treatment as well (p. 382). He argued for the integration of body image research in oncology, especially in cases where the body is literally eaten from within, dispossessing and disintegrating (fragmenting) the image (White, 2000). The integrity of the body is reflected in the integrity of the image.

Whereas language can constitute a barrier to body–image integration, it can also be a useful tool, as examples from oncology and trauma medicine have shown (Cash & Pruzinsky, 2004). Not only can the left hemisphere assist in processing feelings of dysmorphia and body image fragmentation – it can also elucidate spatial body-mapping to the researcher or physician, thus providing valuable feedback to adjust the therapy, both physical and mental. Additionally, body image fragmentation may be caused by flashbacks, memory disturbances, disengagement, time loss and trance, as well as sensory misperception, all of which are detectable and interpretable in words (Maniscalco, 2022).

However, in order for such salutary and restorative interpretation to take place, language must be imbued with concrete content. It is easy to get carried away by contentless, yet symbolically loaded speech. On a personal level, such language is meaningless because it does not advance foster body image unity and the sense of myness. Everything one expresses in language about one's self should have some positive non-symbolic body-self and image-self relatedness. The more abstracted, symbolic, or vague the language, the more it will foster fragmentation of the body image.

Reflective and Pre-Reflective Self

Nave et al. (2021) distinguish between a *reflective self* and a *pre-reflective self*. The former is "narrative" and "involves an explicit awareness of one's perceptual image or mental state," the latter is that of an "embodied presence" in the world, providing the individual with a sense of selfhood and "phenomenal interiority from the external world" (p. 2). Interestingly, Nave et al. (Id.) postulate that it is the reflective self that gives rise to an "enduring sense of identity" because it is only when the individual begins to contemplate his or her own existence (thoughts, motivations, personality, memories or appearance) that the individual begins to "identify" one's self. The quandary that neuro-phenomenological research faces is that contemplations of the self via deep mediative states result in a "global dissolution of the sense of self, and the pre-reflective self in particular" – a state which does not easily subject itself to research (Millière, 2018).

The reflective self and the pre-reflective self may also be understood as the image (which is reflected in the mirror, described and mediated), and the body (which is a physical object, sensually perceived, with definite boundaries). In order to avoid this dichotomy and to partially reconcile the conflicting notions, phenomenology uses the term *living body,* which was first introduced by Husserl (1952/1989), who intended to describe the human body as a fluid entity which permeates the outside world and is thereby experienced by the self. The term "living body" can thus be directly linked to the term introduced in Chapter One, body experience (Sakson-Obada et al., 2016), which refers to the sum of each individual's physiological and psychological functions.

Husserl's phenomenological method stems from Kant's transcendental idealism. Kant had distinguished between *phenomena* (things as they appear) and *noumena* (things as they are in themselves), arguing that, somewhat paradoxically (considering that phenomena are mere images of things), only *phenomena* are knowable and can be known by us (Kant, 1929). "Phenomenal" understanding of the material world stems from George Berkeley's (1685-1753) *Treatise Concerning the Principles of Human Knowledge* wherein he introduced his famous *Esse est percipi* ("to be is to be perceived"), ergo: all material things are only real because we perceive them. Naturally, this statement has many offshoots and may lead to solipsism in one direction, and skepticism in the other.

Kant followed the "idealist" branch. Kant can be interpreted in two (not necessarily contradictory) ways: first, appearances are mental states; second, appearances are things as they appear, regardless of the mental state of the observer. If the observer is observing one's own body in the mirror, the body is being experienced as an "appearance" *embodying* one's self, not as a physical object (Körper). If one closes one's eyes and perceives one's Being, then the body becomes a transcendent fluid mechanism for such perception, in which case the mental projection of this body can be literally anything one wishes it to be.

Husserl's likewise sets apart the world of the image on the one hand, and the material world of the body on the other. While his terms *noesis* (consciousness) and *noema* (objects) do very little to enhance understanding of the two spheres of existence, they do bring the two worlds closer together – after all, consciousness is etymologically derived from Latin *conscire* (to be aware), from the assimilation of *con* "with" (or *com* "thoroughly") and *scire* "to know" (cf. science). Harper (2022) underscored that the meaning of "knowing or perceiving within oneself, sensible inwardly, aware" dates back to the 1630s, and that from the 1650s, the meaning has also implied being "aware (of a fact)" – while the more modern understanding (that of being "active and awake" and "endowed with mental faculties") dates to 1837

(Harper, 2022, par. 2). Further, the affix *ness* denotes an action, quality, or state. Thus, "consciousness of the self" tautologically refers to the "knowing self within the self."

The problem is not merely definitional and linguistic, because language interprets perception and the meaning is transformed (and may even be lost) in interpretation. Everything interpreted becomes an aspect of the thing-in-itself. To interpret is to think, and to think is to be – thus, the "new" *esse set percipi* leads back to the "old" *cogito ergo sum.*[97] Why? Because being is a process, not a syllogistic deduction, and perception is instantly a form of thinking. Even a dog looks at its tail when he perceives being bitten by a mosquito. What is the dog thinking? He is perceiving and reacting – but so is a human who feels pain and pain, after all, is the clearest sign of existence.

The noumenal and phenomenal worlds are thus united in each individual existence. This is one way to understand Husserl's *phenomenological reduction*, perhaps the most facile way. However, such *reduction* can also be interpreted as a process which never ends, because one is constantly self-identifying and (re)creating oneself by means of perception and conscious reflection (thought). No-one can live in the world of things as a thing – one can only exist through action.

Thereby, the body becomes a material anchor for the many images that are constantly being perceived, reflected upon, and projected back into the world. Husserl spoke of going "back" [ruckfrage] to the sense of self, whose "identity is temporarily seated in the sedimented layers of

---

[97] Heidegger (2001) noted that at "nearly the same time as Descartes, Pascal discovers the logic of the heart as over and against the logic of calculating reason," a domain which "belongs to calculating representation" as opposed to "the realm of merely producible objects" (p. 125). While representation (reflection) is a thinking process, the word "calculating" may be misleading in this context.

consciousness built up through our temporal experiences" (Cogan, 2022).

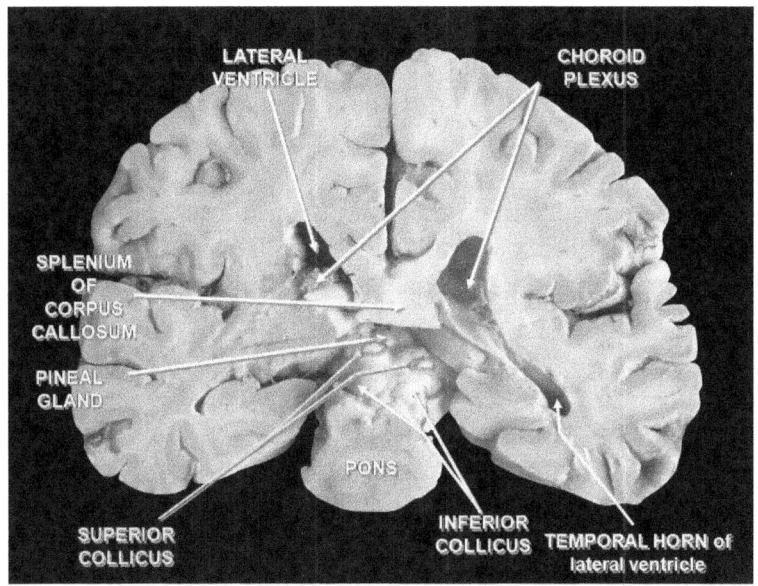

Superior Colliculus[98]

Interestingly, it is those individuals who pause to ask: "Who am I? What is the 'I' that *is,* the *I* that *am*?" that are most at risk of body image fragmentation.[99] No doubt, phenomenological reduction sounds great on paper but, in real life, it lays bare the impossibility of any total and permanent knowledge of the self. The only way to avoid this looming abyss seems to be to define the self along physical and scientific boundaries, in terms of the skeletal structure

---

[98] Attribution: *Superior Collicus* by Anatomist90 - Own work, CC BY-SA 3.0. https://commons.wikimedia.org/w/index.php?curid=19132821 [misspelling original]

[99] Not to mention: "Am I?" and "Aren't I?" or the prescriptively agrammatical "ain't I?" – leading to the ultimate impossibility of self-definition, simply because the *I's* in *me* are many.

and neural pathways. However, even such approach has not been wholly successful, as documented by the research into interpersonal neurobiology, and clinical practice (Siegel et al., 2021).

The superior colliculus is most likely key to body image integration (Damasio, 2010). Its two deep layers (the *stratum griseum profundum* and the *stratum album profundum*) receive sensory inputs from "vision, auditory, and somatosensory pathways" and are associated with motor as well as sensory functions (Zubricky & Das, 2022, par. 1). "There is no other place in the brain," Damasio noted (2010) where "information available from vision, hearing and multiple aspects of *body states* is so literally superimposed, offering a prospect of efficient integration" (p. 89) [italics added]. The superior colliculus receives visual input directly through the optic nerve. It also receives direct auditory input, and "somatosensory projections to the deep laminae" allow for response to tactile stimuli (Zubricky & Das, Id., par. 4). The superior colliculus also receives inputs from the prefrontal cortex "involved in the regulation of attention and distractibility" (King, 2004, as cited Ibid.).

Clearly, the superior colliculus is the prime candidate for the locus of body image integration from *perceived* inputs. While its functions are complex and not fully understood, it has been shown in experiments with rats and rhesus monkeys that damage to the superior colliculus resulted in increased distractibility and disorientation (Edwards & Henkel, 1978; Gaymard et al., 2003). However, no studies have been conducted to-date that would show how the superior colliculus actually contributes to the reflective and pre-reflective formation of the self. It is also still largely beyond human technical and scientific (surgical) capacities to "repair" a defect in superior colliculus, although novel neurosurgical microsurgical techniques have enabled dissection and treatment of tectal gliomas[100] (Lapras et al., 1994; Liu et al., 2018).

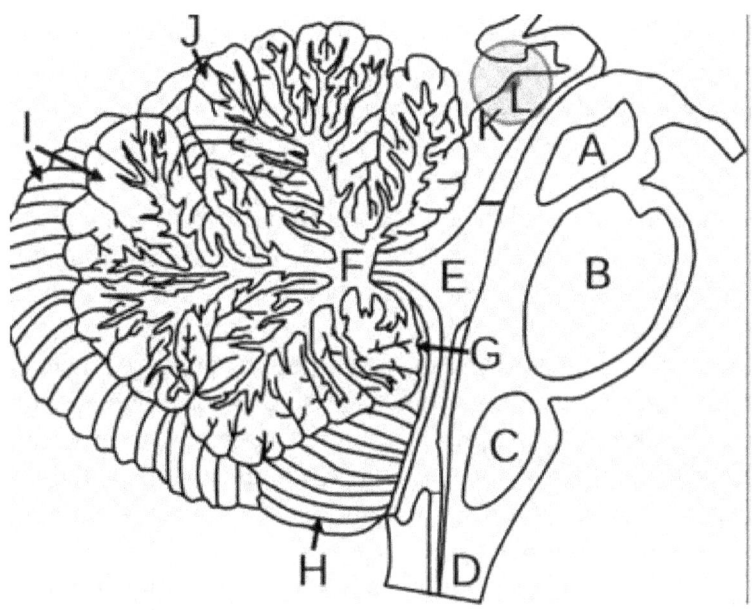

Diagram of the superior colliculus of the human midbrain (shown in dark red) and surrounding regions. The superior colliculus is surrounded by a red ring and transparent red circle to indicate its location. A: Midbrain B: Pons C: Medulla oblongata D: Spinal cord E: Fourth ventricle F: Arbor vitae G: Flocculus H: Tonsil I: Anterior lobe J: Posterior lobe K: Inferior colliculus L: Superior colliculus[101]

---

[100] Glioma is a "growth of cells that starts in the brain or spinal cord" (Mayo Clinic Staff, 2023). The cells in a glioma appear "similar to healthy brain cells called glial cells" which surround nerve cells and help them function; the growth of glioma, however, may become malignant and cause a tumor (Ibid.).
[101] Attribution: *Superior Colliculus* by Svenskbygderna (talk) - Own work, CC BY-SA 4.0. Retrieved from
https://commons.wikimedia.org/w/index.php?curid=90702734

Psychosomatic Correlates: Represented Reality

Psychosomatic correlates of body image boundary dimensions were described in detail by Fisher and Cleveland (1968). Their research confirmed the hypothesis that persons whose "psychosomatic symptoms involve the body exterior" (body image dysfunction), tend to surround themselves with a "protective, defensive wall" (their "Barrier Scores" were high); on the other hand, persons whose psychosomatic symptoms involved the body itself (internal body maladies), scored low on the Boundary Scores (p. 73). This means not only that insecurity about one's body's image tends to lead the individual to the formation of a protective barrier against the surrounding world, to the construction of a more artificial body image (resulting from excessive preoccupation with one's *perceived image*). This body image construct is not directly confirmed by reality (surrounding world), thus it becomes even more fragile than a self-construct stemming from an internal malady.

Yet another paradox stems from the realization that the body-image *construct* directly influences the body itself, its behavior, and self-image. This is because outward tracts from the superior colliculus project into the central gray matter overlying the rostral oculomotor nucleus, as well as areas "adjacent to the contralateral trochlear nucleus and contralateral abducens nucleus" (Zubricky & Das, 2022, par. 6). Represented reality thus turns into projected reality.

The researchers in this field (Fisher & Cleveland, 1968 had borrowed from multiple other sources) considered five diagnostic groups in their research: people suffering from 1) stomach disturbances; 2) ulcerative colitis; 3) rheumatoid arthritis; 4) neurodermatitis; and 5) conversion hysteria. The body exterior (image) was related to everything seen and tangible (skin, muscles, joints); the body interior related to the internal symptoms (1 and 2). Baseline was established by Rorschach. The results confirmed the hypothesis stated in the preceding paragraph. No significant differences between men and women were found.

Consequently, it can be concluded that body-image fragmentation is less marked when there is an actual problem with the body, but becomes more prominent when the image is at issue. When cohorts were shown a short movie (eight scenes, thirty seconds each, of a "projected movement sequence") and then asked about "the dissolution or breaking up of animal and human bodies," the disintegration involving human bodies was invariably more prominent in subjects who scored higher on the Barrier Scores, that is those concerned with the image (appearance) more than with health of the body (Fisher & Cleveland, Ibid., pp. 96-97).

Other tests (verbal association, drawing) indicated that body-image boundaries (barrier) were more firmly established and projected in people concerned with the *image* of their body: the façades of the houses their drew were more elaborate, completed clauses related to the skin more negative, and their verbal associations referred more to the outside, that is to say outer, superficial qualities. Interestingly, when the researchers accounted for Sheldon's somatotypes[102] (i.e., actual body structure and type), the Barrier Scores were found not to correlate to one's somatotype (Cheatham, 1953). This indicates that the image of the body is created regardless of the actual body, and may be entirely absolved of and comprehended as separate and apart from the real, material world.

The image is thus pre-conceived and a person may grow to either cherish or dislike it, similar to the way one

---

[102] William Herbert Sheldon (1898-1977) developed a theory of *somatotypes,* associating body types with human temperament types. The classification is based on the three layers of embryos: the endoderm (which develops into the digestive tract); the mesoderm (which develops into the muscle, heart, and blood vessels); and the ectoderm, which forms the skin and nervous system (Patwardhan, Mutalik, & Tilu, 2015, as cited in Nickerson, 2022).

feels about one's favorite shirt, coat, or dress. For example, White (2004) notes that people who have been diagnosed with cancer will often make decisions about their "appearance-changing cancer treatment" based on how likely such treatment is to alter their image, such as loss of hair or mastectomy (p. 384). Some patients experience skin pustules, bleeding, necrosis, infection, irritable bowels, and other physical conditions which may have a serious impact not only on their body image, but also social acceptance and mental wellbeing. These are all invariably intertwined and interconnected.

The image of the body is crucial in ego formation, which means personality formation (Tovian, 2002). No persona is so strong that it cannot be undermined and disintegrated by its own image. Even slight changes in the body (mastectomy vs. breast augmentation; liposuction vs. gaining weight; hair loss vs. hair growth) can trigger emotional dysfunction or, conversely, may boost emotional stability, which is why reconstructive and cosmetic surgery is able to, quite literally, achieve miracles for people whose body image is under attack – and it little matters whether such attack is real or merely perceived. Persons under stress, PTSD, victims of bullying and harassment, as well as patients who suffer from maladies that are concealed within the body (cancer, urological disorders, etc.), may experience self-doubt, shame, humiliation, and a "damaged self- and body image" (Tovian, 2002, p. 363).

Ogden et al. (2006) noted that revisiting and dealing with such issues of physical dissociation leads to mental compartmentalization and conscious dissociation from one's self-awareness. Individuals develop a "tendency to the dissociation… of functions that constitute personality" (p. 37). Van der Hart et al. (2006) divided dissociation into two kinds: one, in which the individual is engaged in daily activities in an avoidant fashion (basically pretending as if nothing has happened); the other, in which the individual constantly engages in "defensive actions against threat" (cited in Ogden, Ibid.).

Such a bifurcation may sound overly simplistic. Dissociation, much like body image fragmentation, is a complex phenomenon. In dissociation caused by trauma, the individual is reacting to an anticipated threat and forming a *defensive reaction* before the threat arises. At the same time, due in part to body–image fragmentation, the individual "cannot access top-down thinking to inhibit defensive actions" (Ogden et al., 2006, p. 87). In other words, if there is no connection between the body and the image – the body does what it will: dangles in air, curls up in the corner, or goes on mindlessly pursuing some predetermined course... It is not until one acquires the awareness of "what the body is doing" that the capacity and ability to connect the body to the image arises (Id., p. 88). Conversely, it is well known that body-oriented therapies have an immediate effect on dealing with emotional issues. All sympathetically mediated defensive actions are socially projected and communicated attempts at body image reconciliation and mediation.

The question is whether body–image fragmentation can be reconciled at all, or if it is simply a given of the human condition – and, if the latter is the case, whether or not it ought to be professionally addressed at all. Any unanticipated threat prompts individuals to explore their human limitations and question the validity of self-consciousness (Peterson, 1999). There is an *"isomorphic relationship between the state of the internal representation of motivational states and the external world,"* Peterson noted (Id., p. 195)[italics original]. "Isomorphic" means that the structure is preserved on the opposite plane (here, the external state perceived internally, and vice versa). What Peterson argued for was the relationship connecting the world of meaning (image) to the objectified and objectifying self through action, presumably of the body.

This fairly complicated analysis can be simplified by stating that all meaning is meaning-in-context, which is invariably *social*. Therefore, all identity is social. It is universally supposed that there cannot be an identity which is not shared. One identifies as something in relation to something or someone else. Consequently, no image is separable from the body – because the body identifies as something through its image.

Fragmentation of the image is its dissociation from the body, a state that can be accomplished willfully but, more often than not, results from prior traumatic experiences, as well as cultural and social constraints. However, all fragmentation is a matter of perception and, therefore, diagnosable, and treatable. What is more, a fragmented self is not always pathological. It can, in fact, be entirely natural. Peterson (1999) emphasized that entire human existence is constructed around "the strange" and "stranger" in the environment, a "novelty" which may or may not become traumatic, depending on the degree of the perceiving individual's social and cultural accommodation, and circumstances associated with each instance of perception (p. 246). It can therefore be concluded that even fragmentation is not a stable phenomenon but, rather, that it fluctuates and alters in degree, depending on the environment and circumstances in which the individual finds himself.

Human beings represent the image on the Semantic, Episodic, and Procedural planes: Semantic is the final plane of expression (through words); Episodic is inner experience and memory; Procedural is that of social and emotional interaction with the other (environment). While the body (what is and what should be) is a matter of fidelity to an "unquestioned concept of reality," the image is a re-presentation of the once-presented reality (Id., p. 258). The semantic plane of representation can thus assume multiple (even contradictory) forms. As Peterson noted, each level of

196

abstraction from the concrete opens the doors to multiple meanings, interpretations, and reinterpretations of the *idea* that was, at one point in time, the original image. This, however, destroys the stability of the body-as-image and, ultimately, undermines the concept of the self which, as will be shown in the next chapter, surpasses one's body image.[103]

---

[103] For example, recent demonstrations of nudity during various public parades, in which the body is seemingly used as an apparent social protest or counter-cultural statement, are indicative of body image fragmentation: bodies are painted, tattooed, variously mutilated, and treated in self-mutilating ways, indicative of body–image fragmentation, and serious inner turmoil of the individuals who are thus displaying themselves in public. Exhibitionism may also be symptomatic of inner sexual inadequacies and various BDD conditions (Aggrawal, 2015). Silverstein (1996) noted that specifically exposing genitals produces feelings of power and control which enable the individual to overcome inner inadequacies and feelings of shame.

Self-Image and the Sense of Self

The sense of self is a seemingly familiar but also deeply deceptive concept. Stated as: *Self-Image and the Sense of Self*, the title of this chapter posits two planes of the self-structuring consciousness. Human consciousness is structured on these two planes which is one of the reasons why one may speak of the body and the image as often incongruent, even competing, phenomena. Nave et al. (2021) divided the self between the reflective *me* and the pre-reflective *I*. The *Me* appertains to the image (perceptual sense of identity), while the embodied self of the *I* exists as an egocentric realization of *Me* – this *I* reaches beyond perception and can, arguably, be independent of the *Me* whose existence derives from body-image mediation. One is also prone to speak of the self-image as context and environment-dependent, versus the self which is God-given and natural.

The motto to this book is taken from the *Song of Myself* by Walt Whitman, whose *Me myself* is the *I*, the pre-reflective self, the inner core that one is before even understanding what one is:

> Rippers and askers surround me,
> People I meet, the effect upon me of my early life or the ward and city I live in, or the nation,
> The latest dates, discoveries, inventions, societies, authors old and new,
> My dinner, dress, associates, looks, compliments, dues,
> The real or fancied indifference of some man or woman I love,
> The sickness of one of my folks or of myself, or ill-doing or loss or lack of money, or depressions or exaltations,

Battles, the horrors of fratricidal war, the fever of
doubtful news, the fitful events;
These come to me days and nights and go from me
again,
But they are not the *Me myself.*

Apart from the pulling and hauling stands what *I am*,
Stands amused, complacent, compassionating, idle,
unitary,
Looks down, is erect, or bends an arm on an
impalpable certain rest,
Looking with side-curved head curious what will
come next,
Both in and out of the game and watching and
wondering at it.
Backward *I* see in my own days where *I* sweated
through fog with linguists and contenders,
I have no mockings or arguments, *I* witness and wait.
(*Song of Myself,* Sec. 4) [italics added]

The pre-reflexive core Self "witnesses and waits."
What is the *I* waiting for? It is not until Section 24 that Walt
Whitman defines himself as "an American, one of the
roughs, a kosmos." [sic] One is nothing without the
reflection, but also potentially everything with it.
    The power of the *I* is also apparent from the fact that
the self exists as a part of Being, wherefrom it takes its
energy. The "rippers and askers" are just that – ripples on the
surface, askers by the mirror, behind the glass. The deep
remains unseen. But being unseen means being unreflected.
Walt Whitman is called America's National Poet because he
absorbed the reflective *me* of the Nation (the "dates,
discoveries, inventions, societies, authors old and new…
dress, associates, looks, compliments, dues… real or fancied
indifference[s]), and separated it from the *I,* which is the *Me
Myself* standing above, observing, unique in its all-

encompassing wholeness – the God-given Soul of the Nation.

There is a degree of paradox embodied in such symbolism. He is both "in and out of the game" and "watching and wondering at it." The period is significant here because it is a conclusory statement without a conclusion. The period symbolizes a conclusion; but it is only a pause, in which the omniscient *I* "sits and waits." The *I* waits for it to become the self-objectified *Me*. This happens thorough the observation of *the other* (country and its people) and absorption of it.

Walt Whitman was the master of self-objectifying, which means seeing one's self in the other/s, and re-absorbing it through it/them. The sense of self is developed through self-objectification (Rabstejnek, 2015). The term "self-object" describes objects that the individual experiences as part of one's self. According to Kohut (1984) and Kohut and Wolf (1978), self-objects[104] are of two kinds: *mirroring selfobjects*, which refers to those objects that confirm one's "sense of greatness, perfection, and vigor;" and *idealized parent imago*, which refers to the objects idealized by the individual as "infallible, omnipotent, and calm" (as cited in Rabstejnek, 2015, p. 1). These two areas create a baseline tension between ideals and ambitions on the one hand, and what is commonly referred to as "reality" on the other. Thus the dichotomy between *Me* and *Me Myself* runs parallel to that between the body and its image.

---

[104] Kohut used no hyphen. Hyphen is conventionally used with self-though. Rather than using it, Kohut created a new word, by now an established technical term, *selfobject* (see the next page, and Note 105).

Selfobjects and Self-Image

The word *selfobject* was coined by Heinz Kohut (1913-1981), an Austrian-born American psycho-analyst who was primarily concerned with the analysis of the self.[105] His original intention for the selfobject consisted of the function of the object as an extension of the person (Goldberg, 1980). APA (2023a) included an expanded definition, which referred to other people as selfobjects, extensions of one's self. This may lead to psycho-pathological states of dependency, and be characteristic of the narcissistic disorder. It is arguable, however, whether the APA definition is a *de facto* expansion, rather than a *de jure* contraction of the concept.

Everyone knows someone who is attached to an object, such as a car. He will polish the car, talk to "him" or "her" sweetly, and take "them" for a ride. The car is a projection of his ego; but it is also a selfobject to which the persona is attached as a form of substitute for inner lack of former attachment during developmental stages, or even later in life (e.g., during marital difficulties, stressful work environment, finding no-one who will "listen to me and understand me," etc.).

There is a precarious consequence to the expanded definition of *selfobject* which lies in the fact that an individual may consider other people as material objects (of

---

[105] Kohut used *selfobject* as one word. Modern reader may deem hyphenation to be more accurate, especially where the self is portrayed in relation to an object outside of itself by projection or mirroring. *Selfobject* may then be applied to emphasize that the *self* has already adopted and accepted the *object* via reflection. Ergo: to view objects as self-objects is not necessarily pathological; whereas to view them as selfobjects may be a sign of narcissistic personality (see further below). Philosophically, both arguments are valid: the hyphen is used for compounding meanings (compound adjectives) as well as for clarity, to avoid confusion by separating the meanings, e.g., to recover vs. to re-cover, to repress vs. to re-press). *See* the Preface, p. xvi.

a certain determinable degree of utility) or, alternately, may view material objects as animate beings with souls. One should refrain from passing a moral judgment since, in either case, the individual needs an emotional crutch for a reason which is impossible to fully comprehend unless one should spend hours of therapy sessions with the person (or simply hours of listening to them as a friend).

In the context of body image formation, the concept of selfobject is necessarily tied to the projection of one's image onto other people or, conversely, projection of other people as selfobjects onto the perceiving individual.

The above allusion to an "emotional crutch" suggests that, more often than not, the existence of selfobjects is necessary, in order to prevent the individual from suffering the consequences of cognitive dissonance. *The Dissonance Theory* holds that elements of knowledge (cognitions) can be "relevant or irrelevant to one another" and that if two cognitions are relevant to one another, they can then be either *consonant* or *dissonant* (Harmon-Jones & Mills, 2019, p. 1). Consonant means congruent and logically connected; dissonant means either opposite or unconnected. Dissonance leads to psychological discomfort and avoidance of cognition (Festinger, 1957). Thus, people will avoid individuals who project incongruent, dissonant elements which, however, may be a matter of individual judgment (such as a nose ring).

Note to the illustration on the following page:
This photograph was taken from a publicly available image on Facebook, where it was displayed as an example of abhorrent body mutilation. While the immediate impression is that of dissonance, the symbolic elements (actual piercings) are not irrelevant to one another – they may be seen as mutually congruent and expressive of a unified image. Culturally and anthropologically, rings (especially the nose ring) may represent wealth (Berber tribes), sexual pleasure (Ayurveda), marriage (Middle East, Africa, India), rebellion (Western cultures).

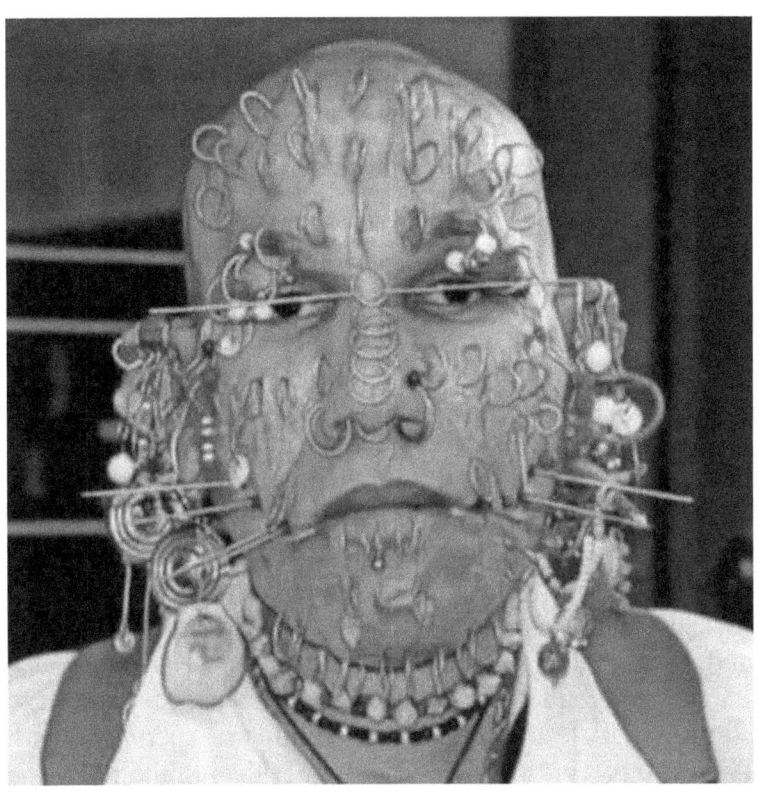

This psychological discomfort increases with the magnitude of dissonance and can be mitigated by either reducing the importance of the dissonant condition, or adding further information that is congruent, or both: "the magnitude of dissonance (and consonance) increases as the importance or value of the elements increases" (Festinger, 1957, p. 18). For example, a bodybuilder suffering from *orthorexia*[106] to the point at which he becomes anorectic or bulimic will feel the following dissonant and consonant cognitions: eating healthy contributes to health – but it also

---

[106] Orthorexia is a fixation on healthy food to such an extreme that it becomes an obsession (cf. *Glossary*, at the end of this book).

limits one's going out to restaurants, socializing with non-bodybuilders; it conditions performance and helps stamina – but it may also decrease endurance and overall health, cause discomfort, headaches, digestive issues, leading to overcompensation (overeating on "junk days"), potentially resulting in anorexia and bulimia; it leads to feeling "good" about oneself – but it also leads to an unhealthy obsession with the body image, social media, perhaps even to the narcissistic disorder.

If an individual creates a selfobject in a famous bodybuilder or model, the conscious decision to copy and follow the selfobject will create cognitive dissonance between the object-image and self-image. Once the decision has been made, the *free choice paradigm*[107] is triggered: the individual will look for confirming information and dismiss or undervalue the information that undermines the selfobject (because otherwise, the selfobject would crack and fragment and, with it, the self itself). For example, learning that a famous bodybuilder in the gym poster has been addicted to steroids will lead the onlooker youth to experiment with these drugs (confirmation bias), rather than to the reject the selfobject. Similarly, learning that a pretty model is anorectic or adheres to a certain diet will lead the individual to copy that particular diet, even if it should directly prompt to anorexia, even bulimia.

Imagine that the selfobject is destroyed – for example, the bodybuilder-model dies of a heart attack caused by the overuse of anabolic steroids. The individual

---

[107] Each former choice affects the latter choice in the same direction. For example, choosing painting A from between A and B, rejects painting B. Subsequent choice between paintings C and D will underscore positive qualities in A and suppress similarities with B (Brehm, 1956). According to the cognitive dissonance theory (Festinger, 1957), when a decision between two similar alternatives is made, a psychological tension (dissonance) is created by the "desirable aspects of the unchosen alternative" and the "undesirable aspects of the chosen one" (Alós-Ferrer, C., & Shi, F., 2015, p. 34).

will consciously strive to adopt the selfobject-of-desire as part of one's own self-image. Whatever effort on the path to perfection has been exerted is and will remain justified – the *effort justification paradigm* states that all dissonant cognitions (puffiness, deteriorating health, BMI weighing heavily on the heart, dieting leading to orthorexia, causing anorexia or bulimia, etc.) are justifiable in view of the overarching goal and, therefore, justified: "No gain, no pain," is the most famous motto among athletes in general, and bodybuilders in particular.

Further dissonance is reduced by increasing the desirability of the outcome, such as appurtenant fame or respect one achieves when one wins a tournament or show. This can be particularly important for individuals with diminished self-esteem and distorted body image, as well as those suffering from various consequences of childhood trauma. These groups largely overlap. For example, bullying or various "rites of passage" are the suffering necessary to validate the individual's right (value) as a member of the given group (e.g., fraternity, lawyers' peer group, real estate echelon of the "chosen," etc.). By the same token, the group's perceived value increases in proportion to the value attributed to the rite of passage. What is more, society stimulates and extols the use of selfobjects: bodybuilders, athletes, models, movie stars… all become highly-paid and acclaimed, despite their personal cognitive dissonances, eating disorders, distorted self- and body images.

The creation of selfobject-of-desire may or may not be a conscious, rational decision. The earliest self-objects are formed unconsciously, even before the rational brain is developed, in conjunction with the attachment patterns (Ainsworth et al., 1978). Irvine et al. (2019) noted that there are complex interactions between neuro-physiological, socio-cultural, and cognitive factors that affect both body image and self-image development, and thus also the attachment to, adoption and use of, selfobjects.

The Triune Brain

Neuroscientist Paul D. MacLean (1990)[108] formulated a model of the brain he called *The Triune Brain* which, although in a highly simplified fashion, helps us understand the process how this happens. Every human being has a rational brain, and an evolutionary brain. The latter consists of the reptilian and the mammalian parts.

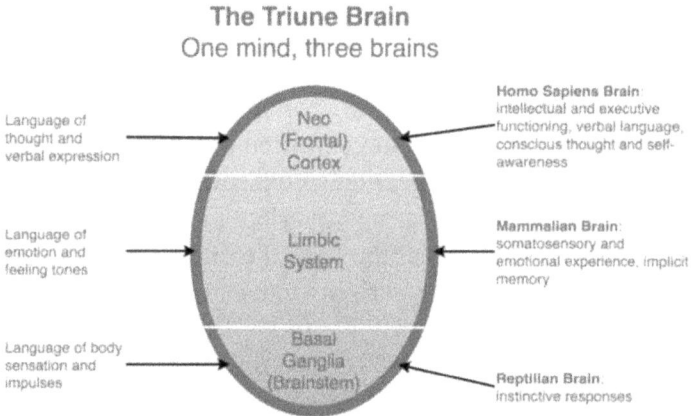

The Triune Brain
One mind, three brains

Language of thought and verbal expression → Neo (Frontal) Cortex

Homo Sapiens Brain: intellectual and executive functioning, verbal language, conscious thought and self-awareness

Language of emotion and feeling tones → Limbic System

Mammalian Brain: somatosensory and emotional experience, implicit memory

Language of body sensation and impulses → Basal Ganglia (Brainstem)

Reptilian Brain: instinctive responses

It is imperative to realize that, as endocrinologists are wont to say, the brain is built "from the bottom up." First comes the ancient animal brain, referred to as "reptilian," which fulfills the basic functions of the body that every newborn can execute. Along with hypothalamus, this brain

---

[108] Paul Donald MacLean (1913–2007), physician and neuroscientist who made significant contributions in the fields of physiology, psychiatry, and brain research through his work at Yale Medical School and the National Institute of Mental Health.

regulates primeval impulses. Hypothalamus,[109] located directly above the brain stem, is the size of an almond and connects the nervous system to the pituitary system, controlling and taking over basic functions and reactions. Trauma and PTSD leave indelible marks on the hypothalamus.

The limbic system (mammalian brain) produces emotions, monitors danger, and social networking. What is more, episodic and long-term memories are located here. The limbic system is shaped in response to experience, which means it is "neuroplastic" and modified throughout the individual's life. As Bessel (2021) notes, neurons that "fire together, wire together" – the brain is formed through action and by use (Chapter 4). The moment children begin to socially engage, experiment with objects, even in the absence of speech, the limbic system responds and the brain grows. The limbic system can also be shaped later in life, by experiences – both positive (love), and negative (e.g., a violent assault).

As Neocortex – the "third brain" – develops, emotions begin to contrast with the rationale, such as the fight-or-flight reaction repressed by the rationalization, for example, that the sounds are not from the machine gun but from the neighbor's 4th of July firecrackers. The neocortex is the "top brain" located in the frontal lobes. Its capacity does not begin to fully develop until about the 1st grade, when the child begins to learn language, and advances in abstract thought and logic.

Neurologically, the self is a constantly projecting mirror: the medial prefrontal cortex (MPFC), the posterior cingulate cortex (PCC), and the inferior parietal lobules (IPL) interminably and fluently process information and interact with one another, in order to form the sense of self

---

[109] From Ancient Greek ὑπό (hupó) "under," and θάλαμος (thálamos) "chamber."

(Delahoy et al., 2022). These regions have been studied in functional magnetic resonance imaging (fMRI) during self-referential cognition composed of direct self-appraisal (thinking about oneself), and reflected self-appraisal (thinking about oneself from a third-person perspective). Delahoy et al. (Id.) discovered a "distinct inhibitory influence" by the left IPL upon the PCC during reflected, compared to direct, self-appraisal which, however, "was accompanied by evidence of greater activation in both regions during the reflected self-appraisal condition" (Ibid.).

Consequently, Delahoy et al. (2022) concluded that the sense of Self is largely a result of "higher order" self-reflection, in the PCC, with the left IPL supporting abstract self-related processes "including episodic memory retrieval and shifts of perspective" (Ibid.). Therefore, neurologically, there is no difference between reflection (input from others) and self-reflection (input from oneself).

This conclusion may be a key piece of information, crucial to the resolution of body dysmorphic issues that originate from the individual's environment, mircrosphere (family), attachment patterns, and possible transference.

What this research did not capture, however, is the fact that even in the ultimate loneliness, Man reflects upon the world, as sundry unique, yet universal, examples from *belles lettres* show us: one may be as insulated as the Prisoner of Chillon or as self-insulating as Hamlet, yet may instinctively form a reflective Self in the environment into which the individual is *thrown*. Barack Obama's youthful "quest to belong" may be cited here as a case in point. This quest, however, is far from unique among American youth (Schamberg & Barker, 2007, par. 1).[110] Indeed, the natural

---

[110] What was unique in former President Obama's upbringing was that he grew up outside of the United States, in Indonesia, and had biracial parents. His home environment was unstable, and did not provide him with sufficient *grounding* "to belong" to a culture (or religion, for that matter). In his education and formative years (through his grandparents),

instinct of a human being is to fight insulation, even where the Power of Will dictates otherwise, for Man is a ζῷον πολιτικόν, political animal, as Aristotle said, and needs social contact for self-fulfillment – but also for self-definition as an individual.

The states that characterize self-boundary (the sense of location, agency, first-person perspective, attention, body sensations, and affective valence) are subjective and can only be self-reported. This poses a significant hurdle to any quantitative analysis and investigation. Such research can be conducted behaviorally, with focus on self-representation through conduct, specifically moral action, and action with respect to value and valuation within a given environment (Chu & Vu, 2022).

---

he is largely a product of White Anglo-Saxon culture which, the fact which he has resisted and refused to accept, in order to belong to what he feels is his true background. The attempts to express himself and "to belong" were largely relegated to his body-image formation: drug and alcohol abuse, anorectic behavior, sexual self-doubts, etc. These are often related comorbidities in such situations and under similar circumstances (the similarities to formative years and upbringing of many suburban youth from unstable families or one-parent homes cannot be overlooked).

The Gap between Reasoning and Understanding

A Path to Moral Self

In their discussion of Kohlberg's stages of moral development, Chu and Vu (2022) noted that the ability to reason "does not necessarily foretell whether people act morally" because there is a "gap" between reasoning and understanding (p. 246). In other words, the frontal cortex is often puzzled by what the limbic system is feeling and unable to quite account for the overacting ADHD amygdala.

This "gap" is similar, and may even be commensurate, to the gap between self-reflection and body image mediation. It is questionable whether an individual can behave morally in the absence of environmental factors. What meaning would such behavior have? Arguably, however, what is worse is when the individual lives in this "gap," not being able to reconcile the self-reflected body image with the environmentally mediated image (the image of the body and self which is mediated to the individual by the environment). Likewise selfobjects may become self-projections.

Looking at an individual who inhabits this gap, one is reminded of Hannah Arendt's statement that, sadly, most evil is perpetrated by those who cannot decide between Good and Evil (Malden, 2020). It is in this gap, that a strange "absence of thought" lies, which enables the individual to perpetrate evil – precisely because there is an indeterminate (thus irresponsible and irreproachable) self. A person who is not self-aware is not legally responsible for his actions because the law holds such an individual not capable of culpability. In other words, there is no conscious self to hold culpable. Sadly, the same absence of self is present in trauma-related disorders, dysregulation, and various dissociative reactions induced as consequence of enduring negative affects that forestall body image mediation.

Can it be really said that there is no self unless, in some form, self-reflection is present? After all, in meditation, the goal is to take possession of the physical boundaries (the body) and to dissolve them, in order to achieve a higher state of consciousness. This heightened consciousness is of the soul without the body. Body dissociation and depersonalization accompany mediation. In fact, the success of meditation is evaluated in the estimated degree of body dissolution, the ability to "float" and "dissolve," thus abstracting oneself from the physical world: "There's a sense of giving up on the holding on. But then there's no need for more effort—you just give up" (Nave et al., 2021, p. 14). A "sense of agency" remains, but it is used wholly on dissolving the body and, ultimately, the agency itself – the participants' descriptions of their mediative experience was even marked by "the decreased verbal use of the first-person pronoun and of active verbs," clearly showing a willful abstraction from, and abandonment of, the self (p. 17). The fact that the dissolution of the body consists of assumption of other forms and spaces indicates that any self, in order to exist, needs a form, albeit such a form may become an *image* (that is to say not necessarily a tangible, living organism). Compare the following descriptions captured by Nave et al. (p. 15), all made by professional meditators without any underlying psychological conditions, selected specially for the research:

"My attention shifted to being more in a space that…is also the body but also around the body. It's not the universe, just around the body…like some pleasant cloud, and its edges…not clear where it ends."

"The sense of body boundaries is beginning to diminish and there's a less defined sense of intimacy

211

or belonging that's experienced somehow in relation to the room's boundaries."

"It's as if I'm present in all of space altogether, like all of the space that my consciousness surrounds in this moment... It's like my presence is something much bigger than, say, just where my body is located. Rather, who I am is present in a very large space, large at least like, say, a building, or something like that."

The objects the self assumes are those of perception "or of imagination" (p. 16). Imagination appears to increase the dynamic dissolution process and agency. At the same time, however, the awareness of the sense boundaries "de-reifies" the solidity of the body-self and "potentially reveals its dependence on attention, affect, mobility, intersubjectivity, and other factors" (p. 23). The insight into the *body-self* is thus elicited through the *image-self* (literally any object one imagines one's self can apprehend and occupy), which starts and ends with body image but invariably also passes through the stage of *no-self* (Gethin, 1998).

Nave et al. (2021) noted that deep meditative Self Boundaries (SB) dissolution "resulting from intense or highly skillful practice" of meditation "can be especially useful in deconstructing the more persisting structures of self-experience," including the "fundamental duality of subject and object" (p. 23). This means that meditation can help coalesce the body and the image where the two are dissonant, discordant, dysfunctional, or fragmented. Some researchers advise, however, that (much like hypnosis) unguided meditation or meditation practiced by amateur meditators, may result in attentional dis-engagement and lead to the destabilization of meta-awareness (i.e., awareness of being aware of the awareness of the self). The latter basically means that the person "drifts into mind-wandering" which amounts to no more than absence of coherent thought.[111]

Meditation facilitates the focus on Being, as opposed to Having. The first is dynamic; the latter, static. Much like a moving body becomes motionless in a photograph, the self requires a vehicle to achieve stability (Bonomo, 2016). Conversely, this vehicle becomes the home of the agency which could be called Pure Being, outwardly projected by self-actualizing action. If this action is good (in pursuit of virtue), one becomes good and lives a worthy life, and vice versa (Aristotle, 1999, Bk. 1, Chpt. 7, Sec. 15-17). The *agens* of this action cannot be located outside oneself, as this would tend to the life of *having*, not the life of *being*. As Emerson (1841) counseled: "Do not seek yourself outside yourself." (p. 13; *see* note 31, supra). By logical implication, this means that the self-image is not an image but the original.

Blasi (1983, 1995) portrayed the self as the mediator of moral reasoning. The self, as defined by Blasi (Ibid.), is tripartite: 1) the moral self (moral values that define self-identity), 2) self of personal responsibility (determining action following moral judgement) and 3) self-consistent self (expressing uniformity of judgement and action). All these components can only be formed and considered with respect to action and judgment, which means only as functions of the environment they inhabit. Human self can neither grow nor form itself without environmental input.

---

[111] It would be inadvisable to discuss a subject one is not familiar with, has not researched, or practiced. As the reader may have discovered by practice, "mind-wandering" appears to be an omnipresent first "stage" for all those who embark on the journey of meditation. The mind passes through the elements that bind it in the material world (the body being one such element) before it is free to focus on the self (and the image of the body), akin to a ship jettisoning offal, in order to achieve buoyancy. Focus on the self (executed, for example, through a matricular mantric sound or formula) has the potential to realize pure *Being*, as opposed to being-in-the-world defined as *Having* (Fromm, 2006).

213

From Veblen (1899), to Lasch (1979), to Bloom (1987), the accrual of this "environmental" self can be traced as a complex of factors working in synergy, away from the sense of self to the self-image as a persona. Haiken (1999) poignantly noted that a growing sense of public anonymity, competitiveness, and a "far less forgiving" (business) society gave rise to a conventionally subjugated self-image which is presented, reflected, and re-presented as a "personality" – a "quality of being Somebody" in the world (pp. 91, 100). In view of such depersonalizing pressure, it is no wonder that some selves become the public image (apparently losing the original entirely), while others interpret the unity of self as uniformity, leading to existence devoid of essence, or, as Ralph Waldo Emerson had poignantly noted, "hobgoblin of little minds" (Emerson, 1841, p. 7).

The Birth of Modern Self

The Voice

The birth of modern self as a persona is closely tied to the change in the paradigm of the self as a result of the birth of psychology as a modern science. The origins of modern psychology can be traced to Descartes' dualism, which divided the body and the mind into two competing phenomena: "I think therefore I am" presupposes self-reflection (thinking) as the primary mode of being. In other words, arguably, the pre-reflective *I* does not exist, until the *Me* arises and "embodies" it with Light of Life.

Cherry (2022) argued that William Battie's *Treatise on Madness*, published in 1758, should be considered the groundbreaking work of psychology. Appendix A provides a rough chronology of modern psychology. This began with experiments with memory, and attempts to measure and quantify the self. The next stage was that of introspection and self-reflection (dissection of dreams, thoughts, and visions); closely followed by the behaviorist view that the self is defined through conduct which forms it. Subsequent holistic approach (gestalt psychology) embraced both behaviorist and self-reflective psychologies but differed from them in that it underscored "higher values" of morality, including love, and the meaning of Being. The holistic "we are what we mean" would not be a statement readily agreeable to either Sigmund Freud or C. G. Jung. On the other hand, if William James were to be considered the more portentous founding figure of modern American psychology, then the will to be and the intent to shape the self, including one's body image, would certainly prevail.

Where the will and intent are insufficient, modern psychologists do not hesitate to contact a professional in the field who embraces more radical body-oriented methods. As Edgerton (2006) noted, it is the improvement of an

215

individual's self-image which is "often the principal purpose and benefit of plastic surgery" (p. vii). Plastic surgery has had an ongoing relationship with body image. It is a form of art as much as science and, for its significance in the impact on self-image, shall be dealt with in a separate chapter.

Regardless of what lies in the individual's genetic makeup, there are few who are satisfied with *the status quo*. Both self-image and a sense of self as an inborn identity are malleable and constitute one of fundamental human freedoms of choice. As James (1896) pointed out, the problem arises from the fact that individuals incessantly search for an "objective certitude" with respect to truths that they believe (p. 9). If one believes in the primacy of the image over the body, one will seek assurances in the body, even for the beliefs affirming the image (and vice versa).

Some psychologists have referred to this phenomenon (the dialog with the inner self) as "the Voice," perhaps for lack of other descriptive terminology but also perhaps because it is what often actually happened to their patients. Maine and Kelly (2005) quoted a case of an anorectic who described *the Voice* as "a mean little guy" in her brain who was telling her "that wrong was right, up was down, and that no matter what I did, I was fat, ugly and worthless and people didn't like me" (p. 122). Of course, *she* realized that it was not true but this realization did not deter "the Voice" from leading her "through a carnival fun house" filled with "mirrors that distorted every aspect of my life and who I am. Every day, I felt, The Voice was shouting lies in my ear, and I believed it" (ibid.) [italics mine, capitals original, punctuation added].

While the phenomenon of hearing "the Voice" is often linked to trauma and childhood abuse (Anketell et al., 2010; Shevlin et al., 2014; Van Der Hart et al., 1993, 2006; Waters et al., 2012), it need not be pathological. It is often self-mediated, which means it can be strengthened or diminished by individual's behavior and efforts, as well as through social adaptation. Emotional and social isolation, including shame, self-blame and the inability to express these emotions have been underscored as predictive of various comorbidities and psychopathologies connected to the occurrence of the Voice. These often lead to the formation of a *false self* which seemingly adapts to an ongoing traumatic situation or residual traumatic experience (Young, 1999). Consequently, one's self may splinter into two or more different co-reacting selves.

A *Dialogical Self Theory* was proposed by Perona-Garcelán et al. (2008, 2015) where the self is disintegrated into different voices, each offering a perspective based on values apparently inconsistent with the individual's history. The researchers (Ibid.) argued that the causes of dissociation here are multiple, including: an interruption in the integration of experiences into the self, loss of perspective, coupled with the increasing distance between the *Me Myself* and the *I* positions, and *derealization.* The voices are overwhelmingly negative and work in synergy, shaping the deformed worldview of the individual who, slowly but surely, loses the grasp on reality.

However, the creation of a voice need not be detrimental or destructive to the individual. It can be a useful coping mechanism. It is only detrimental where it impairs social contact or prevents the individual from seeking reinforcement (such as therapy). It should also be noted that the Voice may have unexplained causes (masking the traumatic experience from which it originated), in which case it may be unpredictable and, ultimately, detrimental to the individual, leading to body image fragmentation.

The Sense of Self: Satisficed Self

The true self is that of the Ego, the "kernel of instinctual dispositions" (Bollas, 1987, p. 51) with the Id as an "organizing principle" and Super Ego as an overseer (Kohut, 1971; Ogden, 1992a, 1992b). Should this extrapolation appear too Freudian, hence dated, to the modern reader, let it be known that Freud's genius lay exactly in this analysis: to divide and separate the essence (soul) and the existence (body) of the human being is improper unless one realizes that both mental and physical actions are united in the "I" of the person which governs all experiences. Watson (2014) noted that the division is that of different levels of consciousness which connect fluid and constantly morphing situations into a palpable "topography" of the mind (p. 2, note 2).

Therefore, the sense of self is a composite which mirrors the world. This mirror may sometimes show distorted images that the individual perceiver absorbs as real and starts believing in them. For example, the Voice the anorectic patient heard (described above) was perfectly real to her. Indeed, who could tell her otherwise – but herself?

Her conscious acceptance of the voice is far from unique. Indeed, James (1896, p. 9) described the new self as "the way we face" the world, focusing on an aspect of the mirror-image, which is to be distinguished from the natural self. The *natural self* is "metaphysically dependent on the body from which its states emerge and upon which they supervene" which, however, also means that it "survives no longer than the body does" (Ganeri, 2015, par. 2). The natural self is a precondition for the self-consciousness of the self-reflective self.

At the same time, this self-reflective self-searches for the "inner 'truth' of an individual" and creates "internal psychic structures" that arise under the influence of various "cultural narratives" (Baker-Pitts, 2015, p. 105): "She cannot detach herself from the cultural lens any more than she can detach herself from a rejecting parent," said Baker-Pitts (Id.) of a daughter brought up by a mother whose predicate was that the daughter "will feel better" when she "looks better" (p. 107).

The divergence from the natural self is particularly poignant where the individual's various "self-states are not received, acknowledged, and reflected back by caring figures" (p. 109). This is particularly important in forming healthy attachment patterns during childhood (Ainsworth et al., 1978). Nonetheless, it can be just as critical during adulthood, especially for a formerly traumatized adult. In cases of crises, the individual reverts not to the natural self but, rather, to default cultural narratives for protection: for example, current cultural narratives may betoken that that changing one's gender identity will make the trauma or crisis go away, or that obtaining a large tattoo will provide the individual with more security in social contact.

Cash and Fleming (2004) emphasized that social feedback is always reciprocal, accompanied by the phenomenon of *attributive projection* which makes individuals infer that others see them the way they see themselves. *Confirmation bias* then tends to affirm them in their beliefs, resulting in what is perceived by them as self-protective cognitive processes and behaviors, such as dressing down, avoiding eye contact, or even avoiding society altogether.

Not only does the attributive projection affect how individuals experience body image, but it directly affects their experience of everyone else, contributing to other individuals' confirmation biases. Since the process is always reciprocal, each individual taken for what they *believe* they are, which is what they are believed they are. Consider how this phenomenon functions in certain professions, such as law or real estate, where the ego and self-assured *image* creates a similar assurance in the client (confirmation bias, not necessarily based on evidence). Meanwhile, the *sense of self* (the *I* behind the *believed* Ego) may be very insecure, craving attention and constant self-assurance.

Therefore, the sense of self is ultimately based on what behavioral organization and behavioral decision theories refer to as *bounded rationality*. Bounded rationality states that all individuals decide by intent, rationally, considering optimal solution, which may not be perfect but is the best one under the circumstances. Simon (1956) established the term *satisficing* for this adaptive decision-making. He stated that all "organisms adapt well enough to 'satisfice'," but that they "do not, in general, 'optimize'." (p. 127). A "satisficed" individual is satisfied at a certain level of needs. Further, where decisions appear to be emotional, individuals still in fact act rationally because they are goal-oriented and adaptive. With respect to body image, rational adaptation may be procedural, limited by the environment (how the image is mediated), and substantive, limited by the boundaries and limitations of the body itself. In any case, the sense of self is a satisficed self, adapted to current requirements with the satisfaction of specific, current needs.

The Sense of Self: Dissatisficed Self

The term *Napoleonic Complex* originated with Alfred Adler (1917) who, however, spoke of the "feelings" of inferiority, not a "complex." The word "complex" was created by journalists and propagated by cosmetic surgeons of the renown of Jacques Maliniak, Henry Schlierson, and Jerome Webster, to advance their field (Haiken, 1999). The word "complex" implies feelings of inferiority which may be real (such as a physical deformity) but that may also be merely perceived, or even "imagined" (p. 118). Whether real or perceived, such feelings require that the individual self act so as to satisfy them.

Feelings of inferiority often stem from social and cultural experience of the individual who tries to adapt, responding in accordance with the precepts of the *Bounded Rationality Theory* (BRT). For example, Knapen et al. (2018) observed that height in men is clearly linked to status and nutrition but (which is a less well-known fact), also to intelligence. In their studies, men who felt shorter (both, in absolute terms, and by relative comparison to a taller opponent) kept more coins and, therefore, were judged to be more selfish than men of an average height. Interestingly, this reaction was not observed when the opponent (of a short man) was significantly above the average height. Knapen et al. (2018) concluded that "life experiences" as well as physical strength (not measured by the researchers in this survey) may have "affected" such interactions (p. 1143).

It may also be concluded that confirmation bias and BRT can be applied comparatively. Where comparison is extreme, the sense of self is less dependent on BRT analysis.

The Self must clearly behold both, the image and the body, negotiating the subjectivity of the sameness, and the difference – both in oneself, and in others. How such negotiation works in real life may be observed from the interaction between a military commander who told

Napoleon Bonaparte that he "felt uncomfortable being so much taller than his Emperor," to which Napoleon allegedly replied: "You may be taller, but I am greater" (Donker & Burmanje, 2012, p. 53). Arguably, such a statement is not a sign of overcompensation for a perceived deficit but, rather, of a healthy integration of it. Therefore, the subjectivity of the sameness and the difference of the otherness is not always coincident to the difference between the cohesive self and the fragmented self (Kohut, 1987).

Analyzed according to the BRT, if the more accurate interpretation were to be that of Napoleon's overcompensation for a perceived deficit, BRT would apply and a sense of self be formed as a "satisficed self." On the other hand, if the man questioning Bonaparte was much taller, therefore exempting comparative confrontation, BRT would not apply, and Napoleon would be displaying a satisfied (as opposed to *satisficed*), healthy self. In any case, the image is mediated and the mirror-input reflected – it is only the degree of mediation and commensurate individual perception which matters.

The Modern Self: Conclusion

Baker-Pitts (2015) concluded that where body image integration cannot be achieved, people reach out for help, most often in the form of cosmetic surgery or therapy. It is not uncommon for therapists to refer their patients to plastic surgeons. Unlike in the past (when only reconstructive surgery was seen as legitimate and the "charlatan" cosmetic surgeons were viewed with opprobrium), plastic/cosmetic surgery is seen without any stigma today, as a profession on an equal footing with all other medical fields, if not higher. One may go so far as to observe that having a cosmetic procedure done is indicative of self-improvement and maintenance of a healthy image. Such healthy image is often

222

depicted as a "going concern" which gives a person "an inner lift" (Haiken, 1999, p. 152).

The term *going concern* was used by the editor of the *Vogue* magazine in 1961 with reference to the woman herself – or her-*self*, rather (Ibid.). Going concern is an accounting term which means that a company is "financially stable enough to meet its obligations and continue its business for the foreseeable future" (Kenton, 2021). In other words, the body image has become a commodity over and above that of the sense of self.

What is more, the sense of self is often shaped and formed by the mediated image, image that is no longer in the sole personal possession of the individual. Rather, it is a marketable artefact, similar to a photograph, even an icon or an avatar on social media. Even where it had been intended as an artificial going concern (in order to safeguard the natural self), it ceases to function as such, once it is thrown into the world and (socially or otherwise) marketed. Needless to say, all forms of such marketing are transformative of the *me,* though not always of the pre-reflective *I,* the *Me Myself.* However, they are not all destructive, and many are merely means for the individual to survive, forming the image in order to satifice the self.

Reconstructing the Image and the Body

To the initiated, the word "reconstruction" may trigger a red light warning: Derrida is coming, beware! Some tenets of the deconstructivist and structuralist philosophies have been discussed above. The chief reason is that one may analogize and view the text–meaning relationship as parallel to the body–image relationship, an analogy which is helpful to the understanding of various body image concepts and maladies. Literary critics select and examine various parts of the text, re-examine them in different contexts and environments, and then interpret the author's vision and the meaning of the text. Structuralists believe text is composed of signs which have culturally-bound meanings based on opposition (such as male and female). Deconstructivists believe that no such opposition is present. Rather, text consists of objects that have varied values and whose hierarchy is unstable, if it exists at all. Both views have their place in body-image analogies.

Psychiatrists and psychologists approach the diseases of the mind (body's image) as related to a particular condition of the body itself, symbolic of a deeper issue, the individual's history, and the environment they live in. For example, in BDD, one body-part may loom larger than all others and be subjected to body-self-deconstruction (destruction and reconstruction of the part-image of the body). The etiology (causes), nosology (classification), and symptomatology (effects) are diagnosed on case-by-case basis, very much like the author's intent, symbolic meanings, the type of text (genre, register), and the effects on the reader (observer). Psychologically speaking, re-construction means literally rebuilding and restructuring, whether the psyche, or the body. This reconstruction may require that the given be destroyed first and the image (psyche) accommodated, or the other way round.[112] Where psychologists and psychiatrists are helpless, plastic surgeons smile and beckon.

The "father of modern plastic surgery," Gaspare Tagliacozzi (1545–1599) of Bologna, Italy, focused on reparative cosmetic surgery in individuals maimed during various duels, street brawls, or physically ravaged by diseases. It was Tagliacozzi who pioneered the method of nasal reconstruction in which the flap from the upper arm is "gradually transferred to the nose" (Haiken, 1999, p. 5; Stark, 1975). The following oft-cited quote from Tagliacozzi is as true today as it was 500 years ago:

> We restore, rebuild, and make whole those parts which nature hath given, but which fortune has taken away. Not so much that it may delight the eye, but that it might buoy up the spirit, and help the mind of the afflicted. (Tagliacozzi, 1597)

As apparent from this quote, from the start, the emphasis in cosmetic surgery has been on the reconstructive, not esthetic domain. The aesthetic impact of a successful surgery was intended to "buoy up the spirit" and "help the mind." The reconstruction has always been that of the spirit (image) through the body – simply because the body is easier to change than the mind. The change is immediate, with lasting results. But, one had better measure twice before he cuts!

From among the pioneers in plastic surgery, Sir Charles Bell (1774–1842) stands out for his focus on carefully "measuring" and charting blueprints before

---

[112] One may speculate that to re-construct something created by God has always been perceived as something abhorrent and sacrilegious. It may be for this reason that cosmetic/aesthetic surgery was, for many decades, if not centuries, denigrated, and relegated to the position of quackery and disrepute.

making the cut. His practice encompassed both cosmetic-esthetic domain of the mind as well as the reconstructive sphere of the body. It was during the Napoleonic wars, that Bell noted how socially disabling gunshot wound injuries in the face were. In 1814, he published a *Dissertation on Gunshot Wounds* which included a series of diagrams of facial injuries French soldiers had suffered in Spain and at Waterloo. It was this focus which gave rise to modern plastic surgery.

Sir William Arbuthnot Lane (1856-1943) followed in Bell's footsteps. Lane established the Cambridge Military Hospital, and convinced the Queen to set up a hospital at Sidcum in Kent which would specialize in maxiofacial surgeries and other deformities suffered by the veterans of World War I. From a handful of experts in the field, Lane chose Harold Delft Gilles (1882-1960), a young otolaryngologist from New Zealand, to head this hospital. Posted to France in 1915, Gilles had witnessed first-hand horrific facial wounds and deformities caused by shrapnel, gunshot, and gas. These horrendous body-scars became image-scars marring and distorting the body image of the sufferer, altering his social life forever.

Harold Delft Gillies deserves a longer aside here. Gilles standardized over 11,000 surgical techniques and, in 1946, performed one of the first successful phalloplasties on a transgender man, on whom he "formed a new penis from the patient's existing skin and tissue" (McInnis, 2022, par. 1). In 1915, Gilles volunteered to serve in the Royal Army Medical Corps. He was posted to Wimereux, France, where he met Auguste Charles Valadier, a dentist who went on to pioneer groundbreaking maxillofacial surgeries.[113] Gillies also watched and assisted Hippolyte Morestin (1869-1919),

---

[113] Lat. *Maxilla* – jaw + *facial* – face: surgery on the face, head, neck, mouth, and the jaw, including cleft lip and palate reparative surgery, and reconstructions of deformities caused by tumors and various types of cancer.

"the Father of the Mouths," who became famous treating surgeries of the jaw and face with skin grafts and flaps.

Aldershot (popularized by Rudyard Kipling's poem Gunga Din) became the center for reconstructive surgery in England in 1916. On January 11 that year, Gilles established the first plastic surgical unit in Aldershot (McInnis, 2022). When Lane set up the Queen's Hospital in Sidcum (called Queen Mary's Hospital as of 2022), with over a thousand beds available on-site and "dozens of surgeons devoted to improving the techniques of reconstructive surgical practices," Gillies moved there, in order to cooperate with other surgeons, such as Rubens Wade and Ivan Magill, pioneers of endotracheal anesthesia (Ibid.).[114]

In 1920, Gilles published a training manual, *Plastic Surgery of the Face*, which illustrated sundry skin graft techniques, body tubes, and prosthetics. He later practiced at St. Bartholomew and faced unavoidable criticism for performing cosmetic surgeries, in order to improve patient's psyche, ego, and body image. During World War II, Gilles again performed reconstructive surgeries on soldiers. These included surgeries on the pubic area and reconstructions of penises, which led to Gilles' becoming the first expert in sexual reassignment surgery (called "gender affirmation surgery" as of 2022). His first patient, Laurence Michael Dillon, was a transgender British doctor, on whom Gilles performed 13 surgeries, from 1946 to 1949.

Gillies also became a founding father of the British Association of Plastic Surgeons, and its first Chairman on November 20, 1946. In 1948, the BAPS began to publish

---

[114] Insertion of a rubber or plastic tube into the trachea, in order to sustain patient's supply of oxygen, and to administer anesthetics to the patient. In the endotracheal technique, a tube is passed through the mouth (orotracheal intubation), through the nose (nasotracheal intubation) or through a tracheostomy opening (tracheostial intubation). The tube may also be maneuvered through the glottis by the so-called "blind" technique, using a laryngoscope (Sadove, 1947).

The British Journal of Plastic Surgery, which has become a renowned standard in the field. In 1957, in collaboration with David Ralph Millard, Jr., Gillies published *The Principles and Art of Plastic Surgery*, volumes I and II, a thrilling summary of Gilles' lifetime experience and a guiding textbook for many future plastic surgeons. Gilles was awarded the degree of Honorary Fellow of the Royal Australasian College of Surgeons, the American College of Surgeons, and the Royal Society of Medicine, London.

In 2005, the Association of Plastic Surgeons, founded by Gillies, changed its name to the British Association of Plastic, Reconstructive and Aesthetic Surgeons, or BAPRAS, finally granting full recognition to plastic and cosmetic surgery. This change constituted a tacit but crucial acknowledgement of the significance of the connection between plastic surgery and psychology.

It is not by coincidence that a parallel can be drawn between the advances in plastic surgery, and psychiatry. Returning to the roots, although there is no direct evidence that Alfred Adler (1870-1937) studied the psychological impact of World War I injuries on the psyche of the veterans of that war, his linking the negative impact of feelings of inferiority to substance abuse in weaker or socially disadvantaged individuals clearly demonstrates that similar causal mechanisms are in force here as in cases studied by Bell, Gilles, and even Tagliacozzi – mechanisms other than upbringing and heredity.

The fact that rhinoplasty pioneered this parallel development is likewise not coincidental – the nose is the most prominent feature on the human face, and emphatically also indicative of the person's racial origins (Haiken, 1999). The "reigning cultural norms of beauty" demanded an absence of "racial or ethnic stigmata" (p. 177). Thus, while many World War I veterans were still "walking their flaps" in Sidcup,[115] the contemporary Jewish comedienne and actress Fanny Brice had, as contemporary papers put it, "cut off her nose to spite her race" (p. 182), thereby spearheading the development of plastic-cosmetic surgery from what was till then a purely reconstructive focus of the professionals, to the cosmetic-aesthetic domain. Though she was publicly mocked in the 1920s, by 1936 even most serious and reputable surgeons, such as Vilray Blair, proclaimed it a worthy effort to change the shape of "the pronounced Jewish nose" for "social or business reasons" (p. 184).

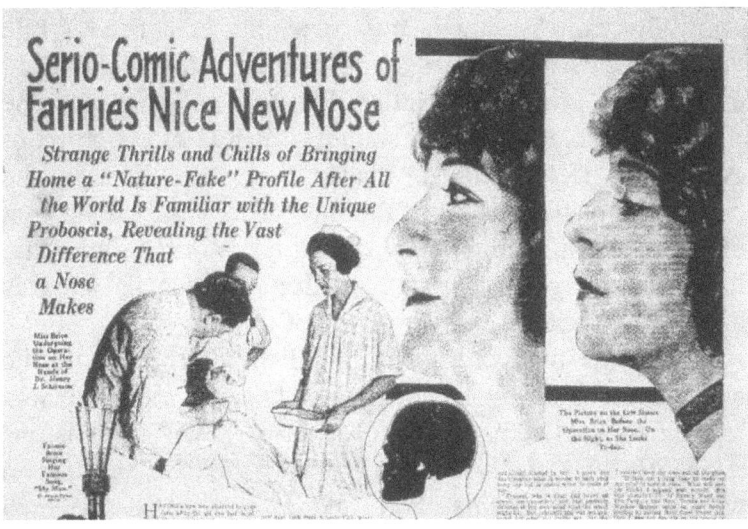

The Sandusky Register of Sunday November 25, 1923, on "Fanny Brice and her New Nose."

---

[115] "Walking the flaps" refers to moving the flaps of skin from a healthy part (e.g. the chest) to the affected part (e.g. the face), in order to cover the injury with a "new" flap of skin. The skin must remain connected to the rest of the body for perfusion because otherwise, it would die.

Brice's procedure photos are distinctly different from pre- and post-results of procedures performed at Sidcup: below, compare the pre- and post-reconstruction photographs from Sidcup, cited by Gillies as an example of the principle: "Restore normal tissue to normal position." The end results are dramatic,[116] but also dramatically indicative of the similarities and differences between a reconstructive surgery and one that is purely "cosmetic" Bamji (2013). The differences are apparent: a reconstructive procedure is primarily focused on functionality and use. Many of the soldiers suffered debilitating injuries to the face, primarily from shrapnel and machine gun fire. While improvements in anesthesia and treating infections "meant that these gruesome battlefield injuries had become survivable," they often left soldiers "unable to eat, drink or even speak" (Klein, 2018). What is more, the collapse of the facial features (e.g., loss of the jaw, nose, ears, etc.) meant maimed body image, thereby loss of one's original identity. In such cases, the reconstruction of facial features necessarily meant a reconstruction of the self.

While many surgeons found the cosmetic, and the reconstructive fields irreconcilable (because medicine was "meant to heal rather than to beautify"), with the rise of television and Hollywood movies, American (and soon world) culture became more and more visually oriented (Haiken, 1999). In 1926, surgeon John Staige Davies asked: "What is the ethical difference between doing an abdominal operation and removing wrinkles from a sagging face?" (Ibid.). His response was that the abdominal surgery was medically necessary while the wrinkle removal was "simply decorative." As his colleague Vilray Blair stated at the time, a true member of this honored profession would not belittle it by "catering to the vanities and frivolities of life" (Ibid.).

---

[116] Courtesy of the Royal College of Surgeons, London.

However, as has been noted above, mere ten years later, in 1936, his opinion changed dramatically.

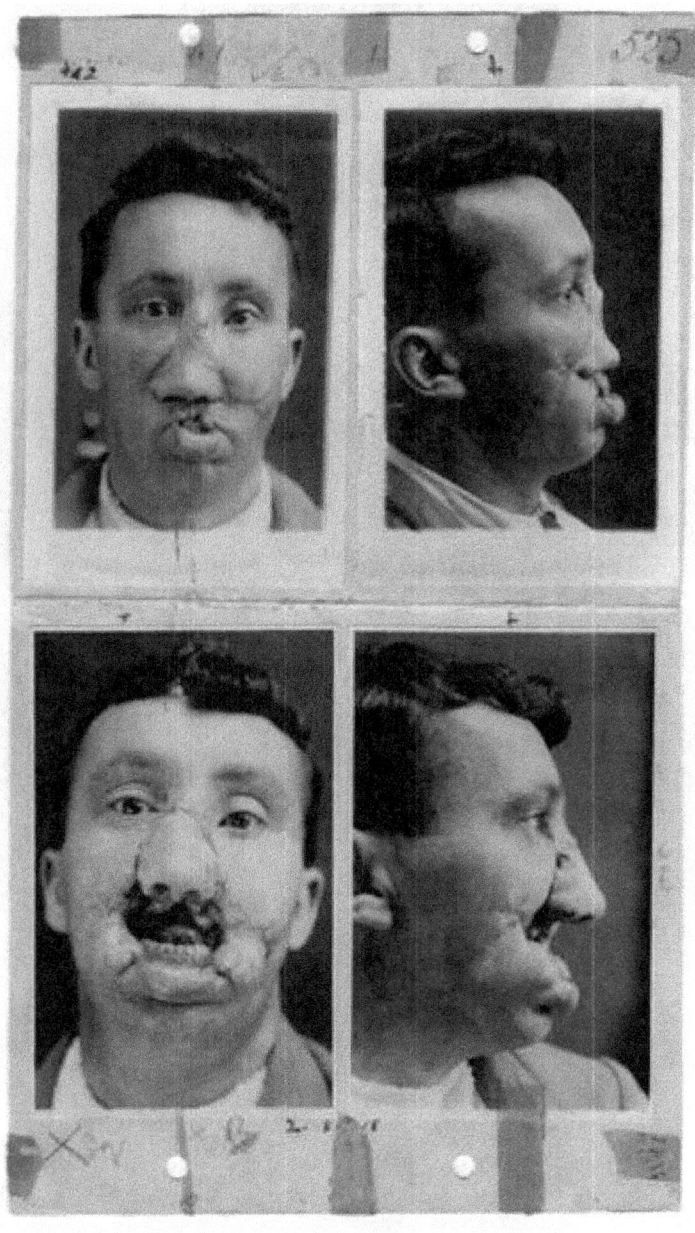

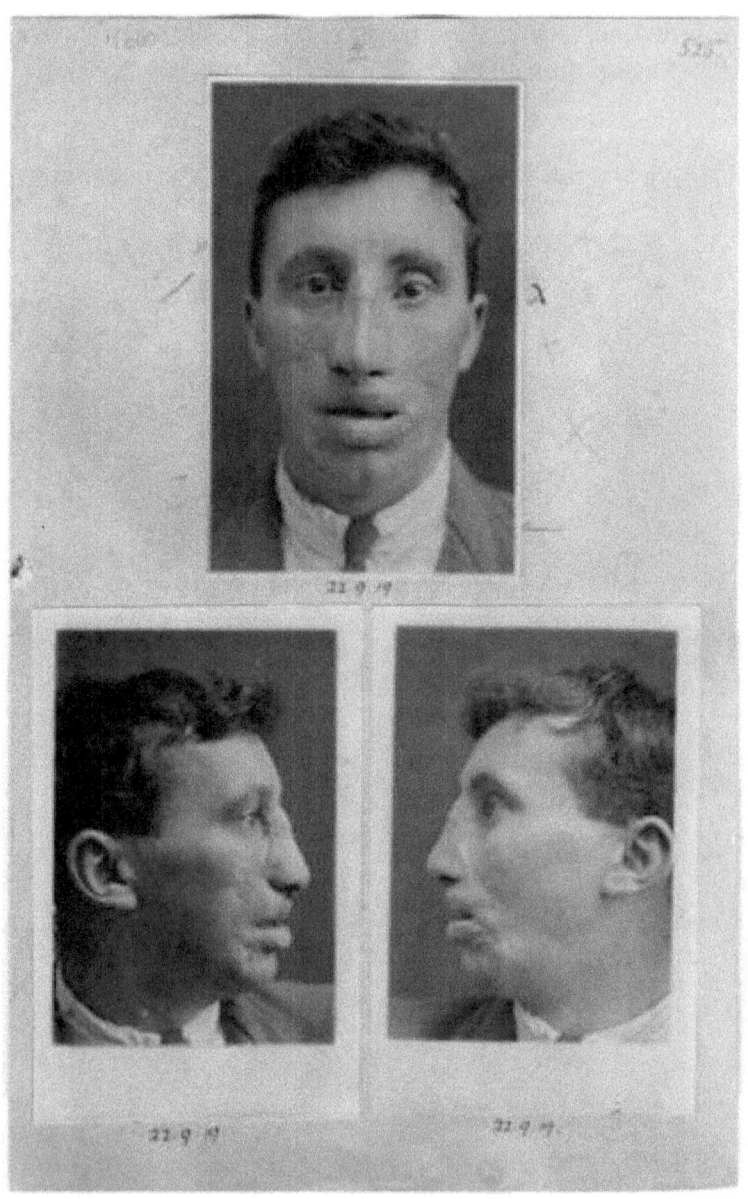

Note to the pre- and post-op images depicted above:
On his return to England, Gillies set up a special ward for facial wounds at the Cambridge Military Hospital in Aldershot, and even "sent his own casualty labels to the field hospitals in France," in order to "make sure that men with such injuries were sent directly to him" (NAM, 2022).

This dramatic change was paralleled by advances in psychology, in particular the rise of the "inferiority complex" phenomenon which was found to have resulted from either an actual or an imagined physical or psychological deficiency (Adler et al., 1917; APA, 2022). The "imagined" deficiency may appear as a visual deformity to the subject individual, although it may not appear so to others. The fact that the individual imagines and perceives a deformity does not make it any less disfiguring than a real physical deformity would be. Why then should the surgical procedure on the one be any less ethical than on the other? Why should one be called "cosmetic" and the other "reconstructive?"

Still, the classification was perpetuated, in part because many cosmetic surgeons were availing themselves of experimental methods and materials, such as paraffin injections, sponge rubber and gutta percha ground in a spinach grinder, and other "variety of foreign materials" described by Charles Conrad Miller (1881-1950) in his groundbreaking 1907 volume entitled *The Correction of Featural Imperfection*. Among these, Miller listed: "bits of braided silk, bits of silk floss, particles of celluloid, gutta percha, vegetable ivory, and several other insoluble foreign materials" which were used to repair "facial contour defects" (Rogers, 1971, p. 267).

By the onset of World War II, two thirds of all patients who visited Dr. Jerome Webster's offices came there for purely "cosmetic" reasons, driven by racial and ethnic concerns, as well as the normative pressures of beauty (Heiken, 1999, p. 187). Hollywood wannabes were routinely advised to "get a nose job before going west" and television experts' first question would invariably focus on some visual characteristic of the individual, commonly the nose, lips, cheeks, and the profile of the face (Id., p. 188). By 1950, cosmetic surgery became a necessity imposed by the "tyrannical reality" of modern life (p. 146). While the visible

233

marks of this reality were wrought in the face, sometimes (though not always) by skilled surgeons, the invisible marks in the soul were also asking for treatment.

When drawing parallels between the development of cosmetic surgery and psychology, Sigmund Freud's (1856-1939) treatise on *Fetishism* stands out for its focus on the nose, contemporaneous with the rise of rhinoplasty: Freud (1927) described a patient with a "certain sort of shine on the nose," which the venerable psychiatrist interpreted as a "glance at the nose," perceptible only to the patient, which originated in his childhood and had, as interpretations of virtually all bodily phenomena in Freud invariably had, sexual connotations. The nose has frequently symbolized the phallus, and has sometimes been associated with the conception. Book (1971) points out that "[a]natomically and physiologically, there have been a number of reports, both in lower animals and man, linking nasal function and sexual activity" (p. 450). Interestingly, studies assessing motivation for rhinoplasty "have uncovered in some applicants significant unconscious themes of heterosexual conflict" (Ibid.). The rise of psychiatry, its primeval Freudian slant, and the rise of rhinoplasty as a cosmetic-reconstructive procedure are more than coincidental. The imagined deformity of the "shiny nose," for example, or the perceived social handicap of Fanny Brice, and the actual deformity of the Aldershot patients portrayed in the pre- and post-operative photographs (above) all impact body image and self-image of these individuals in similar ways, often to comparable degrees. Their experiences are often deep, lasting, and socially scarring.

Therefore, although the distinction between reconstructive and cosmetic surgical procedures continues to be made by both professionals and laymen, in terms of the impact on body image and self-esteem, there is little difference. Sometimes, the boundaries are blurred even in the same procedure. For example, is mastectomy due to breast cancer a reconstructive or a cosmetic procedure when the patient decides to have her breasts enlarged in the same surgery by the same expert? It could hardly be said that one is more ethical than the other.

Individuals are always seen and judged by other individuals, and any departure from what is considered "normal" is usually feared or laughed at, subjected to scorn and opprobrium, which is why many subcultures and countercultures have always existed in human history – in order to unite those who share various abnormal and anti-cultural biases, such as the Diggers and the Levellers, Bohemians, Beats, Goths, various non-conforming sexual identity groups, and many others (Condor-Fisher, 2021). The transformation of the body through piercings, tattoos, extreme muscular growth, and other non-surgical practices serve not to reconstruct the body but, rather, to express the self by altering the image – mostly, by sending a message of identity with (or opposition to) someone else. The body is a medium on which the idea of the self is written.

Tattooing subcultures are a fine case in point. The same has happened with the tattooing industry which has repeatedly happened in fashion – and which has also taken place in cosmetic surgery, namely that the subculture was assimilated into popular culture (Perraudin, 2018).[117] Unless the tattoos are of an extreme nature, or at completely socially unacceptable places (often importing criminal allegiance), no member of the popular culture will pause to express outrage or disgrace at seeing a tattooed man or woman today – although there were times (in not so distant past) when

---

[117] This does not happen with counterculture movements. While subcultures exist within the larger society and recognize their norms and rules, counterculture members never do (e.g., polygamists, punks, hippies). Thus, a counterculture can never become pop-culture, unlike a subculture. Members of a subculture share cultural history, linguistic, ethnic, culinary backgrounds, and influence the main culture, its behaviors, beliefs, and values.

such outrage would not only have been expressed, but been expected as affirmative of proper behavior, morals, and the norm.

It ought to be noted that in recent years, social media have played a significant role (similar to that of the television and movies in the 20th century) in commercializing and popularizing subcultures, and even countercultures. Often, what used to be considered abnormal or unnatural or immoral has entered center stage and become the norm in many spheres of modern society. The image of the self has become omnipresent and predominant, malleable, and freely "photoshopable." The inner self is turned completely outward into the image-self, which is objectified, and over which the original owner loses control. The inner self no longer matters – it has been destroyed, reconstructed, and objectified.

Danger arises that with the reconstruction of the body, the image is swept into the pop-culture or sub-culture much like some infirm sediment on the banks of a stream enters the current and gets carried far away from its original birthplace, only just to be deposited in the dark, at the bottom of a mighty river, which accommodates many but is true home to but a few. The self of such image-oriented individuals still longs for intimate relationships, and to belong, but it remains solitary and identity-deprived. Under the pretense of obtaining all, there is none.

Consider the story of Prisha Mosley. Mosley was a troubled child who suffered from anorexia, obsessive-compulsive disorder, borderline personality disorder, anxiety, and depression. She looked like a skeleton: "I could stick my whole hand in my stomach between my rib cage... my hip bones were sticking out really bad, my hair was falling out and my skin was gray. I made everyone sad," she confided (Bolar, 2022, par. 6).

After several suicide attempts, she was hospitalized. "I just hated myself and my body," Mosley said (Id., par. 8).

Two years later, at 15, she "discovered transgenderism" and was wholeheartedly welcomed into this community. In order to belong and be accepted, she began to identify as a male. She was approved for surgery, underwent hormonal treatment, and double mastectomy.

What played a significant role in her "transitioning" was not only the advice she received from medical professionals, but also the influence and pressure from the subculture of transgenderism, which has become increasingly popular in recent years. She was suddenly accepted and extolled. Her suicidal ideation ceased. Her "self" was affirmed. Suddenly, someone was interested in her as an individual. The body became the means of acceptance and blending with what appeared to be a powerful mainstream culture. Apparently, this identification of *the self* with *the other* accomplished what no therapy could.

It took her several years to realize that she had made a mistake and (in her words) had been "emotionally manipulated" (Ibid.). At the time the interview was published, ten years after she had first embarked on hormone therapy, she was transitioning back to female.

How could this happen?

The desire to belong is one of the most fundamental human needs (Maslow, 2011). Maslow observed that successful, self-actualizing people have been "satisfied in their basic needs" first, before other needs arose (Hoffman, 1988, p. 154). Belongingness is one of the needs that cannot quite be ranked as a "lower" need because the human being always craves to belong among a particular society of his peers, relevant to the increase in his knowledge and life experience. Conversely, ostracism is one of the oldest and harshest of human punishments (Condor-Fisher, 2021). The body can be both a means to meet the desire to belong, but also a means to ostracize and reject the self. When the body is "reconstructed," so is the image.

Significantly, the image appropriates the self and resides in the body. There is an outside image and the inner image of the self. Where these two are in sympathetic arrangement, the person has little or no body image problems. That is one of the reasons why the veterans of World War I needed reconstructive-plastic surgery – in order to align their social image and their self-image.

However, there is also the inner image of the self which only the subject individual can see. It is in the person's best interest that it be aligned with their social image, in order to live a full and meaningful existence. One cannot very well live their entire life in disguise – or, if he does so, he causes himself immense suffering, and his life will have but miniscule meaning compared to what it could have had had he lived a life of his real self. That is why reconstructive surgical procedures that would have been characterized as "cosmetic" 100 years ago, can be termed reconstructive today. Where the need to belong is fulfilled only superficially, the inner self suffers and is prompted to self-destroy. Self-mutilation, self-punishment in the form of starvation or purging, even participation in extreme sports in complete disregard of life are often taken with subconscious desire to end the suffering caused by the fragmentation of body image.

There is another type of reconstruction which does not alter the self but is desirable nonetheless, because it creates a more successful social image. For example, by altering her nose, Fanny Brice certainly furthered her career in Hollywood – without necessarily altering her self-image. It is difficult to assess such cases objectively but, in Brice's case, judged by her interviews and her subsequent public and private life, the surgery had no negative (fragmenting) impact on her body image.

Wolf (2002) noted that "PBQs" (Professional Beauty Qualifications have become "BFOQs" (Bona Fide Occupational Qualifications) in recent years, in spite of the legislative effort to move the tide in the opposite direction: Title VII of the 1964 Civil Rights Act in the United States, and the 1975 Sex Discrimination Act in Great Britain (p. 28). Breast augmentation surgeries and tummy tucks, even facelifts and many other facial enhancements, can be listed in the same category. Surely, a curvaceous, busty girl with a youthful face will find more employment opportunities than her less surgically endowed peers in a vast majority of occupations. Even where such should not be the case, a mere increase of a notch or two in self-esteem will shore up sufficient reasons to go under the knife.

The judiciary did not always side with the legislative branch on these issues. For example, in *St. Cross v. Playboy Club of New York* (1972), the New York State Human Rights Appeals Board determined that a woman's "beauty" was a "bona fide qualification for employment" (p. 32). The fact that the ends are sometimes achieved by the business paying significant sums in purported damages (e.g. to male applicants, so that the business could employ only females) indicates that sex, youth and beauty have never lost their marketability (*Grushevski v. Texas Wings Inc.*, 2009).

On the other hand, in *Dothard v. Rawlinson*, 433 U.S. 321 (1977) appellee Rawlinson (hereafter appellee) filed action with the Equal Employment Opportunity Commission, and ultimately brought a class action against appellant corrections officials challenging the statutory height and weight requirements and a regulation establishing gender criteria for assigning correctional counselors to "contact" positions (positions requiring close physical proximity to inmates) as violative of Title VII of the Civil Rights Act of 1964, inter alia.[118]

---

[118] Rawlinson filed this case after her application for employment as a "correctional counselor" (prison guard) in Alabama was rejected because she failed to meet the minimum 120-pound weight requirement of an Alabama statute, which also established a height minimum of 5 feet 2 inches.

A three-judge District Court decided in appellee's favor. Based on national statistics (comparative height and weight of men and women), Alabama's statutory standards would exclude over 4% of the female population but less than 1% of the male population. Therefore, the court found that the appellee showed a prima facie case of unlawful sex discrimination, which appellants had failed to rebut. The court also found the challenged regulation impermissible under Title VII as being based on stereotyped characterizations of the sexes and, rejecting appellants' "bona fide occupational qualification" defense under §703(e) of Title VII, ruled that being male was not such a qualification for the job of correctional counselor in a "contact" position in a maximum security penitentiary for men in Alabama.

Here, although the correctional facility requirements were concerned with the body and its physical dimensions, the implied concern was with the image. An unbiased observer would surely ask how is a 120-pound woman of 5ft 2 going to tackle street-weathered criminals twice or even three times her size. One may even venture to argue that if beauty is the domain of the feminine, then strength is the domain and province of the masculine – hence the image that beauty projects, or strength it portrays, necessarily pertain to body image. Arguably, both are also equally objectively measurable: in beauty or strength contests, statistical surveys, measurements of symmetry, proportions, weight(s), etc. Every alteration of the body and its proportions will then be reflected in the image it projects, the image which impacts not only the observer but, above all, the observed individual. Therefore, there can be no reconstruction of the body without reconstructing the image, therefore the self. The body can either precede or follow, but it cannot be altered independently of the self.

Is it not the case that, where the legislative and the judiciary assume contradicting (if not contradictory) stances on the issues of beauty, image, employment qualifications, etc., such as in *St. Cross* and *Rawlinson*, one begins to perceive a degree of mass body image fragmentation? If the judiciary implements the decisions stamped by the legislative branch, and has the power of review, then it functions as a mirror to the national image. It also makes the decisions that are implemented in real-life situations, which would indicate that it is concerned with the conduct of the Nation's body. In ideal cases, there is a complete congruence between the body and the mediated image – the laws are implemented as written. In cases of fragmentations, the laws are subjected to the new precedent or deemed invalid and the legislative branch is challenged (by political pressure, which means social pressure, originating from cultural body-image mediation) to rewrite them, or to make new laws. Personal, interpersonal, and national body images live in constant interaction. They are all constructed and reconstructed, to ensure that there is but minimal friction and fragmentation. It may even be postulated that where the Nation's body–image (body-versus-image) appear fragmented, in the sense delineated above, it will negatively impact the personal (interpersonal) and individual body images. Conversely, a nation made up of fragmented selves cannot have a healthy National Self, the Soul of the Nation is ill and desires healing. Here, there is nothing a cosmetic surgeon can do; and perhaps the less he does, the better.

Soul of the Nation, Nation's Body Image, and Personal Identity

The phrase "Soul of the Nation" has been considered in the context of body image and individual identity above (*see* pages 140, 200, and the conclusion to the previous chapter). It purports to embody the national identity, and the spirit of the nation. However, a discussion on the "Soul of the Nation" would be incomplete without pausing to consider the *body* of the Nation and its *image*, as two entities that interact, to form and reflect the body image of each individual citizen.

The body is generally understood as the people that compose the nation. The image is the intangible embodiment of the national identity, expressed in the national symbols, characteristics, and pride in the Nation. It is both the people (nation) themselves that project and interpret belongingness to the group of a particular national identity, and other peoples and nations that mediate this image of nationhood. There are great similarities between the national body image and that of each individual identifying with that nation.

The body image of the nation is shown and projected symbolically. A nation cannot dress itself uniformly, nor can it behave in a certain uniform fashion at all times. Yet, the principle *e pluribus unum* (out of many, one) prevails: each individual has the nation's passport or identity card (driver's license), and is governed by the laws of the nation. The nation is united by its symbols and its common language. In the United States, the symbols of the Flag, Anthem, Bald Eagle, Statue of Liberty, Liberty Bell – all symbolize the concepts on which it was founded and uniquely distinguish it from other nations. The Nation is represented as the bearer of Liberty Enlightening the World. What is more, each state within the Union has its own Flag, and unique distinguishing symbols derived from its geographic location and peculiar historical circumstances that gave it rise: the tree, bird,

242

animal, and flower that best represent and capture its identity within the Union.

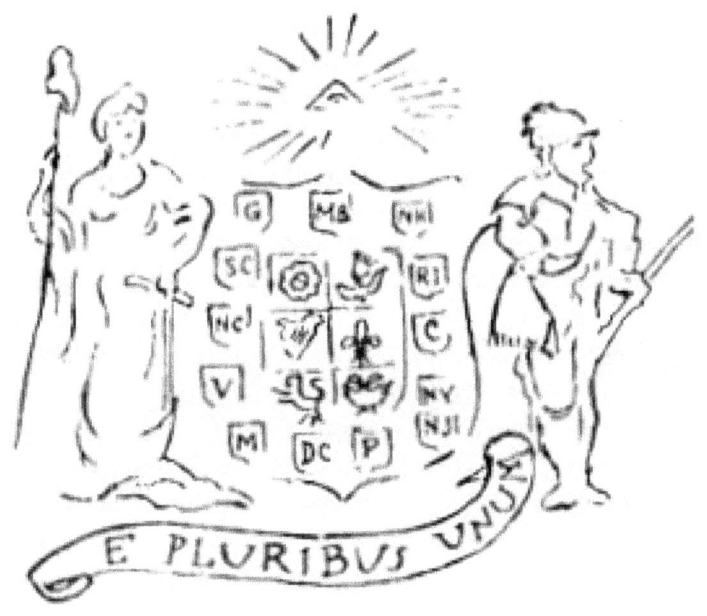

Restored version of Du Simitière's original
1776 sketch for the Great Seal.[119]

The original description stated that the seal was supported by an American soldier "compleatly accoutred [sic] in his hunting Shirt and trowsers [sic], with his tomahawk, powder horn, pouch &c. holding with his left hand his rifle gun rested" (Great Seal, 2023a). The committee (consisting of Dr. Franklin, Thomas Jefferson, and John Adams) replaced the soldier with the Goddess of Justice.

---

[119] Pierre Eugene du Simitière (b. Pierre-Eugène Ducimetière) (1737–1784) a Genevan-American member of the American Philosophical Society, naturalist, American patriot, and portrait painter.

The Goddess of Liberty is portrayed "in a corselet of armour [sic] alluding to the present Times," which means revolutionary times, signifying the fight for freedom of the Colonies: in her right hand, she holds the "Spear and Cap" and with her left, she is "supporting the Shield of the States" (Ibid.).[120] To the left of her, and left of the shield, stands the Goddess of Justice, with a sword in her right hand and a balance in her left hand. The Eye of Providence shines above and on them "in a radiant Triangle whose glory extends over the Shield and beyond the Figures" (Ibid.). Here is the 21st century full color artwork realization of the description:

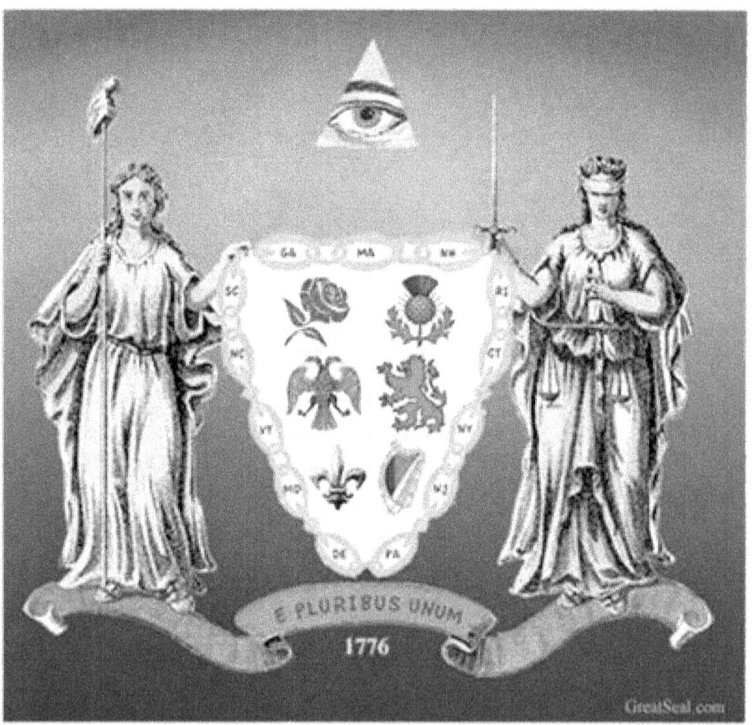

---

[120] So-called Phrygian cap, formerly the *pileus,* a brimless felt cap symbolizing slavery.

The Shield contains symbols of the "Countries from which these States have been peopled" (Great Seal, 2023b), namely: the Rose for England, Thistle for Scotland, Imperial Eagle for Germany, Lion for Holland, Fleur-de-lis for France, and the Harp for Ireland. The Shield is enlaced with a "Border of thirteen shields linked together by a golden Chain" containing initial letters of each of the "thirteen independent States of America" (Ibid.). Certain differences may also be found when compared to the previous model: Liberty is not wearing a "corselet of armor," the symbols of the countries are in a different order, the description does not specify a blindfold on Justice, and the Light doesn't "extend over the Shield and beyond the Figures" (Ibid.).

The expert staff of the Great Seal (2023b) characterized the image as "America's first selfie" (par. 5).[121] It is said to encapsulate not only the origins of the United States, but also its purpose and character. As such these symbols, and the Seal *in toto*, constitute the *dress* of the Nation, of each state of the Union, and the Union itself. *Dress* is used as a technical term here, borrowed from intellectual property law, where it means "the commercial look and feel of a product or service that identifies and distinguishes the source of the product or service" (Justia, 2023). A *trade dress* usually includes distinctive characteristics (*look and feel*) which set the product apart from other similar products. The shape (product design, such as the shape of the Coca-Cola bottle) may be considered its *dress*.

---

[121] The word *selfie* was officially introduced into English by the Oxford English Dictionary in 2013. APA invented another word, *selfitis,* for the obsessive-compulsive disorder characterized by the incessant need to take "selfies." The positive effects on an individual taking selfies and posting them on social media are mainly those of increased self-esteem, and communication of the self with desire to belong. Both such effects can be also seen in the publicity given to the national symbols with regard to the associations and "self-esteem" (standing) of the Nation.

The similarities between this intellectual property dress and the human dress or costume are more than coincidental. The trade word *dress* had been chosen because it expresses the way a product is "dressed" to represent the brand. As has been discussed above (*see* p. 40 et seq.), each individual's daily dress is a compromise between the custom of the day and the expression of personal individuality and independence, displaying the person's gender, socio-economic status, occupation, even interests, hobbies, and affiliations.

It is remarkable that the dress of the American Nation was altered at the very inception. Most notable of these alterations is no doubt that of the substitution of the female figure of Goddess Justice (or Lady Justice, in common parlance) for the male figure of the soldier. Goddess Justice contains a far more expansive symbolic value than a soldier ever could. Ancient Egyptians revered *Ma'at*, Justice "carrying a sword with an ostrich feather in her hair" (Swatt, 2011). She had no scales but weighed the hearts of the dead, in order to decree judgment upon them. The ancient Greeks revered *Themis*, as the organizer of the "communal affairs of humans, particularly assemblies" (Ibid. par. 2). For her ability of clairvoyance, she became one of the oracles at Delphi. Neither Ma'at nor Themis were blindfolded but the very opposite – they were portrayed with a sharp vision. They also did not need a sword because Justice was decreed by consenting to the Oracle's judgment. It was the Roman Goddess of Justice that was handed down to us blindfolded, "evenly balancing both scales," and wielding a sword (Ibid. par. 3). Burnett (1987) noted that she was also variously portrayed with the fasces[122] and an ax (symbols of judicial

---

[122] Fasces is derived from Latin *fascis,* meaning a "bundle" usually of wooden rods, often with an axe, symbolizing power in general (Etruscan civilization): while one stick is easily broken, many rods, tied together, will withstand great power. Specifically, in ancient Rome, fasces were the symbol of magistrate's power and jurisdiction. The *fascinus* of

authority) in one hand, and a torch or flame in the other (symbols of truth).

The sword is clearly a symbol of power, but so is the ax with the fasces. One may argue that the sword symbolizes military power while the fasces with the ax stand for magisterial and legal power. There are thirteen fasces on the wall end of the Lincoln Memorial, representing thirteen original colonies, with the Bald Eagle perched above; and the Memorial itself has 36 Doric columns, representing the states of the Union at the time of the Civil War. Fasces hold the weight together, and each is necessary to support the other and the structure itself (National Park Service, 2023). The female representation of power gives it an added dimension of safety, custom, social order, and proper procedure – although, sometimes, all the representations were surpassed by the ultimate one – "the will of god" (Finley, 1978, p. 78).

In terms of national personifications, the female figure usually represents the continent, land, or a country: Colombia, Britannia, Germania, Hibernia, Hispania, Helvetia, Polonia etc. The city and the state are also traditionally female. By contrast, the male figure represents the citizenry (the nation itself): Uncle Sam, John Bull, Deutscher Michel, Russian Ivan. The male figure is blunt, direct, somewhat naïve, self-assured, and persistent. The female figure is more reserved than the male, but of noble bearing, representing wisdom. The costumes are also different: apart from the soldier's trousers, there is a marked difference in style. The robe Goddess Justice is dressed in is a sumptuous, sixteenth century gown which, however, has very un-sixteenth century short sleeves reminiscent of the older, Italian woven costume (Boucher, 1965/1987). It appears to be made from gilded silk, indicating wealth and

---

Goddess Vesta is also used to alight the sacred hearth. Therefore, in the female province, a single *fascinus* is not so much the symbol of power but, rather, the symbol of life and safety.

prestige. On the other hand, Goddess Liberty is dressed in a plain, austere robe, whose origins can be traced to the Byzantine Empire. It is altogether proper and fitting that she be dressed thus, symbolizing the rise from slavery to freedom, the virtue of poverty, and the pride stemming from personal independence.

It is important to note that both figures are representative, that means concerned with the image they project, not with the body they possess. The body is used as a symbolic vehicle. They are wearing sandals characteristic of the old Roman Empire (resembling *calceus senatorius*, the sandals of the Roman senators) and their bare hands are grasping the instruments of power and self-identity. They are not positioned in any sexually suggestive manner. If anything, the figures are motherly and matriarchal. The sum total of the body image here is the concern with ethical norms, and the imposition of and devotion to order which, in the American literary canon, has traditionally been the province of the feminine. At the same time, it is the order they impose that they are subjected to themselves. It is perhaps not coincidental that the Goddess of the home, hearth and family, Vesta, has been portrayed as *Phallic Mother* by the 20th Century psychoanalysts, perhaps because of the stick (*fascinus*) with which she would alight the sacred fire (Schroeder, 1998).

They eye above them is the Eye of Divine Providence, to which the Declaration of Independence refers in its last sentence: "And for the support of this Declaration, with a firm reliance on the protection of divine Providence, we mutually pledge to each other our Lives, our Fortunes and our sacred Honor." The eye appears as a superior symbol of light ("glory") above the figures, importing the presence of God.

The original design was altered in 1782. William Barton (of the third Great Seal Committee) suggested that the pyramid signifying strength and duration, and the omniscient eye (the eye of Providence) be stamped on the reverse side of the Great Seal: "A Pyramid of thirteen Strata... In the Zenith, an Eye, surrounded with a Glory" (Great Seal, 2023c).[123]

Wherever there is an eye, there is an observer. With the observer comes the observed. The symbolism of the mirror and the body image is thus complete. It is inextricably intertwined with the Seal. The Nation represents itself through the most fundamental values: Liberty, and Justice. At the same time, it is circumspectly observed by the all-seeing eye. These values are the gifts of Divine Providence, the Providence embodied in the figures of the two Goddesses and, through them, transferred to each member-state and member-individual of the Nation. The imposition of Order is more than a percept of Justice – it is a part of the makeup of the individuals that form the Nation.

All member-individuals then reflect and project back the image by interpreting it, not only in words but, above all, in conduct, thus forming certain national characteristics: audacity, forgiveness, Puritan ethic, etc. By virtue of individual and collective mediation, the symbol is transforming as to each individual, and transformative of itself. Note, for example, the various forms that the personification of America in the figure of Columbia has taken by comparing Columbia personified as the Goddess Liberty, actually wearing the Phrygian cap.

This poster was created during World War I, likely after the sinking of Lusitania (May 7, 1915). Columbia is reaching in by reaching out: she is the mirror-image of the Nation being mobilized to take part in the world conflict, to defend the universal principles of liberty which it espouses and embodies. She is dressed in the American flag, her top has no sleeves and her lower body is dressed in baggy pants

---

[123] *Glory* is the heraldic term for rays of light. *Deo Favente*: with God's Favor. *Perennis*: Everlasting.

which a modern observer would likely refer to as "gym-pants." She is not only the symbol of progress, as the older Columbia had been, but also of emancipation and personal independence.

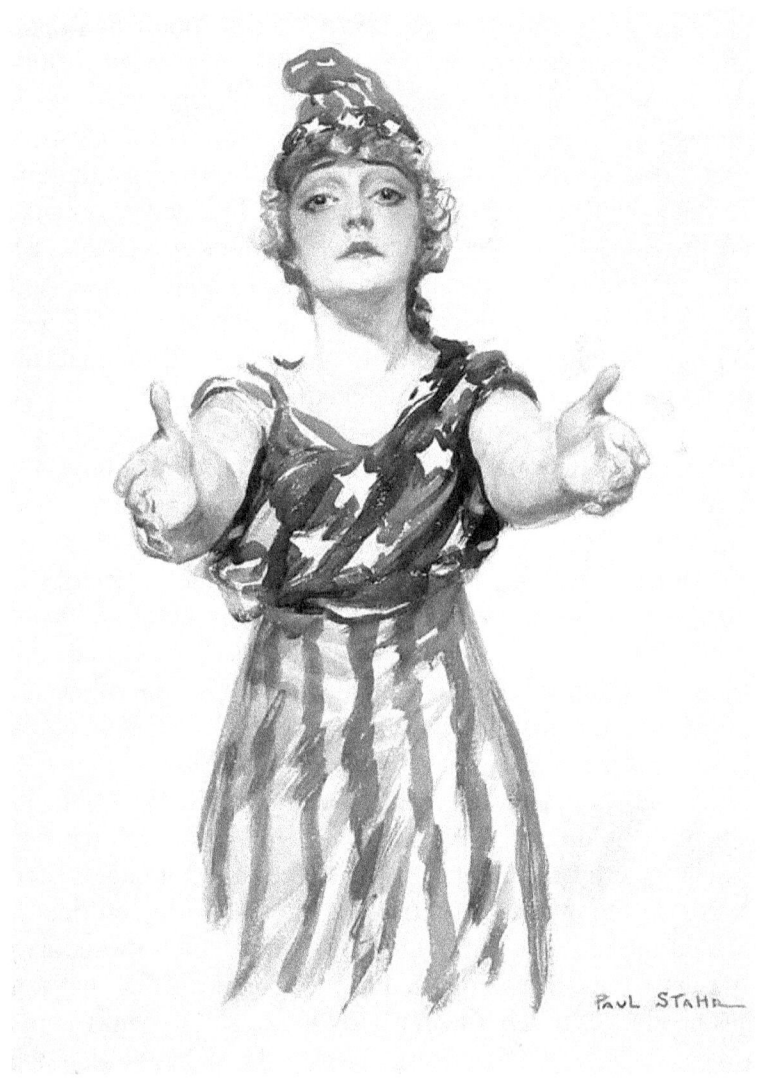

By contrast, the older Columbia, famously depicted in John Gast's painting entitled *American Progress* (1872), rises up as the leader of the westward-moving crowd of settlers. She is one of many, yet standing above them all, carrying the token of progress in the form of telegraph lines across the Western frontier, in order to fulfill *manifest destiny*, the destiny of ever-expanding frontier which, in the American mind, was not to be closed with its physical extinguishment announced by Frederick Jackson Turner before the American Historical Association in Chicago in 1893, mere twenty years later.

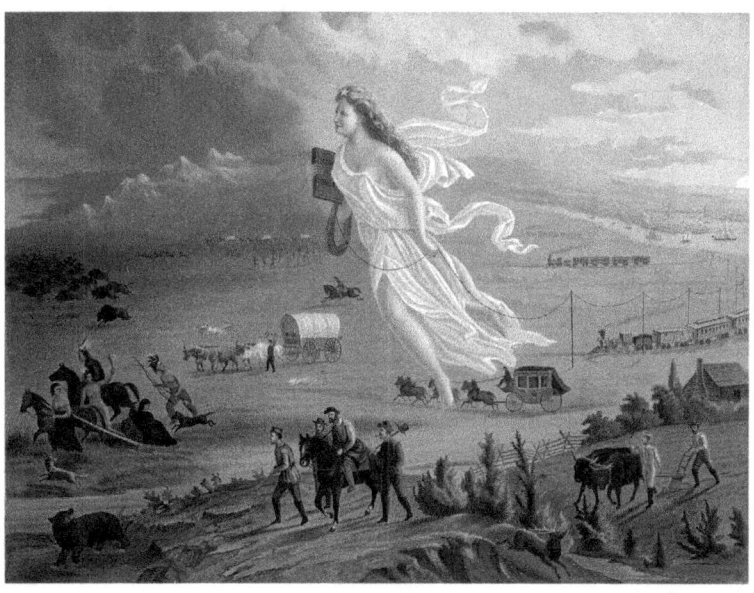

Note that this Columbia is dressed in a much more traditional and feminine fashion, resembling the Goddess of Liberty from the Grand Seal. She is young, pretty, and sensuous. In her right hand, she carries a book entitled *Common Schools,* the symbol of enlightenment and progress. There is no *fascie,* no stick or any other phallic symbol of power. Neither is there any Phrygian cap as part of her attire. Rather, her hair flows freely and sensuously, caressed wildly by Zephyr, the western wind, symbolic of the Romantic spirit of hope and boundless opportunities and, with them, also an unbounded and "borderless" body image. Her forehead is adorned with a "Star of the Empire" (Crofutt, 1873).[124] The star symbolizes both guidance and protection (the Star of Bethlehem), as well as progress, hope, and excellence, the five-pointed star (*see* detail below).

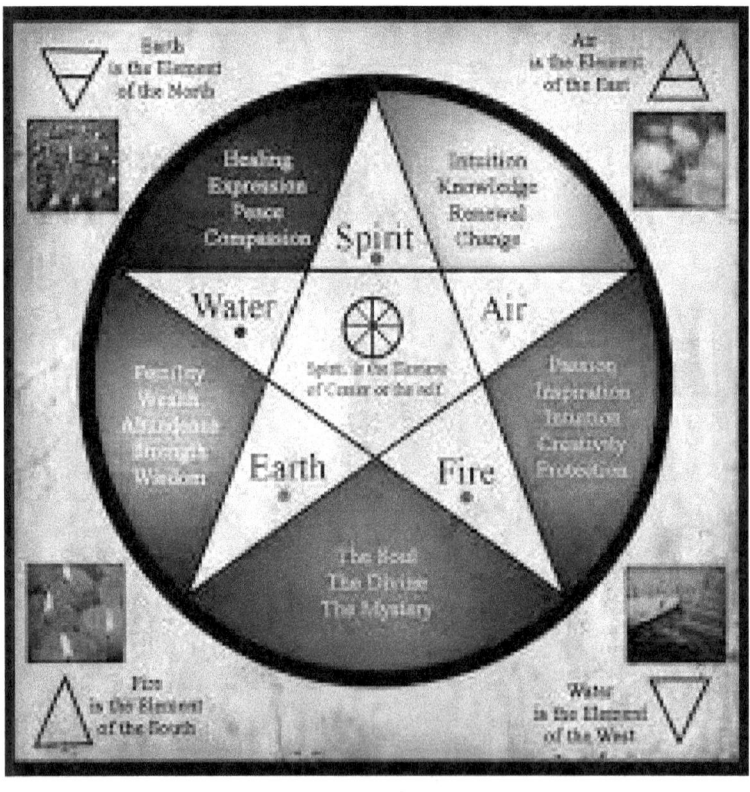

---

[124] Publisher George Crofutt distributed the painting as a print with his magazine, *Crofutt's Western World*. The original description is attributed to him.

252

The five-pointed star is a divine symbol of unity of the body and the image: the oneness it represents is the whole of the top (human spirit/image) united with the four elements (the body). Conventionally, the five-pointed star imports the connection between the Human Spirit and Mother Nature, and it also symbolizes the "incarnation of Jesus Christ" (Egret, 2023). In other words, it also *embodies* the spirit.

Consequently, the portrait of Columbia in Gast's *American Progress* is that of the *image* of the *body* with the representation of body image unity in the center of its forehead. Its message is: I am the body which is the image that embodies. Although, logically speaking, the reasoning is circular, spirituality defies logic: one must believe in order to embody (the belief). The belief, however, is irrational by nature. Therefore, there is a complete unity of the body and the image.

The star depicted above also represents other ideas (images): it stands for the five wounds of Jesus (Holweck, 1912), thus advancing the Judeo-Christian Tradition of the Republic, and it signifies the power of the spirit over the four elements of the universe (which may be interpreted as superiority of the image over the body), as opposed to the reversed pentagram, "with two points projecting upwards," which is a symbol of evil because it "attracts sinister forces" by overturning "the proper order of things" (Waite, 1886, p. 136).[125] The painting also coincides with the official adoption of the pentagrammic star (in 1873) as the symbol of the order of freemasons called The Order of the Eastern Star, established in 1850 as the Masonic Appendant Body open to people of faith, men and women alike. Its tenets embrace the five knightly virtues, traded from early

---

[125] It is said to represent "the goat of lust attacking the heavens with its horns, a sign execrated by initiates" (Ibid.). Note: "to execrate" means "to curse" (from Latin *execratus*: *ex* "out" + *sacrare* "to devote to").

253

medieval times: generosity, friendship, chastity, chivalry, and piety (Eastern Star, 2023).

Freemasons were among the most notable surveyors and builders in America. The process of surveying, mapping, and building can be characterized as embodying the image, giving it a form. Some of the best well-known names of the American Revolution were Masons: Ethan Alien, Edmund Burke, John Claypoole, William Daws, Benjamin Franklin, John Hancock, John Paul Jones, Robert Livingston, Paul Revere, Colonel Benjamin Tupper, and others. Of the 56 signers of The Declaration of Independence, eight were known Masons and "seven others exhibited strong evidence of Masonic membership," and of the forty signers of the Constitution, nine were known Masons, "13 exhibited evidence of Masonic membership," and "six more later became Masons" (Harici, 2006, par. 5). Further, Lafayette was a Freemason, as was the majority of the commanders of the Continental Army, most of George Washington's generals and the first President himself. The Boston Tea Party was planned at the Green Dragon Tavern, also known as "Freemasons' Arms" (sometimes dubbed "the Headquarters of the Revolution"), and George Washington himself was sworn in as the first President of the United States by Robert Livingston, Grand Master of New York's Masonic lodge. Also the cornerstone of the Capitol was laid by the Grand Lodge of Maryland (Harici, 2006).

American national body image has been, to a great degree, portrayed by Freemasons, their skills and wit which stemmed from the thoughts and philosophies of the Enlightenment: rationalism, empiricism, and the scientific method. It is therefore understandable that personifications of the Nation do not separate the body from the image but, rather, attempt to unite them. There is no dichotomy, no hesitation, no staring in the mirror, asking oneself: Is this who I am? Somewhat paradoxically, one might say, because the periods in history when these images were created were largely characterized by turmoil, revolutions, wars, and other upheavals. In view of the need for national unity in these harrowing times, however, the seeming paradox dissipates.

The unifying symbols were also buttressed by the principles of Protestant ethic imbued in them. According to Max Weber (1920/2002), the way to salvation is to live an ascetic, purpose-oriented existence, focused primarily on accumulation of material worth. Protestant ethic is rooted in rationalized, organized, ascetic life, subjugated to "the *concept of the calling*" (p. 40) [italics original]. Vocational competence and proficiency are manifested by material success. At the same time, this material success detracts from the bodily needs (asceticism) and projects the aspirations to higher values. Thus, while the apparent focus is on the body (material), it is the image that is the ultimate goal. Transcendentalism and Protestantism are inextricably intertwined and imbued in virtually all symbols and symbolic images: be it the grasp on the instruments of power and freedom (The Great Seal), or purposeful marching westward across the continent (Columbia in the *American Progress*), or raising the arms to connect with *the other* (WWI Columbia), or even in the finger, sharply pointed at *you,* in fact addressing the *Me Myself* of the Nation (Uncle Sam).

As to the latter, while Uncle Sam is also "wearing" the pentagram, it is on his hat, not on his forehead, as is the case the Columbia, thus part of his costume, which includes the Stars and Striped ribbon adorning his hat. Uncle Sam also does not symbolize the Nation, but only the United States' government. In fact, the symbol was coined during the War of 1812, from the letters "U.S." stamped on barrels with supplies which were sent to the soldiers by the meatpacker Samuel Wilson (1766-1854). The U.S. stood for the United States, but soldiers interpreted it as "Uncle Sam" (History.com, 2023). The image was popularized by the famous political cartoonist Thomas Nast (1840-1902), who gave Sam the white beard and stars-and-stripes suit, familiar to the reader today (Ibid.).[126]

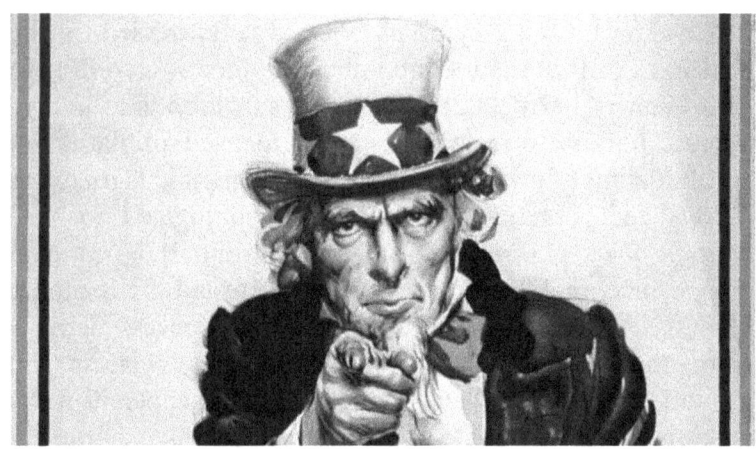

Matthews (1908) noted that the original idea (which gave rise to the image) was mainly negative, referring to the belligerence and cheapness of the U.S. government – the supplies were lousy, Uncle Sam was a war-hawk who cared little for his people, and "did not pay well" (p. 34).

The image of Uncle Sam depicted above was created by James Montgomery Flagg (1877-1960). In this particular version, Uncle Sam has a tall top hat on, is wearing a blue jacket, and his right index finger points straight at the viewer (History.com, 2023). This version is perhaps best known as a key recruiting poster during World War I, in which context the index finger is typically interpreted as casting responsibility on the Nation.

---

[126] Nast is also credited with the modern image of Santa Claus; the donkey as a symbol for the Democrat Party; the elephant as a symbol for the Republican Party; and the downfall of New York City's Tammany Hall machinery, caused by his caricatures of the Tammany leader William Tweed vis-à-vis the then NYC mayor Fiorello La Guardia who ran to end Tammany Hall corruption.

However, the index finger is capable of importing broader and more comprehensive meanings, often as the symbol of authority, ambition, and pride (Kinz, 2023).[127] In astrology, the index finger is connected to Jupiter, husband of Juno, God of Light, the sky and the weather (Ganesha, 2023). It represents welfare and the laws of the state, which is also why this image can be interpreted a demand to obey. As a consequence, the meaning of Uncle Sam is radically different from the meaning of Columbia by Stahl (depicted further above) with her outstretched arms and an ardent, impassionate stare cast at the viewer.

Nevertheless, it is obvious that the image of the body carries a meaning both as a whole, and in various parts: eyes, hands, fingers, posture, etc. All these body parts symbolize and project meanings that, in the case of the national symbol, both address the nation, but are also co-written, co-created and spoken-to. Therefore, there can be no personal body image of a citizen of the nation wholly devoid of the national body image of the nation the citizen is belongs to. The national and individual identities are co-dependent and co-created.

In view of such findings, it is appalling that the American Psychological Association has not conducted any survey and analysis of the subject. There is a plethora of surveys on mental health, stress, depression, racism, and other topics, all of which show bias toward personal and interpersonal focus in the microsphere and mesosphere, not focus on the problems related to macrosphere and the Nation (APA, 2023c). Clearly, however, how one feels about belonging to the Nation bears upon how one feels about oneself and one's personal identity. A recent survey from the Associated Press-NORC Center for Public Affairs Research found that political leanings are decisive where one's National Identity is concerned: Republicans are "far more

---

[127] *See* also *The School of Athens*, p. 62 (above).

257

likely to cite a culture grounded in Christian beliefs and the traditions of early European immigrants" as essential to U.S. identity, while Democrats "are more apt to point to the country's history of mixing of people from around the globe" and the tradition of "offering refuge to the persecuted" (PBS, 2017, par. 2-3). 7 in 10 people reported that the country is losing its identity. With reference to identity, the surveyed mentioned the rule of law, the Constitution, and the American dream (Ibid.). However, these ideas are only tangentially associated with the images discussed above, not to mention the daring, far-reaching interpretations thereof, which include the symbols of the Grand Seal as well as the varied meanings of Columbia.

Consider the NBC (2017) poll entitled *What Does It Mean to Be Truly American?* This poll, as well as the PBS poll, cited above, was taken after the election of Donald Trump. The Republican ratings on "National Pride" jumped by 20 points, while the Democrats' evaluation remained very low (22 percent were proud to be American). The top ratings in the poll indicated the importance of Language, Customs and Traditions, Belief, and Birthplace. These are the fundamentals of the National Identity. By the same token, they represent the degree to which each individual embraces his or her personal identity: one's language, the traditions one observes, their faith, and the country of birth (the order cited by the poll).

Interestingly, "being able to speak English" is by far the most important national characteristic. "Interestingly," because other nations speak English, but also "interestingly" because a most recent government survey shows that the number of people in the United States who speak a language other than English at home has "nearly tripled from 23.1 million (about 1 in 10) in 1980 to 67.8 million (almost 1 in 5) in 2019" (Dietrich & Hernandez, 2022, par. 1). At the same time, however, "the number of people who spoke only English also increased" from 187.2 million in 1980 to 241 million in 2019 (par. 2). It might surprise a native-born American that the U.S. government claims that there is "no official language in the United States," and that whoever wants there to be an "official language" promulgated in their state "should contact his or her elected official" (USA.gov, 2023, par. 1).

Customs and traditions have been cited as the second most important national characteristic, regardless of political leanings. These encompass primarily fashion, food, art, sports, and the observance of holidays. Zimmerman and McKelvie (2022) noted that fashion itself is subject to "social status, region, occupation and climate" making it difficult to universalize and define an "American style" – although there do exist certain elements of costume which are generally recognized as prototypically American, such as: the jeans, baseball caps with diverse national teams' logos, the Texan cowboy hat, and cowboy boots (par. 12). One may argue that it is only fitting for a "nation of immigrants" that prototypically American fashion-setters, such as Ralph Lauren, Calvin Klein, Michael Kors, Brooks Brothers, Victoria Secret, etc. are international brands that largely manufacture their goods abroad.

The next item on the what-it-means-to-be-an-American list is cuisine. However, the "typical" American cuisine originated in Europe, and it was also influenced by the diet of Native American tribes. Hamburgers, potato chips, macaroni and cheese, meat loaf, the proverbial apple pie… are considered American, even though they did not originate in America. Various kinds of food thus bring along with them national traditions from abroad, and follow tastes and dispositions which stem from local climates, as well as settlement patterns. For example, the typical "American southern-style comfort food" (fried chicken, collard greens, black-eyed peas, cornbread), popular in Texas and the Southwest, is a "blend of Spanish and Mexican cooking styles" (par. 14).

In the domain of the arts, the United States has been widely associated with Hollywood and the Broadway. It is not an underestimation to say that American television dominates the world, as does American music with its very distinct musical rhythms of the country, gospel, jazz, blues, bluegrass, rock'n'roll, rap, and hip hop genres. It is also through the movies and music that inculturation of language takes place.

As to sport, American football, baseball, and basketball dominate. Although they can all be cited as prototypically American sports, they too have foreign origins. American football (gridiron football) is closely related to rugby and soccer. Rugby had been started at Rugby School in Rugby, Warwickshire, England. It gradually evolved from medieval forms of football, played among towns and cities vying for primacy with an inflated pig's bladder (Rugbyfootballhistory.com, 2023). As to basketball, although it is said to have originated in Springfield, Massachusetts in 1891 (Cooper, 2023), various forms of the ball game with a "hoop" had been present in the Americas (and elsewhere in the world) for over 4000 years, often symbolizing the passage of the sun or the journey to the underworld, mythical struggle ending in death, which was not always merely symbolic (Cartwright, 2013).

American holidays form a major part of the American custom and tradition. Most notably, July 4, Thanksgiving, Memorial Day, Labor Day, Presidents' Day, Veterans' Day, and MLK Day. They all observe important events in the history of the Nation that form the national identity and create a healthy core of what it means to be an American.

In the Pew Research survey cited by NBC (Ibid.), faith was listed after culture and tradition as a separate cultural value but, sociologically, it is inseparable from the other elements of culture and tradition listed above. Traditional religious belief is invariably "manifested through the creation of culture" which devolves around symbolic objects and images (Abdulla, 2018, p. 102). Zimmermann and McKelvie (2022) found that 70% of Americans identify as Christians. According to the Pew Research Center, only 23% have no religious affiliation at all, and only 5.9% identify as "non-Christian faiths (PRC, 2023). However, also only four in ten American also say that the United States "should be a Christian Nation" (Smith, Rotolo, & Tevington, 2022, par. 1). This dichotomy is unremarkable in that it parallels the distinction that every individual makes between (personal) faith and (organized) religion. Religious experience includes "activities of worship and contemplative techniques" that are "embodied in social institutions" (Smart, 1979, p. 34). Personal religious experience is defined in terms of "personal commitment" and "spirituality" (Gschwandtner, 2021, p. 2). Even people without a firm religious belief or adherence are in some ways *spiritual*. Spirituality is a mode of exercising one's innermost beliefs, a "particular way of living out one's religion" (Gschwandtner, 2021, p. 2). The degree to which these beliefs are subsumed or separated from mass religious practices of the region differs from religion to religion, and is accorded different weight even within one religious system, such as the difference between how the Protestants vis-à-vis the Catholics adhere to communal belief and the Church, and how they practice their faiths and exercise their spirituality in everyday lives.

Cultural practices and traditions more than wield incredible influence over the individual's self-image – in fact, they shape it from the earliest childhood: language, customs and conduct of the parents, as well as close friends and relatives, the kind of faith practiced in the native locale, sports, and activities one engages in, the music peculiar to the nation, etc. All these form and shape the individual's self-image. This self-image is thereby closely connected to the national sense of selfhood and what may be termed

Nation's body image – the image that each Nation also projects onto other nations, the way it wants to be seen, the manner in which it practices and exercises its politics. Every aspect of the individual body image and self-image partakes of the national body image, and vice versa: the individual cultural and ethnic diverse backgrounds of the citizenry are united in the body image of the Nation.

Cultural and Ethnic Aspects of Body Image

Both inter-ethnic and intra-ethnic differences may be found across cultures and in various cultural contexts. It is impossible to ascertain and describe them all, albeit certain major differences are well-known and familiar to every body image expert. These devolve of socioeconomic status, sex and gender, peer and parental influences, ethnic identity, and sexual maturation. Body mass index and socioeconomic status are among the more measurable values.

Nonetheless, crucial data must be collected via questionnaires, which makes results dependent on the vagaries of language, and culturally biased. For example, since Asian cultures "emphasize values that promote interpersonal harmony" within the family and the community, there exists a "pressure to act in a manner that does not reflect poorly on the group" – the pressure which leads to the suppression of states, events, and situations that are considered "shameful" by the questioned individuals (Kawamura, p. 244). By the same token, BDD Foundation (2023) reported that shame, and fear of being considered vain were the chief factors in preventing the diagnosis of body image related problems.

It should be noted that Asia has the highest concentration of plastic surgeons in the world, while Japan, South Korea and Hong Kong are the "top spenders" (per capita) on skin care in the world; in South Korea, one of every three women aged 19-29 has undergone plastic surgery (Madan et al., 2018, p. 54). Sociologically, it is the omnipresent pressure from the group, exerted on every individual of that group, to represent the group to the best of their abilities which underscores this emphasis on body image perfection.

While the United States has the largest total number of plastic-cosmetic surgeons, it is South Korea, Argentina, and Brazil that have the most cosmetic surgeons per capita.

The following table shows the total number of cosmetic surgeons, population, and the number of citizens per surgeon:

USA	7000	341mil	48,714
Brazil	5,843	213mil	36,454
China	3,000	1.4bil	466,666
Japan	2,707	126mil	46,546
South Korea	2,581	51.8mil	20,069
India	2,400	1.4bil	583,333
Argentina	2,000	45.2mil	22,600
Russia	2,000	146mil	73,000
Mexico	1,749	127mil	72,612
Germany	1,541	83.8mil	54,380
Turkey	1,300	84.3mil	64,846
Colombia	1,200	51.5mil	42,908

The table clearly shows that while the United States has the highest total number of cosmetic surgeons, South Korea, Argentina, Brazil, Japan, and even Colombia by far surpass the U.S. in the number of cosmetic surgeons per capita.

Hess (2021) listed the following summary of cosmetic procedures per percentage of population, showing trends that correlate to ethnic and genetic roots:

1. South Korea: liposuction, rhinoplasty, blepharoplasty
2. Greece: breast augmentation
3. Italy: Botulinum Toxin Type A (Botox Dysport), and liposuction
4. Brazil: breast implants, and liposuction
5. Columbia: liposuction
6. USA: liposuction, breast augmentation
7. Taiwan: Botox and other wrinkle treatments

Apparently, breast implant surgery and liposuction are the procedures for which there is the highest demand regardless of race or ethnicity. It is certainly not unremarkable from a medical viewpoint that their frequency coincides and that, therefore, they are correlated. Still, non-invasive procedures, such as CoolSculpting (non-invasive fat reduction), Botox injections, soft tissue fillers, and chemical peels have increased significantly more in proportion to the increase in surgical procedures. For example, according to the American Society of Plastic Surgeons (ASPS), while breast augmentation procedures increased by 48% over the last twenty years, the use of Botox injections increased by 845% (GVR, 2023). American Society of Plastic Surgeons reported the following ethnic breakdown for cosmetic procedures performed in the United States in 2020 based on data gathered by the Federal Census Bureau (USAfacts, 2021). These data indicate that the white non-Hispanic group made up 59.3% of the population in 2021 (a marked decrease from 63.8% in 2010). Yet, the proportion of cosmetic procedures performed shows 66% for this group. Hispanic/Latino population makes up 18.9% and is constantly increasing. In spite of their constant increase, Latino populations show a substantially lower demand for cosmetic procedures – only 13%. Black non-Hispanic population constitutes about 12.6%, projecting a very stable representation over the last ten years, and its demand for cosmetic procedure is slightly less, at about 11%. Asian-American non-Hispanic demographics make up 5.9%, which is a noticeable increase from 4.8% in 2010, but the demand for cosmetic procedures among this community is proportionately the highest, 8%.

In conclusion, U.S. statistics show that Asian and White demographics have the greatest demand for cosmetic procedures, while the Hispanics populate the opposite end of the spectrum, with the African-Americans in the middle, being proportionately represented. Arguably, therefore,

Asian-Americans and Whites should display the least body image satisfaction.

94% of all procedures are undergone by women, out of which 45% are women aged 40-54. The list of procedures in the highest demand is as follows: 1) nose (rhinoplasty), 2) eyelid (blepharoplasty), 3) facelift, 4) breast augmentation, and 5) liposuction. Statistics for males indicate: 3) cheek implant, 4) liposuction, 5) ear surgery. Rhinoplasty and blepharoplasty are in the highest demand regardless of sex and race. This is not surprising and only confirms the fact that, regardless of gender, the nose and the eyes are the most prominent, dominant, and important parts of body image in social contact.

White Caucasian and Asian non-Hispanic groups are ethnically and racially as diverse as one could imagine, yet they request the most surgeries of the same type. Arguably, this also indicates the greatest body image dissatisfaction among the listed ethnicities. Another reason may be the facility and availability of surgeries and surgeons, related to the disposable income. Asian communities are among the wealthiest in the United States and are the least likely to live in poverty (Budiman & Ruiz, 2021). However, no statistics are available that would show how this income is spent, or the dissection within the group (the Indian-Asian group has by far the highest disposable income, yet does not appear to make up the greatest percentage of cosmetic procedures).

The fact remains that both, the Asian conformist group-representative mindset, and the White individualistic ego-oriented culture, are equally prone to cosmetic surgery, indicating greatest body image dissatisfaction in these groups. Their motives may be the same, they may overlap, but they may also be widely different. While worldwide media trends alter virtually all local standards of beauty, not all cultural groups are equally susceptible to them.

Oyserman, Coon, and Kemmelmeier (2002) found that industrialized Western societies teach a predominantly *independent* self-construal, while traditional Eastern nations hold an *interdependent* self-construal. This makes Eastern cultures more receptive to the outside influences on the local standards of beauty, and therefore more likely to conform to the patterns normalized by the media (Madan et al., 2018). Cultures high in interdependence have a "desire to not fall behind the group" (Heine and Lehman 1999) and feel "compelled to conform to societal expectations and norms" (Torrelli 2006; as cited in Madan et al., 2018, pp. 13-14). *Interdependent cultures* are also said to be "tight" in that they demand adherence to social norms, while *independent cultures* are referred to as "loose," indicating their tolerance to non-conforming behaviors (Gelfand, Nishii, and Raver 2006; Gelfand et al., 2011).

Analyses conducted by Madan et al. (2018) reveal that members of interdependent cultures are: 1) "prone to conform to their perceived beauty ideals" which results in discrepancy between "their perceived actual and ideal state of beauty" (p. 24), 2) more likely to use appearance enhancing applications and methods, and 3) have "higher conforming tendencies" (Ibid.). This behavior may be attenuated if the interdependent culture is "loosened" (p. 29): the same effect upon an individual member of the tight culture may result when she physically moves into a looser culture (experienced by Eastern immigrants into a Western culture).

Interestingly, however, normative standards of beauty may also be "loosened" in otherwise tight interdependent societies, achieving the same result. It has been shown that pressures to conform to a strict normative definition of beauty leads to stress and anxiety (Fredrickson & Roberts 1997; Milkie 1999), as well as body-shaming and eating disorders (Halliwell and Dittmar 2004; Kim, Young, and Keun 2014). Therefore, it may be expected that individuals who move from an Eastern interdependent culture to a Western "loosely normative" culture but remain subject to the same interdependent normative standards (e.g., through self-imposed linguistic and cultural limitations) actually suffer more symptoms of the normative beauty pressures than either their interdependent peers who did not make the transition or their native-born "loose culture" compatriots who have grown up in a more individualistic milieu, accustomed to these norms.

It has been observed that particularly in the loose normative environments, beauty becomes a "criterion of competition among women" which leads to "antipathy, salience and envy, and manipulativeness and competition" with their peers (Cash & Fleming, 2004, p. 281). Cash and Fleming (Id.) found that women who were "more invested in their own appearance" were "less satisfied with their bodies" and held a "more traditional view of male-female relationship" (pp. 281-182).

Nevertheless, it should be underscored that aspirations to cultural standards of beauty cut across cultures and ethnic groups, and are not unique to loose, individualistic societies. Conclusion can therefore be made that the standards of beauty wield power over individuals far above the normative structures of any given culture or society. This power is underscored by the fact that body image, both female and male, is frequently sexualized and traded as a commodity.

Beauty, Culture, and the Media

Oxford English Dictionary defines *beauty* as "the quality of being pleasing to the senses or to the mind," or "an excellent example of its type," or a "pleasing feature" (OED, 2023). Very similar definitions can be found in other dictionaries, all implying that beauty is something felt and experienced. Such feelings and experiences are fundamentally esthetic and subject to taste. At the same time, there is a universal consensus, dating back to Plotinus, that it is the form and shape that elevate aesthetic perception. Form is a matter of proportionality and unity. A body which is misshapen, deformed, outside familiar bounds and proportions, or disunited in parts and as a whole, is not going to be seen and judged as beautiful.[128]

The classical concept of beauty as a general wonderment and delight began to dichotomize in the fifteenth century, with the advent of the Renaissance woman, her unashamed focus on self-beautification but also self-improvement in other spheres of social enterprise (Eco, 2004/2005). Sartwell's (2022) point of *antinomy of taste* (the emphasis on the taste as being both objective and subjective) is well taken; however, his argument that the subjective perspective had not been apparent until the eighteenth century is easy to disprove.[129] Consider this excerpt from Plotinus (204-270):

> In truth there is no beauty more authentic than the wisdom we find and love in some individual. We should

---

[128] For example, one of the main judging criteria in bodybuilding is proportionality: biceps, neck, and calves should all have the same or very similar measurements, while the waist should be about 1.25 times the circumference of the thigh.

[129] *Antinomy* is a contradiction between two percepts, or conclusions based on the same datasets, that are perfectly reasonable, yet in opposition to each other, thus creating a seeming paradox.

leave aside his face, which may be ugly, nor should we pay any heed to his appearance, but look for his *inner beauty*. But if that does not move you to call such a man beautiful, when you look inside yourself you will not perceive yourself as beautiful either. If you seek beauty in this way, then you seek it in vain, because you are looking for it in something ugly and impure. This discourse is not aimed at all people, but should you too see yourself as beautiful, remember it. (*Eneids: Suprasensible Beauty V, 8*, as cited in Eco, 2004/2005) [italics added]

Without broaching upon the philosophical to any great extent, the fact that the beautiful outside is a reflection of the beautiful inside, and that the subjective perspective is inextricably linked to the appreciation of one's inner self which, by extension, relates to wisdom, is as old as human thought. With that said, up until humanism, we find beauty depicted primarily in the female, divine and supernatural form (Madonna). With the Italian masters of the 15th and 16th centuries, a change occurred and beauty began to assume more profane features. Mona Lisa is a case in point. She is both divine and human. Titian made this contrast even more apparent in his *Sacred and Profane Love* (1514). Here, the two women appear to be the same – their faces are exactly the same, so is their hair, and stature. Cupid is playing with water in between them. The woman on the right is naked, apparently relaxed but is staring at the dressed figure with a mixture of envy, jealousy, and aloofness. The figure on the left is dressed in bridal clothes, unabashedly looking into the eye of the painter-observer.

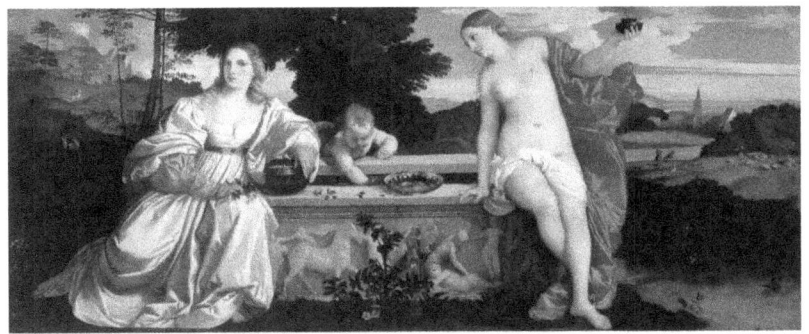

Tiziano Vecelli (Titian): *Sacred and Profane Love* (1514)
"Amor Sacro e Amor Profano"

Indubitably, Titian intended for the painting to display a contrast between the two figures. Yet, one might wonder which one is Sacred and which one Profane here? Would the painting have been entitled *Profane and Sacred* if the figure on the left was to be held as the symbol of the profane? Profane as what? Desecrated, or about to be desecrated, by marriage? On the other hand, is nudity not more profane than some beautiful attire which conforms to all social norms? Also consider Leonardo's study of Salai versus St. John the Baptist discussed in the chapter on *Disrobing the Body,* above. There is no doubt that Leonardo intended to provoke the viewer, but was not his reflection similar in that the figures are the same, and only one of them is clothed? Clearly, Salai is the profane figure, but if the model is the same, are the two not merely two sides (images or representations) of the same Beauty-coin (body)? A major difference would be that Titian's beauties are female while Leonardo's male. Plotinus also spoke of beauty in the male gender, as apparent from the quote above. Notably, all three paintings are dated 1514 – long before John Dryden created the figure of the *noble savage*:

271

But know, that I alone am King of me
I am as free as Nature first made man
'Ere the base Laws of Servitude began
When wild in woods the noble Savage ran.[130]

In Dryden, as in Rousseau and Darwin, the noble savage is a male figure, representing a free Spirit – the same spirit that Plotinus and Aristotle refer to as the Soul. There is no beauty without the soul and, arguably, every Soul partakes of the Beautiful. Could Salai be understood as the Noble Savage giving the finger to the civilized world – even as St. John, in the same human form, points to the Sacred Beauty in Heaven? Does this dichotomy not portray the eternal struggle of the human Soul encased in one material body – which is at the core of every dysmorphic feeling?

Eco (2005/2004) noted that our modern concept of beauty was born in the fifteenth century as a result of several "convergent factors" which included: the discovery of perspective in Italy, the spread of new painting techniques in Flanders, the influence of Neoplatonism on the liberal arts, and the climate of mysticism promoted by Savonarola. Beauty, Eco (Id.) claimed, was "conceived according to a dual orientation that today strikes us as contradictory, but that contemporaries found coherent" – a contradiction which consisted of the contemplation of the perfect (divine) form, and the natural forms portrayed "in accordance with scientifically established rules" (p. 176). Nonetheless, closer perusal of Leonardo and Titian reveals that this contradiction was only too familiar to the Ancient Masters.

What was new that came with the "noble savage" was not the glorification of naked beauty but, rather, the realization that the way human beings perceive and appreciate Beauty is, apart from their individual disposition

---

[130] From *The Conquest of Granada by the Spaniards,* 1672 (Miner, 1972).

and perceptive faculties, also inextricably tied to culture and tradition. Consider the historical painting entitled *The Death of General Wolfe* (1771) by Benjamin West (1738-1820).

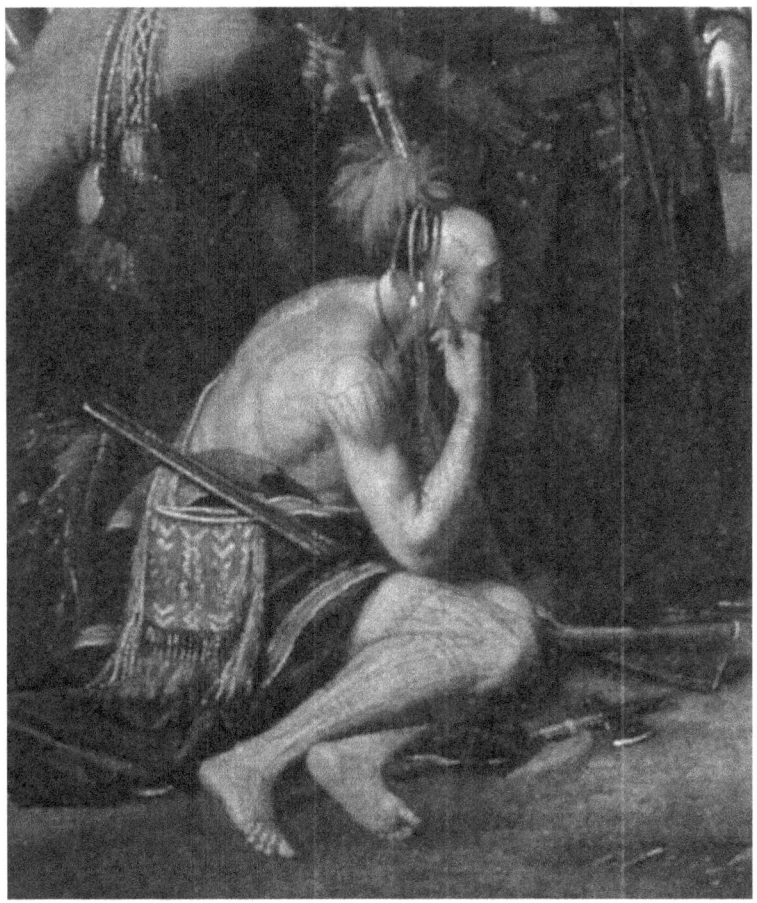

This painting, the detail of which is depicted above, features a native American warrior as a "noble savage" looking on the "civilized" British soldiers as they attend to their dying commander General James Wolfe after the Battle of Quebec in 1759. General Wolfe was idealized as Christ by West (see Michelangelo's *La Pietà*), which makes the contrast even more striking (Fryd, 1995). The Native American figure resembles Rodin's *Thinker* – natural intellect and thoughtfulness emanate from his posture. The detail does not make this quite clear but the native warrior's left hand is touching the dying general's boot, while his hatchet lies on the ground by his right hand. The Native American figure is thus connected with the dying general visually as well as viscerally, which may be interpreted as both enlightening the native to the Christian world (by ritual and allegory) and as the Native recording a crucial moment in history (Abrams, 1985; Pressly, 1985). The Noble Savage has poise, perfect proportions, and tattoos which are proudly on display.

If viewed in light of Titian, which would be the profane Beauty and the sacred Beauty here? West would probably say that it is General Wolfe, whose face is pale and wan, half-way with God. Wolfe resembles the old Madonna while the Savage is off-center left, closer to the observer, larger, and tan in complexion, the color of nature, the sun, and life. Nevertheless, Beauty lies in the eye of the Beholder – the subjective Supernatural and Pure may just as well be reflected in the Warrior who, symbolically, stands for the New Land, uncivilized, therefore unspoiled, and undiluted purity.

Key differences are often made between Western and Eastern traditions. It has been conventionally contended that while the Western world enjoys utility and market-oriented concept of beauty, Eastern traditions appreciate beauty in cultural context, regardless of utility (Sharman,1997). This notion may have been true once but, today, in a globalized economy and computerized world, it would be more appropriate to divide the concept of beauty regardless of cultural background, akin to the division made between the body and its image: there is a realistic, "normal" beauty, with all its natural flaws; and there is an ideal, universal beauty, which can be likened to the ideal body image.

Kant (1914/1790) noted that the *ideal beauty* "cannot be vague" but must be "fixed" and *a priori* there (§ 17), very much like the inner beauty of Plotinus' discourse. Kant blended Reason (the capacity to perceive the beautiful) and Purpose (the meaning of Beauty). At the same time, he stated: *"Beauty is the form of the purposiveness of an object, so far as this is perceived in it without any representation of a purpose"* (Ibid.) [italics original]. This, apparently self-contradictory statement is explained in note 39 to the text, in that the purpose may consist of aesthetic pleasure, such as when the observer has his eyes affixed to and all other senses apparently enthralled by a beautiful sunset.

Pause, to observe yourself observing the Noble Savage at what, after all, is a gory battle-scene. Surely, the beautiful lies not in his bald pate and tattooed torso, nor can it be found in the death of the General. Where then?

Kant distinguished between the beautiful and the sublime, in that the former has a pre-existing form which serves its purpose, but in the latter, the form is indifferent or appears to contradict its purpose. According to this definition, only the *sublime* is beautiful because it defies all purpose and invites the contemplation of the senses, beyond Reason.

The word "sublime" is etymologically derived from the Latin *sublimis*, meaning "elevated" or "lofty" – a compound of *sub* ("under," here: "up to") and *limen* ("threshold" or "boundary"). Morley (2021) noted that, in the Middle Ages *sublimis* was "modified into a verb," *sublimare* (to elevate), used by alchemists to describe "the purifying process by which substances turn into a gas on being subjected to heat, then cool and become a newly transformed solid" (par. 1).

In this context, beauty which elevates should be spoken of as "sublime" with reference to the image of the body. It was

275

Longinus' *Du Sublime* (1st cent. A.D./2006), translated by Nicolas Boileau (1674), which initiated this discussion for the observer-reader of the enlightened world. De Quincey (1838/1968) underscored that there exist marked gender differences in the perception of the beautiful in contraposition to the sublime, "the Sublime corresponding to the male, and the Beautiful, its anti-pole, corresponding to the female" (p. 300). The sublime has been understood as that which inspires a state of "delightful horror," whereas the beautiful has been perceived as "small, smooth and polished, light and delicate, clean and fair" (Ortlieb et al., 2016, p. 206), as something "inspiring us with sentiments of tenderness and affection" (Burke, 1757/1990, p. 39). These percepts have been propounded by Longinus, Burke, and Kant, who were all men, subject to their social milieu and custom. Yet, few have described Beauty with more penchant and accuracy than Dante Alighieri (1265-1321) in *La Vita Nuova, XXVI* (1292-1293) (as cited in Eco, 2004/2005, p. 174):

She pauses by, hearing their praises,
Clad in benign humility;
And, it seems, heaven has sent her
Down to earth to manifest a miracle.
Most pleasing is she to look upon for those who see her,
Through the eyes she sends a sweetness to the heart,
That must be felt to be believed:
And from her lips there seems to come
A sweet sprit full of love that
Says to the soul: sigh.

Beauty is "the sweetness of the heart" that "must be felt to be believed." It is the unity in which the Form (body) speaks to the Soul (image).

The concepts of the sublime and the beautiful cut across genders and cultures. Both women and men possess the capacity to appreciate the sublime, as well as the beautiful. Indeed, many researchers have found that women have scored consistently higher in negative affectivity, associated with anxiety, anger, depression, and shame (Costa et al., 2001; Feingold, 1994; Lynn and Martin, 1997). Contrary to what Longinus, Burke, and Kant postulated (but not contrary to Dante and Leonardo), this leads to the conclusion that women possess the capacity to entertain the sensitivity and understanding of emotions associated with the sublime better than men.

It should also be underscored that the difference lies in the degree of appreciation, rather than in its mode. Therefore, it has more to do with each individual perceiver's background and education, rather than gender or sex. Individuals who are steeped in culture and history, artists, thinkers, philosophers, etc. are wont to being open to the depths and breadths of artistic impressions necessary to digest the sublimity of Beauty (Bourdieu, 1979/1986). What is more, as has been shown by researchers (see below), even a preliminary exposure to a particular concept or form of art prior to testing skews the observers view. In psychology, this concept is known as *priming* (Condor-Fisher, 2021). Thus, an average observer may be primed to perceive the sublime to a greater extent than he or she would ordinarily be able to identify and feel it "unprimed," which is why certain pieces of artwork, including movies, benefit from being introduced by an educated guide.

Further, while the body itself can, under certain circumstances, be perceived as "sublime" (for example by neuroscientists or physicians), in everyday life, it is invariably the animate body and its image that an average human being observes, sees, and perceives, and evaluates in terms of beauty and sublimity. Vera Cruz (2013) pointed out multiple studies showing that beauty equates symmetry in perception, regardless of dimensions, and skin texture (Jefferson, 2004; Kun et al., 2011; Perret, May, &

Yoshikava, 1994; Rhodes, 2006; Rhodes et al., 2007). This means that cultural bias succumbs to the universality of mathematics and physics. Rhodes et al. (2001) further showed that composites of "beautiful faces" (idealized images) were deemed to be more beautiful than the faces that made this composite individually.[131] These two findings are valid across cultures. Therefore, while members of different cultures may value proportions differently, they will perceive symmetry as the main criterion of beauty.

What is more, all cultures consider Beautiful that which is healthy and good, although "healthy" is not always the same – Tahitian "healthy" differs from Parisian "healthy" which is different from Chinese "healthy." In Western world, the correlation between beautiful and healthy results in misleading assumptions of causation, exploited by many marketing companies, media, and the "big pharma."

An average American sees 3,000 commercials every day, and "spends a total of two years watching TV commercials in their lifetime" (Roeder, 2015, par. 3). Britton (2012) noted that these commercials disproportionately affect women, resulting in decreased self-confidence, low self-esteem, and dissatisfaction with one's body image. In several studies conducted over a period of fifteen years, Groesz et al. (2002) found that women had a significantly

---

[131] A fact which was well known to the ancient masters: "I want young people [...] to learn how to ... join the planes together, after which they should learn *each distinct form of every member.* The differences between members are many and quite distinct. You will see that some people have upturned or humped noses; others have flaring ape-like nostrils; others have pendulous lips; some other again are adorned with small, thin lips. And hence the painter should *examine each member carefully*, for faces always differ in some degree..." (from *On Painting: Invention and imitation* by Leon Battista Alberti, 1435, as cited in Umberto Eco's (2004/2005) *History of Beauty*) [emphasis added] Alberti continues to the limbs and poses, noting that "making things look natural" (rather than beautiful) is not the goal of a good artist/painter.

more negative image of their bodies after viewing images of thin women, compared to their assessment of one's body image after viewing images of average-sized or plus-sized models. Similarly, Grabe et al. (2008) noted an increase in body dissatisfaction after *priming* by media exposure, as well as an internalization of the advertised ideal, an internalized belief that the thin body-type represents beauty. Roeder (2015) showed a direct link between such media exposure and the feelings of guilt, shame, and eating disorders, resulting in obesity, isolation, and feelings of helplessness. Thus, paradoxically, the appeal by beauty, for beauty and health, turns against beauty and health.

In the *Feminine Mystique,* her groundbreaking feminist work, Betty Friedan (1963) pointed out that it has traditionally been the homemaker-woman who has been the focus and fodder for the marketing companies, being urged to buy things in order to satiate her restless yearning which, Friedan asserted, turns her into a nameless, vacuous *thing*, longing to be identified and filled. She is urged to buy her identity, her very self, claimed Friedan, subject to the allure of the ideal called the *feminine mystique*. This ideal (which, arguably, in itself corresponds to the sublime, not the beautiful) is presented to her through the camera lens of the *objectifying gaze* which she appropriates as her own, thus further losing her very self, her identity (Gervais, 2013). The camera-gaze is devoid of the mediating function of a human observer. She receives no body image feedback. Rather, the blueprint of an image (what it means to be pretty, beautiful, healthy) is tyrannically imposed upon her. She is pressured to conform.[132]

---

[132] Objectification theorists introduced two terms: the State Self-Objectification (SSO), which is the internalization of the objectifying gaze; and the Trait Self-Objectification (TSO) which is the frequency with which SSO is experienced (Waling et al., 2020). Objectification is environmental, not genetic. It also affects women more than men, and younger women more than older women.

It has been suggested above that the ideal of what is healthy and beautiful is not the same across cultures. Nevertheless, there is hardly a place on earth today without television and its enculturating influences. Obong (2019) bemoaned that this influx of media carries with it not only positive acculturating elements, but also a degree of foreign "bastardization" of the "host culture" (p. 10). Whether through the news, commercials, or the film industry, television disseminates and proselytizes the elements of culture of its origin. Such dissemination may be subtle and entertaining which, however, makes it so much the more disruptive and disastrous to impacted "outsider" cultures. Many authors have opined that cross-cultural influence of the media is not always wholesome and beneficial (Hasan, 2013; McQuail, 2007; Rodman, 2006). Roeder (2015) noted that even on "the island of Fiji, the arrival of television heralded a boom in dieting among women and girls who" prior to this foreign invasion, had not realized that "there was something wrong with them" (para 4).

Nevertheless, it may also be argued that this impact is much less detrimental in cultures foreign to the origin of the broadcast (compared to its "native" culture) because the positive acculturating elements prevail over the negative impact. For example, it may be surmised that people who live in the United States will be much less susceptible to the idealization of American life portrayed in an American soap opera than people living in a developing Country X but, at the same time, the Country X citizens will be less susceptible to the commercial objectification of the female body than native-born American women watching the same programs, simply because, in Country X, there is a greater difference between "real life" and T.V. To this effect, in his *Anthropology of Aesthetics,* Sharman (1997) analyzed the impact of "Western cultural dispositions" on "non-Western" cultures, showing a "critical conflict between form and function in a non-Western context" (p. 181). This, he

280

claimed, is shown by the fact that non-Western artists who manufacture their goods (carvings, paintings, etc.) for tourists do so, in order to please the tourists – without much regard to their own aesthetic judgment. Indeed, the commercialized aesthetic judgment is often contrary to their own tastes, but they create the artefacts for tourist sale anyway, because it is in demand and they need to make a living somehow. In their native environment, when creating for themselves and their own pleasure, there may be refined aesthetics of judgment at play but, Sharman (Id.) noted, it is not of primary importance – the emphasis is always on the preservation of their native feelings and culture, as opposed to foreign tastes, however "refined" those may be. Native art is considered superior by them simply because it is not foreign.

Such feelings would likely be derogatorily labelled nativist and rejected as ethnocentrism if they were presented in any Western culture, or exploited by western artists catering to non-Western tastes in a similarly pragmatic, utilitarian fashion. Needless to say, the term "cultural appropriation" has been created for the same reasons, perhaps spurred by the fear of annihilation of non-dominant cultures.

However well-intended may be, they are largely futile. (Fortunately so, because cultural appropriation of objects, motifs, styles, and artefacts across cultures is manifestly healthy for all cultures – those that receive, and those that proffer such possessions.) Television is only one of the sundry media influencing the perception of beauty and facilitating the dissemination of cultural values across the globe today. Given the ubiquity of I-phones and computers, television may no longer even be the most potent advertising and culturally proselytizing instrument. Social media play an increasingly troublesome role here, mainly because of its addictive propensity and ubiquity of *social comparison* (Mills et al., 2017, p. 147).

Social comparison simply means comparing oneself to other people. Social comparison may take place in front of the television set, vis-à-vis a latest dieting commercial, or when perusing a lifestyle-oriented magazine, and it is particularly prominent on social media where sensational photographs of muscular men and hyper-athletic women stimulate thirst for perfection and idealized beauty across borders and cultures.

Unfortunately, social comparison has also been found to have a negative impact on self-esteem and body image. Tiggemann and McGill (2004) found that women who engaged in social comparison with idealized photographs of thinner women experienced depression and body dissatisfaction significantly more than women who avoided such comparisons. Galioto and Crowther (2013) made a similar conclusion in cohorts of men who viewed idealized images of muscular men. Mills et al. (2017) discussed the role that cognitive processing may have in the "impact of idealized images on mood and body dissatisfaction" and concluded that not enough is known on the subject: why, for example, when women were told to imagine themselves as their counterparts in the idealized pictures, some of them felt better about themselves and their body image, and did so instinctively and naturally, while others reacted negatively, making themselves feel more miserable (pp. 147-148).

Cognitive processing appears to be key in assessing what impact objectification and social comparison have on the individual. Cognitive processing is classified by domains and complexity, with the executive functioning and reasoning taking primacy. The domains are located in different parts of the brain: frontal, temporal, parietal, hippocampus, and others. Since cognitive processing is dependent on culture and environment, it is more difficult for members of a foreign ethnicity (and culture) to imagine themselves as the images in the idealized photographs portraying the in-group native-culture characters. Native and foreign are relative terms. Sociologically speaking, the pro-ingroup views itself as superior to an anti-outgroup (ethnocentrism). Genetics, and race distinctions cannot be obviated, which may be the reason why some individuals, repeatedly placed in situations of social comparison, resort to cosmetic surgery as the only option, modifying their eyes, lips, and nose to fit the advertised profile, sometimes resorting to "skin bleaching" and other outlandish methods, in order to approach the desired ideal.[133] In the individualistic societies, the in-group members may be motivated more by the desire to distinguish themselves (individualized beauty), while in collectivist societies, the desire likely originates from the need to fit in. Cognitively, the need to belong is among the lower needs, therefore, the latter collectivist group member's cognitive processing is more likely to be bottom-up, rather than managerial-style, top-down operation. The concept of beauty may thus be subject to the same peer pressure, but be differently cognitively processed by the individual, with similar results. Consequently, the method of cognitive processing must be taken into account when treating individuals with BDD, ED, and other body image related issues.

---

[133] Fade creams (also called bleach creams) are used by black women to bleach their skin, for example in Ghana, Africa (Jackson & Eagle, 1988). They are said to "contain approximately 2% hydroquinone" which works through "inhibiting the production of melanin when placed on the skin" (Amankwa et al., 2016, p. 67).

Beauty Is But Skin Deep

For good or ill, beauty has been a byword in all languages of the world. The old English proverb about beauty has many parallels, some of which add an extra dimension to the concept of beauty: "Beauty is only skin-deep, ugliness goes to the bone." (Irish saying) "Woman's beauty, the forest echo, and rainbows, soon pass away." (German proverb) On the other hand, the French say: "Beauty has no age." Cultural bias can clearly be perceived from these adages. Nevertheless, the focus in all cultures tends to be on inner beauty, or something else than the "skin-deep" beauty – such as character, honesty, fidelity, devotion, and charm: "Ugliness with a good character is better than beauty" (Nigerian proverb). "Beauty is but dross if honesty be lost" (Dutch proverb). "A woman's polite devotion is her greatest beauty" (African proverb). "Charm is more than beauty" (Yiddish saying). The very concept of beauty is often dismissed as superficial: "Beauty and folly are often companions," say the Italian. "Beauty without virtue is like a rose without scent" (another Danish proverb). "Beauty passes, wisdom remains," is traded among the Kurds. "Beauty becomes a wife, virtue becomes a concubine," say the Chinese. Arabs are very prosaic: "Beauty is power." And so are the Russians: "Beauty is the sister of idleness and the mother of luxury," and: "One cannot make soup out of beauty" (Estonian saying). Nonetheless, the most profound adages about beauty extol it without any reservations: "Everything is beauty, but not everyone sees it" (Confucius). "Beauty is not in the face, beauty is a light in the heart" (Khalil Gibran). Finally: "Beauty is truth, truth beauty,– that is all/Ye know on earth, and all ye need to know" (John Keats).

The "visible beauty" is often the culprit, making Beauty into what it should not be. Thus, two Sicilian sayings place the emphasis elsewhere: "Love, beauty and money are three things that can't be hidden;" and: "April makes the flowers and the beauty, but May gets all the credit." Last but not least, beauty is pragmatically connected with representation of health: "Good health is the sister of beauty" (Maltese saying). Health and beauty are so tightly knit in the human mind that standards of beauty which appear unhealthy (extremely thin models, extremely muscular men and women) are not deemed attractive by the general public. However, this does not mean that they do not have the power to influence and subjugate susceptible individual's cognitive processing.

Culturally speaking, the human skin and appearance are what all languages and all cultures usually refer to and either extol ("Beauty is all the dowery she needs," Sicilians say) or attack ("Beauty's sister is vanity and its daughter lust," as the British saying goes). In this connection (to follow up on the chapter above), Pollock et al. (2020) investigated skin lightening in Africa, throughout Asia, the Middle East, and the Americas, and concluded that "both men and women are frequently targeted" with skin bleaching products, and that these products are reputed to make them more attractive and even "increase their career opportunities" (p. 6). In East Asia, there is a well-known proverb that a "white complexion is powerful enough to hide seven faults" (Li et al, 2008, p. 445). In India, there are significant cultural and sociological differences among castes based on "fairness" of complexion – higher castes (Brahmin) have light complexion, "associated with purity" and "elite status;" while the lowest fifth caste (Dalit, "untouchables") have a darker complexion and are subjected to "social persecution" (Pollock et al., 2020, p. 8). This has always been the case. Thus, rather than blaming the media and western ethnocentrism, the reasons for the preference of light as opposed to darker skin may lie elsewhere. Light complexion offers more room for modification: make-up stands out better on light skin, as do tattoos, and gold. Light skinned individuals have less subcutaneous perfusion, which has traditionally been associated with affluence and light work, as opposed to hard manual labor. Such percepts are valid across cultures and are not necessarily a product (or by-product) of mass and social media influence.

It is not primarily for reasons associated with body-image disorders that the Indian Association of Dermatologists, Venereologists and Leprologists (IADVL), the Pigment Disorders Society (PDS), and other organizations and governments around the world disseminate awareness about, and promote restrictions on, the sale of skin lightening products and ingredients. The desire for lighter pigmentation is ubiquitous regardless of cultural cross-pollination. The focus of some authors on the permeation of "the white culture," globalization, and social media, touting better social acceptance and economic opportunities, is not always justifiable (Singson, 2017, as cited in Pollock et al., Id., p. 8).

What is true, however, is the fact that every individual communicates not just in words, but also by his or her body image – which means, to a significant extent, the skin, and its coverings (clothes, tattoos, makeup, hair and hairstyle, jewelry, manicure, etc.). The skin is where the inner beauty of one's natural self, and the outer beauty of cultural normative self are reconciled, which is also why nakedness is private and socially unacceptable. This topic is further expounded upon in the following chapter.

The Skin and Social Discourse: Tattoo

Skin is the largest organ of the human body and also the most visible one. Four in five patients come to the dermatologist with a cosmetic condition which does not need to be addressed medically (Pohanka, 2001). However, everything on the skin is visible, and often palpable. Even a tiny skin imperfection may feel like a huge problem to an individual. Conditions that are hidden (of psychological nature) may likewise represent themselves on the skin, and vice versa. Costeris et al. (2021) conducted research on patients suffering from acne or eczema caused by psoriasis,[134] and found that all dermatological patients "showed lower self-esteem and lower perceived social support" compared to the control group (p. 14). Conversely, Gieler et al. (2020) posited that it was "experimentally proven" that emotions "get into the skin," and that the "visibility" of the skin as an organ of the human body "bestows dermatology a special position among the various other clinical subjects," thus elevating psychodermatology to an all-important "bio-psycho-social" science (p. 1280).

Whether willingly or otherwise, by accident or nature, the human skin has undeniably formed a medium of social communication for millennia. It has been a canvas for various forms of tattooing and piercing which may reflect social affiliation or its opposite (rebellion, subculture), as well as a punishment or penance (Jablonski, 2013). There is a mention of tattooing in the Old Testament: "You shall not

---

[134] Psoriasis is a chronic autoimmune and non-communicable inflammatory disease of skin and joints. The word *psoriasis* is derived from the Greek word *Psora* (meaning "itchy") and *Iasis* (Gk. For "condition"). One of the causal factors is stress. Its prevalence is 2% worldwide, and 4.6% in developed countries (Dutta et al., 2013). Psoriatic patients suffer from scaly, red, coin-sized skin lesions, most often occurring on the elbows, knees, scalp, hands, and feet. Symptoms include itching, irritation, stinging and pain (Parisi et al., 2013).

make any cuttings in your flesh on account of the dead or tattoo any marks upon you" (Leviticus 19:28). Gershon (2021) suggests that the reason stems from the fact that slaves in Egypt were tattooed as property belonging to the pharaoh, and that the Torah originally banned tattooing because it was "the symbol of servitude" (par. 6). However, also followers of certain deities and priests would willingly tattoo the name of their God or idol on their skin, professing their affiliation (Ibid.).

Since the skin dies away and renews itself all the time (Pohanka, Ibid.), and begins to decompose almost instantly at death and upon burial, it cannot be determined with certainty when people began to apply tattoos. However, remnants of tattoos have been found on mummies from 2,000 B.C. and research indicates tattooing had existed at least 1,000 years before these early findings (Schmidt, 2013; Zhitny et al., 2021).

The very word "tattoo" is of Polynesian origin. It first appears in journals of Captain Cook (1769) as both a noun and a verb, meaning "pigment design in skin" (Etymonline, 2023a, par. 2). It is derived from Polynesian *tatau* which means "a puncture, mark made on skin" (Ibid.). Century Dictionary (1902) refers to tattoos as symbolic markings "found on sailors and uncivilized people" signifying a "sentence of punishment" (Ibid.). Earlier names in English included Jerusalem cross (1690s) allegedly in reference to the "tattoos on the arms of pilgrims to the Holy Land," sometimes also referred to as Jerusalem letters (1760).

Another meaning of the word *tattoo* is that of a "signal calling soldiers or sailors to quarters at night" (Ibid., par. 1). This meaning comes from the 1680s, an earlier citation also notes the expression *tap-to* (1640s), from Dutch *taptoe*, from *tap* "faucet of a cask" and *toe* "to shut," the reference being to the shutting off of the taps of casks for the night. Figuratively, the expression means "say no more" and we also know it as the children's *ta-ta*.[135] As such, it means the final statement or *good-bye* before departure, a meaning which is close to the formerly mentioned *tatau*, associated with deity and death.

A tattoo on the skin has an undeniably definite quality, intended as such by the wearer. Linderova et al. (2019) found that 75% of students who were tattooed reported satisfaction with the tattooing. This inquiry went into the artwork, apparently, because 100% reported that they did not regret obtaining a tattoo. Their motivation was predominantly some "personally important event or memory" (p. 66). The same survey of university students noted a positive correlation "between wearing a tattoo and self-confidence" as well as a connection to personality traits, such as increased self-consciousness, extraversion, and tolerance to other tattooed people. Among the more negative traits, the researchers observed a "lack of sexual attachment" marked by need for attention, and an alleged claim of "uniqueness" claimed by the cohorts (p. 67).

Social representation through tattooing or other permanent marking of or on the skin (scarification, piercing) is a form of social discourse. It is simultaneously a "mark of collective identity," an "intimate expression of personal aesthetics," a "symbol of interpersonal relationships," and an expression of self-identity (Burton, 2001, p. 64). Tattoos thus represent a *"liminal dialogue* between private and public life" (Ibid.) [italics added]. The concept of *liminality* was developed by Turner (1974), who defined it anthropologically as a period of disorientation at the

---

[135] This connotation has not been sufficiently etymologically proven but it would appear to exist, based on the morphological analysis herein. It should be noted that the transferred sense of "drumbeat" is of later origins (first recorded from 1755), and the phrase "Devil's tattoo" (meaning an "idly drumming fingers in irritation or impatience" is further derived from this latter meaning of the word *tattoo* (dated 1803; Ibid.).

threshold (Lat. *limen*) of the rite of passage when the ritual subjects pass through a period and area of ambiguity, a sort of social limbo which has few (though sometimes these are most crucial) of the attributes of either the preceding or subsequent profane social statuses or cultural states (p. 57).

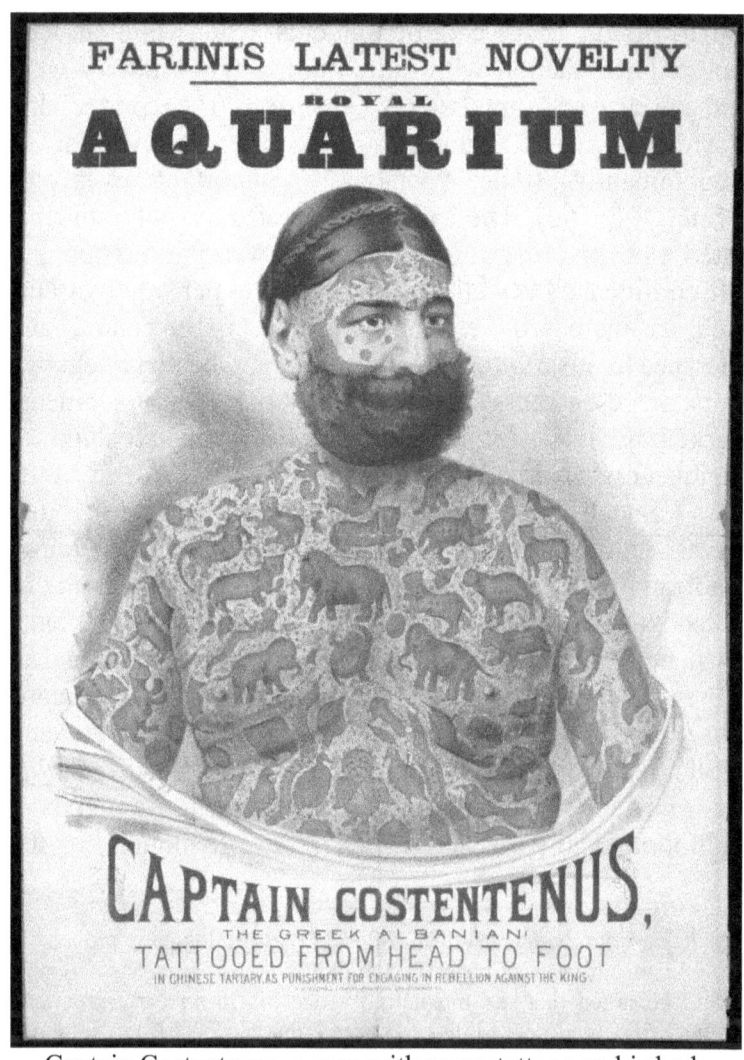

Captain Costentenus, a man with many tattoos on his body. Color lithograph. Public domain. *Welcome Collection.*

This usually happens during a transitional stage (betrothal, pregnancy, death of a loved one) but it may also mark an accomplishment or achievement which opens up new doors for the individual. Thus, although the sign in the form of the tattoo appears to be constant symbol, it is a symbol of development and transition, similar to a change in clothing, from one social status to another, or to a uniform which marks affiliation to a social "tribe." This transition is sometimes tied to a breakup or breakaway from the current social structure, accompanied by a radical modification of economic and social relationships, such as moving out of home, away from one's parents, divorce, adoption, acceptance by a subculture, imprisonment or, conversely, release from prison, etc. Since such events may be socially stigmatizing and traumatic, non-tattooed individuals are wont to view the tattooed ones as scarred by adverse events, therefore less sexually desirable and attractive, less intelligent, perhaps also less healthy, as well as "more rebellious" (Tabassum, 2013, p. 15).

All such markings and even characterizations point to a stage in self-development and self-identification. Individuation always takes place in relation to another group, mainstream culture, subculture, sometimes even counter-culture. Symbolically expressed "biographical stories" are thus placed into social discourse, which they enrich by their presence (Kosut, 2000). Interestingly, although the demand for tattoo removal is on the rise[136] (Ho and Goh, 2015), those who have had tattoos from the past

---

[136] Ho and Goh (2015) reported a constant increase in the demand for tattoo removal. The latest numbers show that the global tattoo removal market size was $4.34 billion in 2021, and it is estimated to reach $12.15 billion by 2030, representing a CAGR of 12.1% (Gitnux, 2023) [Compound Annual Growth Rate]. Motivation for tattoo removal usually stems from the need for employment (new job), or desired acceptance in new social circles.

rarely regret getting it, stating that it marks an important event or person from the past that they still respect and honor (Armstrong, 1991). A tattoo represents "an historical reference point" which also commemorates a certain emotion which is momentary and fleeting, outside the individual's control, but the tattooing of which places it under the control of the individual (Atkinson, 2004; as cited in Tabassum, 2013, p. 21). Therefore, apart from contributing to social discourse, tattoos have an irreplaceable function in regulating personal social equilibrium and mental well-being[137] (Atkinson, 2004; Bell, 1999; DeMello, 2004; Goulding et al., 2004; Kosut, 2000; Wohlrab et al., 2007a, 2007b, 2009).

---

[137] A participant in Atkinson's (2004) study stated that the tattoos were her armor: "I put on this armor and show how I won't lie down and be a victim" (p. 138)

Body Speaks: Body Language

The body image is projected onto the observer through different parts of the body, of which the skin is the most obvious one, albeit the most static and immovable, part, thereby often compared to a canvas. On the other hand, the eyes, lips, hands, and fingers, the face, the way one walks, and one's posture speak actively and fluidly, expressing a variety of body images and creating a discourse with others. Body-language has been developed into a pragmatic science of discourse which is often used particularly by actors, politicians, police interrogators, employment hiring experts, and specialists in many other fields, including movie industry directors, fiction writers and even public at large, in order to "read" the person, or to manipulate one's expression, so as to intentionally convey information about oneself.

The first written work dedicated to body language was published some four centuries ago. John Bulwer's (1644) *Chirologia: or the Natural Language of the Hand* focused on the hand as the organ of expression. Bulwer based his findings not only on personal observations but also on other texts, including "biblical verses, medical texts, histories, poems and orations" (Kuhnke, 2007, p. 12). It should also be noted that the human hand, and the elongated thumb in particular, is what distinguishes the human species from all other animals and what chiefly contributed to the development of the human brain (Fisher, 2017).

Novelists and actors have been proficient in describing body language ever since the novel developed as a genre, and acting as a profession. It was the study of body language and facial expressions in animals, initiated by Charles Darwin in his 1872 research entitled *The Expression of the Emotions in Man and Animals* that gave the impetus to the science of ethology, the study of animal behavior (Fisher, 2001). Darwin himself credited Sir Charles Bell's "discoveries in physiology, published in 1806 the first edition, and in 1844 the third edition of his *Anatomy and Philosophy of Expression*" for his scientific thrust into the till-then little researched subject of body-language (Darwin, 1872, p. 2).

In 1967, Desmond Morris published *The Naked Ape*, where he discussed the signs of aggression, fear, excitement, and other emotions in apes and their similarity to humans. Almost at the same time, Paul Ekman and W. V. Friesen set up what they termed the Facial Action Coding System (FACS) to "measure, describe, and interpret facial behaviors" (Kuhnke, 2007, p. 12). FACS is a "comprehensive, anatomically based system" for describing "all visually discernible facial movement" (Ekman, 2023).

FACS is intended to analyze and break down facial expressions into individual components of muscle movement, called Action Units (AU). Action Units fit into categories of expression which can also be termed facial body images. Ekman (2023) noted that the workshops organized under his auspices have been extensively used by "law enforcement agencies, film animators, and researches of human behavior" (Ibid.).

In the 1960s, Albert Mehrabian, with Morton Wiener, and with Susan R. Ferris, conducted several experiments which resulted in his formulating a "7-38-55%" rule (British Library, 2023). The first finding was that the visual clues (facial expressions) "gave a more accurate result than the audio clues by a ratio of 3:2" (Ibid. par. 3). When a group of cohorts was subdivided into three, and asked to 1) focus purely on the tone of the spoken word; 2) to ignore the tone and focus solely on the word; and 3) to use both the tone and the word to discern the emotion the speaker was trying to convey, it became apparent that the tone of the voice was a "stronger indicator of emotion than the actual meaning of the word itself" (Ibid.). Mehrabian concluded that the total

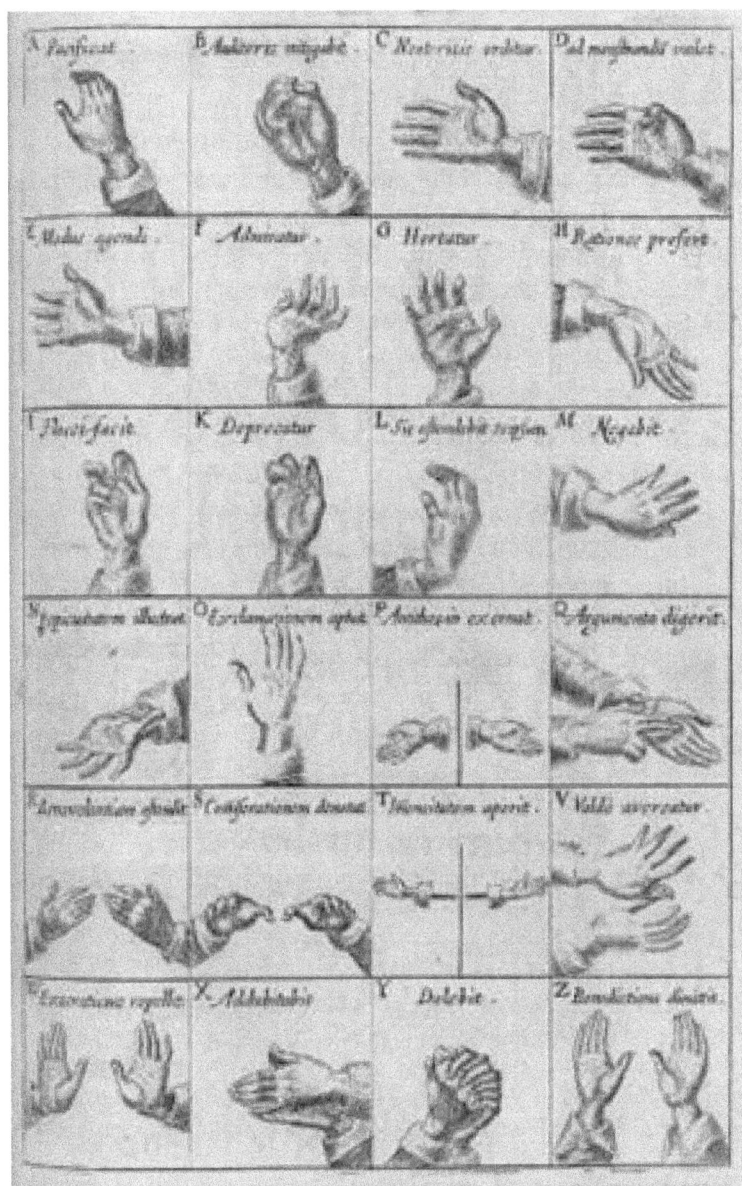

The Language of the Hand, illustrations from John Bulwer's
(1644) *Chirologia: or the Natural Language of the Hand*

perception was composed of 7% verbal liking + 38% vocal liking + 55% facial liking, which indicates that facial expression is more powerful than language itself.

To some, it may mean that body-language speaks louder and better than spoken or written language. Therefore, it could be argued that the presentation of body image is more powerful than any form of linguistic performance, whether descriptive or performative.[138] It should, however, be emphasized that this experiment was limited to single words and simple phrases.[139] Language has powers that go far beyond words used in Mehrabian's experiments. Consider the following passage from Henry James' (1881/2006) *The Portrait of a Lady*:

> He had a narrow, clean-shaven face, with features evenly distributed and an expression of placid acuteness. It was evidently a face in which the range of representation was not large, so that the air of contented shrewdness was all the more of a merit. It seemed to tell that he had been successful in life, yet it seemed to tell also that his success had not been exclusive and invidious, but had had much of the inoffensiveness of failure. He had certainly had a great experience of men, but there was an almost rustic simplicity in the faint

---

[138] Austin (1955/1962) introduced the term performativity into language. Performative language is language which does things, as opposed to language which states things. For example, "I agree" may indicate acceptance of an offer, thus creation of a binding contract. Austin spoke of felicity conditions which must be met for the language to perform a function. Butler (1990/1999) developed this concept in social context, arguing that gender is a social construct created by performative acts. Therefore, performativity should include body language.

[139] The first experiment contained words: "honey," "dear," and "thanks" (to convey liking), "maybe," "really," and "oh" (to convey neutrality), and "don't," "brute," and "terrible" (to convey dislike). The second experiment was based solely on the word "maybe" and different, acontextual tonalities thereof.

smile that played upon his lean, spacious cheek and lighted up his humorous eye as he at last slowly and carefully deposited his big tea-cup upon the table. (Chapter 1, par. 3)

When a skilled novelist is describing the facial expression of a character, the reader will feel and perceive emotions as if the reader was in the room with the character, watching the "clean shaven" expression of "evenly distributed features" filled with "placid acuteness." Whether this sentence should be read in a trembling voice, descriptively apprehensive one, or one filled with anger, or one without obvious emotions, coldly and calmly, does not matter as much as the words themselves and what they *do* to the reader. In fact, the voice would detract from (rather than add to) the image, if spoken by a reader abstracted from the message.

In real life, however, body image, and the message conveyed by it, carry an immediate performative meaning, which is supported by all kinds of circumstantial evidence – from involuntary muscular twitches in the face to the posture, stance, and look, all of which convey meanings. Kuhnke (2007) emphasized that, in order to express the message fully and truthfully, including the emotive and emotional undertones, spoken word should always be supported by non-verbal images, images conveyed by the body. In fact, it is impossible for any human being to do otherwise. The body necessarily becomes part of the message which is also why no people speak like novelists, not even the novelists themselves.

Gestures: Division and Acquisition

Body language can be divided into body parts but it is "reading" all the parts in conjunction that provides the reader with accurate message. Pease (1988) noted that gestures occur in clusters and the congruence (or incongruity) of these clusters provides the reader with cues as to the accuracy and validity of the message. Fingers have very clear meanings, such as "thumbs up" or "thumbs down," a raised index finger (the "accusatory finger"), or the middle finger. So do the hands, palms: turned upward, they are warm and welcoming, indicating sincerity and openness; enclosed into a fist or palms turned down, they suggest conflict or superciliousness. There are gestures that import courtship: a woman crosses her legs, dangling it, touching her thighs, a man straightens his tie. There are gestures of dominance: hands clasped behind one's back, looking up, puffing smoke up; but also of subservience and dejection: looking down, slumping one's shoulders. Nearly everyone is familiar with such gestures and it is not the goal of this book to dissect and analyze them one-by-one. It should be noted, however, that these gestures are of three types: 1) inborn gestures (such as the sucking reflex), 2) gestures learned by habit and imitation (e.g., the nod of the head to express agreement), and 3) reflexive gestures (in reaction to a stimulus, such as squinting or shrinking away from pain).[140]

With respect to inborn gestures, it was the Austrian ethologist Immanuel Eibl-Eibesfeldt (1989) who discovered that even children deaf and blind from birth will smile in the

---

[140] This division was established by Charles Darwin (1872), who gave credit to the following key authors and researchers: Sir Charles Bell (1844) for his discoveries in physiology (first published in 1806); J. Parsons' (1746) *Philosophical Transactions*; and J. Caspar Lavater's *Essays on Physiognomy* (Edited by Moreau, entitled *Conférences*, published in 1820). The volume is freely available as a PDF file online, transl. by Thomas Holcroft. London: William Tegg & Co.).

same fashion and under the same conditions as children born without impediments in these faculties, which led him to conclude that smiling is an inborn gesture (Gomez-Marin et al., 2014; cf. also Gomez-Marin et al., 2011). Ekman, Friesen, and Sorenson (1969) studied facial expressions in different cultures and found that the basic facial gestures showing emotions are similar across cultures. They called this phenomenon *pan cultural displays of emotion* (p. 86). These findings led them to the conclusion that *pan cultural gestures* are inborn, regardless of race and gender.

Regarding the second category, gestures learned by imitation, children acquire these gestures at a very early age by mirroring or imitation (Meltzov et al., 1999; Piaget, 1946). Loucks et al. (2016) conducted experiments in segmentation, memory, and imitation learning; they found that children organized learning segmentally and according to goal priority. As Rizzolatti and Craighero (2004) observed, such learning is advanced by the *mirror neuron* system: watching the parts of one's own body move in action has similar neural effects upon the observer as watching another person perform the action. Vice versa, this also means that perceiving the body of another individual as it performs acquired gestures or movements affects the observer similarly, evoking in them similar body image feelings, including the mood, disposition, and the perceptive ability to achieve and perform certain movements. Therefore, mere observation carries with it the potential to boost (or undermine) observer's body image.

From about the age of 3 to 4 up, such observations are analyzed cognitively, according to inferred goals and intentions, as well as social hierarchy, and segmentation. Zacks, Tversky, and Iyer (2001) speak of a *partonomic hierarchy* (cited in Loucks et al., Id., p. 1906). Since segmentation is "impacted by an observer's top-down expectations" (Ratcliff & Las-siter, 2007) and "his or her semantic knowledge" (Zacks, Speer, Vettel, & Jacoby,

2006), the level of cognitive development and the stability of self-image as a neural system govern and regulate the extent to which the observed conduct is memorized and acquired (Loucks et al., Ibid.). One might add: "if any," for where the conduct is deemed undesirable, the individual observer rejects it, and may consciously decide to avoid imitating it (Wykes & Gunter, 2005, p. 85).

The rejection of particular gestures or images is more subject to inductive learning than imitation. Inductive learning proceeds from elementary pieces of information to a conclusion. Inductive learning means learning by adduction of facts, which is by gathering and bringing forth of information. It is also a means and process through which "patterns and regularities in the stream of experience are identified" (Whitebread & Bingham, 2013, p. 5). It is through inductive learning that patterns are constructed and reasoning about them applied. Generalization of knowledge and image apprehension (e.g., "this is what a boy should act like," "this is what a girl should look like") take place as a form of environmental adaptation, commonly referred to as experience. Knowledge of words to name things is a matter of inductive learning. This means that the child's environment is analyzed inductively. Once this is done, objects may acquire symbolic representations, including the gestures learned by imitation, such as crossing one's arms as a sign of communication barrier, or giving a wolf-whistle to a pretty lady as a sign of admiration and an expression of sex appeal.

The third category of gestures, reflexive gestures, is composed of three subcategories: gestures reflexive in themselves (such as shirking away from danger), reflexive behaviors (behaviors reflecting states or judgments of value), and reflective learning patterns. While reflexive behaviors reflect upon the individual and collective subconscious, it is in the areas of the latter two reflective behaviors that anthropology found its "keystone" (Davies,

2007, pp. 254-272; Engelke, 2018, pp. 10-15). Schwandt (2001) defines reflexivity as "the process of critical self-reflection on one's biases, theoretical predispositions," and "preferences" (p. 224). It includes emotional and cognitive processes related to "social reality" (Davies, 2007, p. 224). Reflexivity is a process of body image mediation in social context, and reflexive behavior is of extreme social, cultural, and ethnographic-anthropological importance (Malinowski, 1922/2005).[141]

Reflexive behavior in body image context is a behavior that modifies and reflects upon one's body image. For example, standards of beauty for women in female-oriented (fashion, etc.) magazines, and the standards of power and strength in magazines whose readership is predominantly male, stimulate the social discourse on body image and trigger the analyses of the self in relation to the other, and of the current self in relation to the past and future selves. Much like the body images, this behavior is fluid and complicated by the fact that both beauty and power are subject to socially postulated norms and values (Foucault, 1980; Wolf, 2002).

Finally, it should be noted that gestures are perceived and understood along four levels (Yamatova et al., 2017):

- Cognitive level, consisting of thoughts and beliefs about the body;

---

[141] The word "reflexive" is more appropriate in this context than the word "reflective." The latter refers to one's "reflecting" upon the journey and learning, while the former emphasizes the implications and context of one's learning about the self through the world (which involves reflexive pronouns, and reflects the relationship to an outside object or person, in logic termed a *reflexive relationship*). In sociology, *reflexive thinking* is a well-established term, which refers to the questioning of established position, order, hierarchy, and the self in the world. Of course, such thinking involves reflection. As pointed out in the text, one may also *reflect* upon one's body image, behavior, and social context.

- Perceptual level, consisting of perception of the size and shape of the body, and individual body-parts;
- Affective level, describing feelings about the body image and its message; and
- Behavioral level, which is the response to the message, consisting of the attempts to modify it (e.g., by checking on, altering, or trying to conceal it).

Each of these levels has its 1) inborn, 2) habitual or learned (acquired), and 3) reflexive components, as indicated above. All of these levels take place simultaneously and may be conscious or subconscious, usually a combination thereof. For example, when two men meet to speak about business, they reflect their mutual agreement through body language: simultaneously (or in tandem) raising the cup of coffee, stepping up or down with the same leg, mirroring each other's stance, making similar hand gestures (e.g., placing hands on the leg or knee, one on top of the other). Some of these *reflexive mirroring* gestures may be made consciously, as signs of mutual respect, others are largely subconscious, and may follow the progress of negotiations. Women typically use more facial gestures and are better able to "read" them than men, a finding which shall be further elucidated in the following chapter (Pease, A., & Pease, B., 2004).

Male versus Female Brain

The human brain has been analyzed in various experiments and by various methods, using the following approaches (Sabbatini, 1997):

- Volumetric measurements of brain parts, wherein a region is selected and computer tomography employed to assess its volume and thickness.
- Functional imaging, via PET (Positron Emission Tomography), fMRI (functional Magnetic Resonance Imaging), or Brain Topographic Electroencephalography. These methods are used to research which areas of the brain are activated during the performance of various special, linguistic, motoric, and memorization tasks.
- Post-mortem examinations of brains, during which the brain is excised and sliced, in order to assess quantitative differences (e.g., the number and form of neurons, thickness and volumes of brain regions, etc.)

Although the brain size and its volume are governed by the size of the body irrespective of sex or gender, there are subtle differences between male and female brains which reflect on the formation and perception of body images. Reportedly, women have significantly larger parts of the brain dedicated to gesticulation and reading emotive expressions than men. Zaidi (2010) found that the two major areas related to speech, Broca's, in the dorsolateral prefrontal cortex, and Wernicke's, in the superior temporal cortex, are "significantly larger" in women: MRI studies showed that women's Broca's area was 23% larger, and Wernicke's 13% larger than the same areas in men (p. 40). Speech areas are closely tied to the reading and producing of gestures, especially in women because female brains employ both hemispheres in this area while male brains do so selectively – listening and the reading of gestures take place only in the left hemisphere in men (Shaywitz et al., 1995).

Zaidi (2010) also found that women have a "more acute sense of smell" and a larger deep limbic system, which enables them to be more "in touch with their feelings" and provides them with a better ability to "express their feelings" (p. 39). The corpus callosum (a large tract of neural fibers that allows the free flow of communication between both hemispheres of the brain) is larger in women, compared to men, which means that women use both hemispheres more fluently, creating "more synapses between the two sides of the brain" (Bishop and Wahlsten, 1997, as cited in *Ibid.*), thus giving women the apparent ability to perform several tasks at the same time.

Differences between the two genders exist in the hippocampus, amygdala, and neocortex – areas associated, respectively, with learning and memory, emotional perception, spatial reasoning, and language (Juraska, 1991; Lenroot & Giedd, 2009). Male and female hippocampi have different anatomical structures, and react differently to stress and emotions. Adjusted for total brain size, the hippocampus is larger in women than in men (Goldstein et al., 2001).

By contrast, Frederikse et al. (1999) found that the Inferior-Parietal Lobule (IPL) is significantly larger in men than in women but that this difference is limited to the left region. Notably, the left IPL size correlates positively with mathematical abilities, understanding of time and speed, ability of three-dimensional perception, and imagination. The right IPL (where male vs. female differences were not observed) is connected to the understanding of space and the "relationships between body parts" (Zaidi, 2010, p. 39).

Since the IPL processes information from the senses and spatial location of different body-parts, it is crucial to body image perception and formation. It would therefore appear that both men and women are equally susceptible to body image disturbances and the processing of relationships between the body image as one whole as it relates to different body-parts.

It has also been found that while the male cerebral cortex possesses more neurons, the female brain contains a more extensive network of neuropile (Rabinowitz et al., 2002). The *neuropil* or *neuropile* is defined as the space between neuronal and glial cell bodies[142] which is comprised of "dendrites, axons, synapses, glial cell processes, and microvasculature" (Spocter et al., 2012, p. 2918). Rabinowitz and Courten-Myers (1999) demonstrated that the male cerebral cortex showed a 15% higher average neuronal density than did the female cortex. This comports with other studies which found that, given similar average cortical thickness of the female and the male brain, the female cortex possesses "more neuropil, larger perikarya, and/or more astrocytes" (p. 48).[143] Physiologic measurements have also demonstrated higher brain perfusion and metabolic rates in female brains than in male brains (Anderson et al., 1994; Esposito et al., 1996; Gur et al., 1995).

Given this clearly sexually dimorphic cerebral cortical cytoarchitecture, it is reasonable to assume that the female brain perceives body image and individual body-parts with more acuity than the male brain. This may, in turn, result in proportionately unfavorable impact on body image perception by the female brain, as well as increased

---

[142] Neuroglial cells (referred to *glial cells* or *glia*) are different from nerve cells in that glia do not participate directly in synaptic interactions and electrical signaling but do function as supportive mechanisms for neurons. There are about three times as many glia as neurons in the brain. They are smaller than neurons, and lack axons and dendrites. The term *glia* is derived from the Greek word for glue (Purves et al., 2001).

[143] *Perikaryon* is the cell body of a neuron, containing the nucleus. *Astrocytes* are specialized glial cells that contiguously tile the entire central nervous system (CNS) and exert many essential complex functions in the healthy CNS.

sensitivity to body image manipulative mechanisms, such as social media, magazines, and mirroring among their peers.

The most consistently reported differences between male and female brains relate to spatial and linguistic abilities, and are seemingly unrelated to body image perception: men are said to "excel in mental rotation and spatial perception," while women "perform better in verbal memory tasks, in verbal fluency tasks, and in the speed of articulation" (Zaidi, 2010, p. 42). This finding comports to the fact that women are reported to be invariably better at *mirroring* and establishing rapport than men. While such conduct and perceptive behaviors can be learned and intentionally emulated, the fact that the female brain performs instinctively better in this area than the male brain is supported by the scientific evidence of better perfusion, more neuropile, larger perikarya, and more astrocytes in the female brain, as noted above.

Bao et al. (2005) have noted that sex differences exist in the propensity to depression, and the incidence of stress-related psychological disorders, which impact women more severely than men. Wang et al. (2007) used perfusion-based functional magnetic resonance imaging (fMRI) to measure cerebral blood flow (CBF) responses to mild to moderate stress in 32 healthy people (16 males and 16 females). Significant differences were found between the female and the male brains: stress in men was associated with CBF increase in the right prefrontal cortex (RPFC) and CBF reduction in the left orbitofrontal cortex (LOrF), a "robust response that persisted beyond the stress task period" – whereas the same stress in women "primarily activated the limbic system, including the ventral striatum, putamen, insula and cingulate cortex" (p. 227). Salivary cortisol was significantly increased in men, but not in women. Salivary cortisol levels indicate higher blood pressure and glucose metabolism due to psychosocial stress.

The Limbic System

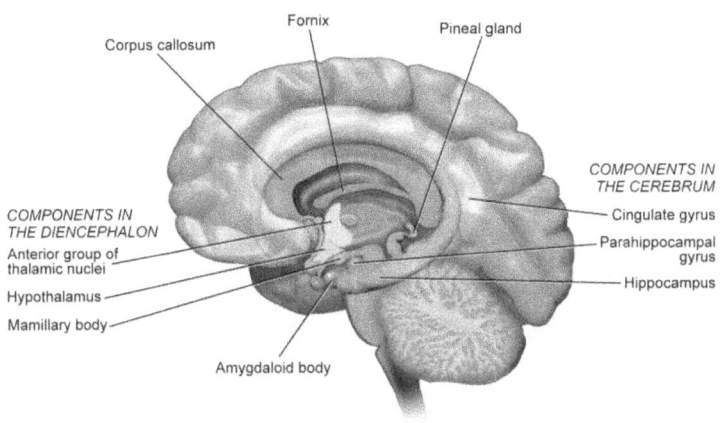

The Limbic System (Blaus, 2014).

A pattern of sex-specific prevalence rates in certain mental and physical disorders has been well documented[144] (Holden, 2005; Kajantie & Phillips, 2006; Kudielka & Kirschbaum, 2005; Lundberg, 2005). This pattern is in part caused by genetic differences (Kolbinger et al., 1991), and in part attributable to the effects of sex hormones (Otte et al., 2005). In general, it can be concluded that men respond to a stressor by the familiar "fight-or-flight" reaction, while women employ a "tend-and-befriend" tactic (Taylor et al., 2000). The former is outside-oriented, the latter is inner-

---

[144] Men are "generally more susceptible" to infectious and cardiovascular diseases, more likely to display aggressive behaviors, and more prone to abuse alcohol and drugs; while women display a higher incidence of "autoimmune diseases, chronic pain, depression, and anxiety disorders" (Wang et al., 2007, Abstract). Regarding cortisol effects, mentioned above, Otte et al. (2005) found an increased cortisol response (associated with Alzheimer's disease, depression, diabetes, metabolic syndrome, and hypertension) to be higher with age, and three times higher among older women than among men.

bound, oriented to the self and the closest circle of friends. It is therefore reasonable to assume that projection, self-projection, and introjection are defensive mechanisms that will be more frequently found in women than in men.[145] Theses defensive mechanisms are particularly important in the context of body image and various social stressors, such as dieting and fashion advertising.

Emerging evidence in social cognitive and affective neuroscience corroborates such findings and conclusions. It suggests that women react to social stimuli as stressors differently than men – in particular, women are affected where the stressor is interpersonal rejection or ostracism versus an achievement-related situation, which affects predominantly men (Cyranowsky et al., 2000; Stroud et al., 2002). The researchers considered solely neurological processes. Social background, education, and individual-specific conditions were not factored in.

McWilliams (2011/2020) noted that in both projection and introjection, there is a "permeated psychological boundary between the self and the world" (p. 111). While the original, Freudian definition of projection states that certain desires and feelings which cannot be accepted as one's own are (subconsciously) *projected* on an outside object-person as a form of ego's self-defense, projection can also be conscious and employed as a strategy to point away from one's own vulnerability and insecurity. This is common with bullies and frequently found in certain professions, regardless of gender (Condor-Fisher, 2021).

Nevertheless, whether conscious or not, while temporarily mitigating anxiety, projection is eventually very likely to result in dissociation, loss of self-control, and *ego*

---

[145] It should be noted that no scientific studies have been conducted in this area to-date, no doubt because individual circumstances and developmental conditions play a major role in ego formation (Klein, 1932/1960; Freud, 1920, 1921, 1923). Such circumstances and conditions are not very well scientifically testable and verifiable.

depletion (Baumeister, 2002). Baumeister et al. (1998) found that ego has limited resources and that it can be emotionally drained or depleted by lack of motivation, and tasks involving extreme self-control.

In body image terms, this means that any projection of the self, any disturbance of the psychological boundary between the self and the world, will have a transforming impact on one's body image, which is likely to be overwhelmingly negative, accompanied by a loss of self-control and ego depletion, resulting in various body image related problems and conditions. Zaidi (2010) noted that the "sections of the brain used to control aggression and anger responses are larger in women than in men" (p. 49). This means that women are likely to be affected by projection and introjection related disturbances of the world-self boundaries more deeply and extensively than men.

Arguably, projection could also be employed as a conscious *offensive* mechanism, akin to projective identification, during which the self maintains contact with the projected object-person, idealizes the self-projected object (such as a bodybuilder, movie star, or pop-artist, etc.) forming an unshakeable bond with them. In this case, the mechanism is *offensive* because it is intended to stimulate one's ego to growth and its force-field points out.[146] Even here, however, projection has been causally associated with narcissistic personality disorder, borderline personality disorder, and paranoid personality disorder (Etchegoyen, 1985). Gabbard (2004) pointed out that projective identification is necessarily a form of transference with all its underlying undesirable qualities, including self/ego fragmentation, thus also body image fragmentation. This fact has been widely confirmed (Feldman, 2004; Gabbard,

---

[146] Here, one should distinguish between the person; their behavior; their needs, beliefs, values, and abilities; and the environment. Lewin's (1951) Force Field Theory has its applications in this context, and the vector analogy may be helpful to visualize defensive vs. offensive projection.

309

1996; Joseph, 1989; Ogden, 1979; Spillius, 1992). What is more, Etchegoyen (1985) underscored the importance of "primitive mechanisms," such as envy, in projective-introjective identification (p. 3).

In conclusion, several distinguishing characteristics can be clearly identified: women use language and gestures more extensively than men in social contact and situations that call for manipulation of information, and in relationship-building. Functional MRI studies also showed that female brain is active in both hemispheres in visual, oral, and gesture manipulation, while the male brain only employs both hemispheres in complex situations (Gorbet & Sergio, 2007). Brain lateralization is task-dependent. While men performed better than women in mathematical and spatial tasks; women "showed a more homogenous pattern of memory," which means that women operated equally well with directional as with spatial cues (Piccardi et al., 2008, p. 127). There are no significant differences in brain structure but male brains have "nearly 6.5 times the amount of grey matter related to general intelligence" compared with women, whereas women have "nearly 10 times the amount of white matter related to intelligence" compared to men (Zaidi, 2010, p. 43). Consequently, women think more with their white matter while men with their gray matter. Neither this conclusion nor the size of the brain correlate to the IQ or to the ability to rationalize and resolve problems. True, at the age of 20, a man has about 176,000 km of myelinated axons in the brain, compared to a woman's 149,000 km, but in women's brains, the neurons are "packed in tightly," closer together (p. 37). As a result, some women even have "as many as 12 percent more neurons than men" (Ibid.).

Therefore, while human brains can be divided into two different types based on sexual dimorphism, with differences in volume, density, and certain operational aspects, all human brains are structurally the same.

Gender Dysphoria

Gender Dysphoria (GD) is a "marked incongruence between one's biological gender and experienced gender" (Yousafzai, 2022, p. 375). Since genderqueer, no-gender, and other-gender individuals are subsumed under this category (see below), GD should be further differentiated into Gender Dysphoria Proper (GDP), for individuals who have undergone sex reassignment surgery (SRS), and Gender Dysphoria General (GDG), for all other individuals with gender dysphoric conditions. All of these groups are sometimes referred to a "transgender and gender diverse" individuals, abbreviated as TGD (Silveri et al., 2021). Thus, "TG" is often distinguished from "GD," which includes other forms of gender dysphoria. GDP and GDG subclassification would be helpful for purposes of social understanding and research, and may also have justifiable clinical implications, as individuals in these subgroups do not always appreciate the "transgender" label.

Individuals with GD often face harassment, bullying, violent physical attacks, as well as discrimination at work (harassment, and termination because of their gender identity), and prejudice in the form of decreased job opportunities, healthcare access, and various other social activities. James et al. (2016) noted that the rate of attempted suicide among transgender individuals in the United States is 40%, which is almost ten times that of the general population. Clements-Noelle et al. (2006) noted that the victimization of transgender individuals was directly correlated to a history depression, substance abuse, forced sex, gender-based discrimination and victimization – factors which were all "independently associated with attempted suicide" (p. 54). James et al. (2016, p. 15) further reported the following data:

- Nearly one half (46%) of TGD respondents were verbally harassed in the past year because of being transgender.
- Nearly one in ten (9%) respondents were physically attacked in the past year because of being transgender.
- Nearly half (47%) of respondents were sexually assaulted at some point in their lifetime and one in ten (10%) were sexually assaulted in the past year.
- More than one half (54%) experienced some form of intimate partner violence, including acts involving coercive control and physical harm.
- Nearly one-quarter (24%) have experienced severe physical violence by an intimate partner.
- Nearly one-third (31%) experienced at least one type of mistreatment in the past year in a place of public accommodation.
- One in five (20%) respondents did not use at least one type of public accommodation in the past year because they feared they would be mistreated as a transgender person.

What is more, Grosse (2021) noted that transgender individuals "may also be stigmatized within the LGBTQIA+ community itself, which might lead to further social isolation." They face "frequent legal and ethical concerns," often from "professionals" (such as attorneys) who sense their insecurities and take advantage of them, as well as pushback (Ibid.). Systemic disadvantages against this community within the institutional and bureaucratic machinery have been well documented (Allen, 2020). For various reasons, the targeting of LGBT individuals "for bullying and violence" is present from their early childhood (Grosse, Ibid.), often because the bullies have the ability to sense their weaknesses and vulnerabilities (Condor-Fisher, 2021).

Transgender Etiology

In modern history, many psychiatrists and mental health professionals have sought to understand this problem and define it, often coming up with different descriptive terms which purported to label transsexuals as suffering from a serious mental or psychological derangement, such as: "conträre sexual empfinding" [sic] (1869, Westphal), a "paranoid sexual metamorphosis" (1894, Krafft-Ebing), a "psychological inversion" (1916, Marcuse), "auto-gyne-philia" (1989, Ray Blanchard), etc. In 1966, Harry Benjamin coined the term "transsexual," and in 1969, John Money described the alteration of sexual identity as "gender reassignment" (Capetillo-Ventura, 2017, p. 54).

In spite of much of the media spotlight and publicity, GD remains a rare condition. The latest available data indicate that there is approximately one million transgender (TGD) people in the United States, which 0.29% of the population (Meerwijk & Sevelius, 2017). This number was counted by comparing the birth gender with self-identified gender, including genderqueer and otherwise non-conforming individuals, thus it refers to GDG.[147] Taking into consideration only the individuals diagnosed with GDP, then, according to the American Society of Plastic Surgeons (2023), 16,353 individuals underwent sex reassignment surgery in 2020, which is 0.0047% of the U.S. population.

On the other hand, it is possible that the following groups also suffer from some form or degree of gender dysphoria: patients with anxiety, depression, bipolar affective disorder, conduct disorders, drug abuse, identity dissociative disorders, borderline personality disorders,

---

[147] The term "gender dysphoria syndrome" (proposed in 1973) includes transsexualism and other gender identity disorders. Gender dysphoria is used to describe the resulting dissatisfaction of the conflict between gender identity and assigned sex. As explained in the previous chapter, not all gender dysphoric individuals should be classified as transgender.

diverse sexual disorders, and intersexual conditions; transvestites, cross-dressers, male and female homosexuals; and people with bodies of androgynous nature (often due to various inborn endocrinological conditions). Although most of these categories will not be suitable candidates for SRS, the associated body image disturbances should be addressed accordingly and, where gender dysmorphia is found, the approach should be attentive to individual needs, and should consider all physical, psychological, and social implications in the treatment.

While only openly trans people, people undergoing transition, and gender nonconforming people identify as "transgender" for statistical purposes, Meerwijk and Sevelius (2017) argued that there are people of either social gender classification that identify under the standard two categories of sex/gender (i.e., as a man or a woman), who may, in fact, be transgender. The researchers noted that comparative numbers may also belie facts, especially internationally, because "differences in social acceptance affect the number of individuals who are willing to self-report a transgender identity" (p. e7). Nevertheless, given that a vast majority of these individuals are counted by the ASPS as those that have had the SRS, the GDP classification, in view of the rarity of this condition, is fully justified.

Etiologically, it has been speculated that the body image is imprinted in the brain as a map (see previous chapters of this book) and that the states of homosexuality, androgyny, or transsexualism are inborn, perhaps caused by the mother's hormonal dysbalance, stress, and other factors (which may be both genetic and environmental). Since these body-schemas or maps are irreversibly imprinted in the brain, all that modern science is able to do is to accommodate the body, not change the mind. Therefore, in cases of gender dysphoria or gender identity disorder (GID-GDP), and solely in these cases, provided that all other options have been fully explored and exhausted, the one long-term effective treatment is SRS.

With respect to cerebral differences, Allen and Gorski (1990) showed that the *darkly staining posteromedial component* of the bed nucleus of the *stria terminalis* (BNST-dspm) in the human brain is highly sexually dimorphic. The volume of the BNST-dspm was "2.47 times greater in males than in females" (p. 698). This region contains concentrates gonadal steroids, and is "anatomically connected to several other sexually dimorphic nuclei," which are also involved in sexual behavior. Kruijver et al. (2000) found that, regardless of sexual orientation (whether heterosexual or homosexual), men had "almost twice as many somatostatin neurons as women ($P < 0.006$)," while the number of neurons "in the BSTc of male-to-female transsexuals was similar to that of the females ($P = 0.83$)" (p. 2034). On the other hand, the neuron number of a female-to-male transsexual was "found to be in the male range" (Ibid.). The same conclusion was reached by Zhou et al. (1995). This number was not influenced by hormonal treatment or sex hormone level variations in adulthood. Therefore, researchers concluded, the brain of transsexuals is *neurologically reversed* and "the brain and genitals may go into opposite directions" which "point[s] to a neurobiological basis of gender identity disorder" (Kruijver et al., Ibid.). In other words, "size, innervation type and neuron number agree with gender, and not with genetic sex" (Capetillo-Ventura, 2017, p. 55).

Reasons for sexual differentiation are complex, and even though researchers contend that "the period where the human hypothalamus' structural sexual differentiation occurs is between 4 years of age and adulthood," such differentiation is "based on processes already programmed in the middle of pregnancy or during the neonatal period" (Ibid.). No studies exist on the influence of socialization and upbringing in this regard but, given that many transsexual individuals "come out" during post-puberty or even adulthood, having been brought up in their respective socially "proper" gender roles, it appears that no degree of socialization is able to "rewire" the neurological setup of the brain. In fact, Capetillo-Ventura et al. (Id.), concluded that:

Psychotherapy with the objective of "curing" transsexualism, in order to get the patient to accept oneself as a man or a woman, is useless with the currently available methods. The transsexual mind cannot be changed into a false gender orientation. Every attempt there that has been to do so has failed. The transsexual mind cannot adjust to the body, thus it is logical and justified doing the opposite and trying to adjust the body to the mind. Besides psychological orientation, this help has been given through two different therapeutic means: hormone medication and surgery (p. 57) [quotes original]

Gender Identity and Body Image

Gender identity is one of the core aspects of one's personality and social functioning, inextricably tied to the formation of one's body image. Deogracias et al. (2007) found that the "gender identity patients had significantly more gender dysphoria than both the heterosexual and non-heterosexual" individuals (p. 370). Body dysphoric feelings correlate with eating disorders which means that all individuals suffering from GD are at an increased risk for ED and associated comorbid conditions, such as depression, anxiety, substance abuse, risky sexual behaviors, and suicidal ideation. Studies concluded that LGBTQIA+ individuals suffer from eating disorders and disoriented eating behaviors at greater rates than their peers (Parker & Harriger, 2020). Advice and analyses regarding ED offered here (see below) should therefore be perused by these individuals and their trusted loved ones with a special interest and an eye keen on discerning individual-specific vulnerabilities.

Particular attention should be paid to the fact that ED in TGD individuals usually serves the purpose of fitting in with the gender of identification. Thus, MtF GD individuals diet in order to achieve a more stereotypical female (thin) body image, while FtM GD individuals use steroids and exercise in order to be accepted in their male gender role. The internalization of the stereotype is even greater with TGD individuals (compared to their "normal" peers) because they find it harder than "normal" population to fit in. Nagata et al. (2020) concluded that many transgender youths, regardless of their gender identity, diet and suffer from ED because restricted intake of calories suppresses their inborn secondary sex characteristics – girls cease to develop breasts and menstruation, boys remain thin and cease to develop musculature and a strong, masculine bone structure. Many researchers noted that TGD individuals

317

intentionally use food intake restrictions, dieting, purging, and laxatives, in conjunction with excessive exercise, and other ED behaviors precisely for this purpose (Diemer et al., 2015; Griffiths & Yager, 2019; Jones et al., 2015, 2018).

Clinical considerations must therefore include related comorbidities (Grosse, 2021). Once the individual is suffering from ED related to GD, no regular and common ED treatment will be effective, unless and until the underlying dysphoric feelings are adequately addressed. Nagata et al. (2020) emphasized that TGD individuals ought to be diagnosed in the same fashion and the same approach to ED be used as that with athletes and sexual minorities. However, in GD population, unlike in athletes, the body image is the ultimate goal, thus separating the diet from the body image is, arguably, impossible. Not surprisingly, therefore, cross-hormone therapies have been found to be effective in treatment of eating disorders in transgender individuals (Jones et al., 2018). Grosse (2021) also argues that such therapy "might lower the risk for developing eating disorder pathology" when used prior to puberty.

Current therapy for GD consists of a guided affirmation of identity and support in the transition process. However, Spivey and Edwards-Leeper (2019) underscore that, in spite of its popularity and prevalence, there is a "dearth of empirical data on gender-affirmative psychological interventions designed to reduce the forms of psychological distress experienced by many transgender youths" and that future empirical studies and "research on affirmative psychological care for transgender youth" are "urgently needed" and must "focus on clearly articulating which youth could benefit from psychological interventions and why those interventions might be effective" (p. 343).

Positive psychology interventions, increase in social connectedness, enhancing personal strengths and values, but also dealing with the TGD individuals' families and intersectional family therapies have been effective in minimizing comorbidities and maximizing the effects of transition therapies (Golden & Oransky, 2019).

Malpas et al. (2021) noted that common clinical strategies have moved from pathologizing transgender individuals to affirming interventions, especially with youth. The strategies currently used include: (1) providing various psychoeducation, (2) allowing space for families to express reactions to their child's gender, while emphasizing the protective power of family acceptance, (3) giving families opportunities for allyship and advocacy, and connecting them to transgender community resources, and (4) centering intersectional approaches and concerns (Ibid.). Future research should examine the efficacy of family-based interventions that incorporate these clinical strategies and collect quantitative data to systematically determine their effect on psychosocial outcomes.

Nevertheless, even after treatment and coming out, LGBTQIA+ individuals may remain confused about their past, their sexual orientation, and how they fit into society. This means that depression, GD, and ED associated comorbidities may remain a problem for them and the need for support will continue. Researchers currently focus on TGD individuals, but there is a significant number of genderqueer and nonconforming people who do not fit traditionally established social categories. These categories ought to be dealt with separately, not lumped together as one "TNB" (transgender and non-binary), as many researchers have been prone to do (Tebbe & Budge, 2022). Indeed, there is no "one fits all" treatment advisable in this area.

Muscle Dysmorphia

Muscle Dysmorphia (MD) is a body dysmorphic disorder characterized by pathological preoccupation with one's muscularity (H. G. Pope et al., 2000). The term *bigorexia* has also been introduced, although it is misleading because "being big" is not the goal of MD afflicted individuals (Cunningham et al., 2017). Rather, it is the desire to be lean, proportionate, and physically fit, although, taken to the extreme, the latter is often compromised and traded for size.

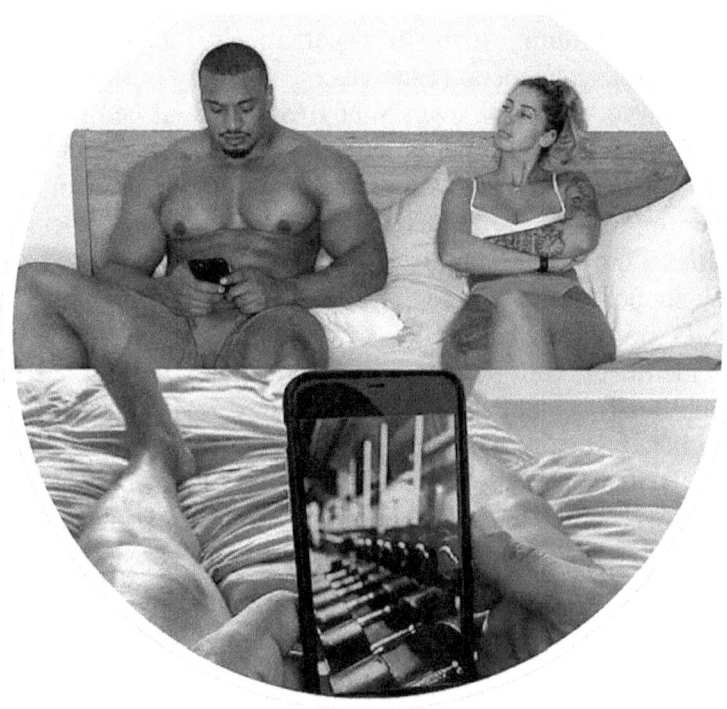

Diagnostic criteria for Muscle Dysmorphia
(H. G. Pope et al., 1997)

A. Preoccupation with the idea that one's body is not sufficiently lean and muscular. Characteristic associated behaviors include long hours of lifting weights and excessive attention to diet.

B. The preoccupation is manifested by at least two of the following four criteria:

    a. The individual frequently gives up important social, occupational, or recreational activities because of a compulsive need to maintain his or her workout and diet schedule.

    b. The individual avoids situations where his or her body is exposed to others or endures such situations only with marked distress or intense anxiety.

    c. The preoccupation about the inadequacy of body size or musculature causes clinically significant distress or impairment in social, occupational, or other important areas of functioning.

    d. The individual continues to work out, diet, or use ergogenic (performance-enhancing) substances despite knowledge of adverse physical or psychological consequences.

C. The primary focus of the preoccupation and behaviors is on being too small or inadequately muscular, as distinguished from fear of being fat as in anorexia nervosa, or a primary preoccupation only with other aspects of appearance as in other forms of body dysmorphic disorder.

Compte et al. (2015) found the prevalence of MD among young males to be as high as 7% of the population. There is a direct correlation to steroid use, body image dysmorphia, and related comorbidities, such as eating disorders (Davey & Bishop, 2006; Morgan, 2008; Olivardia, Pope, & Hudson, 2000). Although eating disorders among men, as opposed to women, have a different direction (i.e., toward muscularity and size, not thinness), eating disorders in both sexes are directly related to the individual's desire to conform to gender-related norms regarding masculinity and femininity (Griffiths, Murray, & Touyz, 2015). Cunningham et al. (2017) cited a study which concluded that 44.1% of "severe body image pathology" related to "muscularity or small body build" among male adolescents, compared to 4.3% among their female peers.

Since MD is a recent phenomenon, sometimes referred to as *reverse anorexia nervosa,* there are not many studies of clinical samples which would provide guidelines for effective treatment. This is further aggravated by the stigma associated with eating disorders among men (Griffiths, Mond, Murray, & Touyz, 2015; Griffiths, Murray, & Touyz, 2015). Steroid use is one detectable factor which can be used to determine the likelihood of MD in both men and women (Cunningham et al., 2017). Psychiatric comorbidities include a lifetime prevalence of mood disorders, anxiety, but also other non-muscle related BDD behaviors, such as preoccupation with one's hair, skin, and appearance-fixing behaviors which are usually associated with ED in women. Pope et al. (1997) argued that MD is directly related to these behaviors and is therefore a form of compensation for a perceived body image deficiency or insufficiency.

Bridges (2009) defined this phenomenon as striving for *gender capital* and "hegemonic idealization," a phenomenon which is contextually significant in "the distribution of cultural status" (p. 83). Bridges (Id.) also found that, despite disparate physical locations, all the bodybuilders surveyed by researchers "occupy one 'field' with a set of transferable capital, an aesthetic disposition, and tastes" (p. 84). Biographical accounts of bodybuilders are similar and, purportedly, the "use" of their bodies to gain social capital is likewise similar Crossley (2004, 2005). The transferability of gender capital means that men who belong to this community will find themselves in familiar circles in practically every gym and at every venue, thus fulfilling their needs for belongingness and self-actualization (Maslow, 1970).

As the illustration above indicates, this need is a desire that supplants other needs and desires, paradoxically including the sexual desire for a partner. The paradox rests in the fact that a significant part of the gender capital for men is their masculine status and desirability as males. By now, nearly everyone in this community or interested in these issues has heard Arnold Schwarzenegger in *Pumping Iron* speak about how "pumping iron" gave him the same pleasure as having sex, thus he was "cumming every day in the gym" (Butler et al., 1977). Arnold's rather surprised, amused visage in this conversation further imparted the unexpectedness in the realization that a whole new "social world" is formed through the individual body and body-reflexive practices, which may partially (or even completely) substitute the customary rites and rituals (Connell, 1995, p. 64).

Pumping Iron became an iconic milestone in the world of male hegemony. The expression of power and unapologetic maleness was a backlash against the rise of the Women's Movement (so-called *Second-Wave Feminism,* following Betty Friedan's 1963 publication of *The Feminine Mystique*). The rise of powerlifting and the use of steroids became widespread and popular during this time, even as "strong bodies were no longer necessary for economic advantage" (Kimmel, 2006).

While professional bodybuilding is a domain of but a few hardcore individuals (certainly few in comparison to other sports, such as swimming, soccer, or football), it is one of the individualistic performative sports founded on displaying one's body and, in particular, gender. The body image is molded and transformed to the best of its potential. This body image is but a fleeting snapshot of the self-in-time, which is a result of a long period of training, dieting, water manipulation, and camouflage in the form of color, oil, and makeup. What is more, the body is cast in a near-perfect pose, carefully practiced, and performed. It is this body image snapshot which is being awarded the prize. This perfect image dissipates as the bodybuilder moves into the off-season stage, putting on weight and eating "normally" again.

Even so, though, this perfect body image, this pose-in-time, remains on posters, in magazines and social media as a paragon of perfection which, in fact, is but a situational transformation representing, among other things, the gender capital of its wearer. As such, it functions as a form of cultural currency – the snapshot of the real self becomes an aesthetic icon, which has taken on both the postulates of social hierarchy and status (male muscular hegemony, coyly sublime female beauty), thus becoming a *model body image* for others to emulate.

While some yearn to re-produce the perfect image as beautiful and desirable, others reject it as unattainable or even unattractive and objectionable. Objections are raised on many grounds, from health to aesthetic function to philosophy, as the argument has been advanced that being preoccupied with food and body image 24 hours a day is the epitome of the *narcissistic disorder*.[148] Some of these

---

[148] Narcissistic personality disorder (NPD) requires more than focus on the self and self-improvement. People suffering from NPD must meet the following criteria: 1) an inflated view of the self, 2) a lack of warmth or empathy in relationships, and 3) the use of a "variety of strategies for

objections are unfounded, others less so. Nevertheless, muscle dysmorphia is rarely one of them. What is more, the projection of independence and the puissance associated with the male gender and its currency, awes and attracts (though not always sexually) females as well. Associated comorbidities (such as social isolation, drug abuse, depression, and eating disorders) are either ignored or proudly accepted as indelible part and parcel of this new identity.

From an ethnographic viewpoint, however, far from being self-serving or perfunctory, body-reflexive practices actually weave the fabric of society. While the gym forms a special world and environment, in which size and muscularity take the highest rung on the ladder, the gym sub-culture is projected onto the world outside, be it in the picture of naked Putin on his horse or Donald Trump proudly wielding his "big hands" in front of "Li'l Marco's" face, not to mention the by now legendary Arnold-Conan wielding his sword (the symbol of masculine power), in order to slay some fire-spewing mythical monster. Such powerful, often strong, and fearless muscular body images create status and transform context, advancing the innermost human need for self-actualization. Such is the survival of the fittest projected on the screen, indefinitely multiplied and reproduced, emulated to death.

---

maintaining the inflated self-views" (Campbell & Baumeister, 2006, p. 423).

Orthorexia Nervosa

Although mentioned elsewhere, *orthorexia nervosa* (ON) should be cited here in particular, as a comorbid condition of MD. The term *orthorexia* is of Greek origin, from *orthos* (accurate, straight, valid, correct) and *orexis* (hunger, appetite). ON is symptomatic of being obsessed with eating healthy food. It was first defined in 1997 by Steven Bratman, an "evangelical…impassionate…Hindu influenced" acolyte of "raw food" and sauerkraut (Bratman, 1997, par. 1-4). Orthorexia includes people who follow certain diets, fear, and shun unhealthy fatty foods, and behave in a ritualistic manner in food preparation (Brytek-Matera, 2012). Majority of researchers of ON are concerned with its pathological form, especially considering that ON is ranked as similar to anorexia nervosa, bulimia nervosa, avoidant-restrictive food intake disorder, as well as obsessive-compulsive disorder (Lasson et al., 2023).

It should be emphasized that eating healthy and enjoying it is not ON. It may turn into ON when food turns into an obsession, causes anxiety, and limits one's social life. Those who suffer from ON are devotedly concerned about what they are going to eat through the day, take excessive time and caution in preparation and planning of food, and feel guilty when they misstep or skip meals. While this may describe pretty much all competitive bodybuilders prior to a show, very few bodybuilders follow such diets throughout the year. What is more, with bodybuilders, food is a means to an end, not the end in itself.

Brytek-Matera (2012) noted that some people are "terrified of unhealthy food" because of their genetic predispositions, have a perfectionist personality, unrealistic expectations, or suffer from various social pressures (p. 57). However, these conditions can hardly be lumped together as one causal factor. Women are reported to be at a higher risk for ON than men (Ibid.), and the at-risk groups include the same individuals as those who are at risk from other eating disorders: adolescents, people with BDD, and athletes – but also physicians and medical students (Fidan et al., 2010), dieticians (Varga, & Máté, 2009), as well as performance artists (Athanasaki et al., 2023). Performance artists constitute a particularly vulnerable group, as their propensities in this regard overlap with various forms of body and gender dysmorphic disorders. Body image disturbances have been associated with ON and may be included in the standard assessments.

Individuals with MD were also found to often report a lifetime history of an eating disorder other than ON, including anorexia nervosa (AN), bulimia nervosa (BN), and binge-eating disorder (BED) (Olivardia et al., 2000). It has even been suggested that one disorder may lead to another, such as that during the treatment for AN, in successfully striving to gain weight, the individual transitions into a muscularity-oriented disorder, characterized by MD and ON (Murray, Griffiths, Mitchison, & Mond, 2017). Interestingly, but not surprisingly, the individuals with MD share eating disorder psychopathologies with AN individuals, although their physiques tend to be polar opposites of each other (Griffiths, Murray, et al., 2015; Mosley, 2009; Griffifths et al., 2016). For this reason, it has been suggested that MD is a subtype of BDD (Murray et al., 2010).

Androgenic Anabolic Steroid Use and Abuse

The use of androgenic anabolic steroids (AAS) and other performance enhancing drugs is common among individuals with MD (Griffiths, Murray, Mitchison, & Mond, 2016). Olivardia et al. (2000) found that nearly one half of the individuals in whom MD was detected also abused steroids, while in the control group (where no MD was detected), only 7% did.

Anabolic Steroids Commonly Used by Athletes	
Oral anabolic steroids	**Injectable anabolic steroids**
Oxymetholone	Nandrolone decanoate
Oxandrolone	Nandrolone phenpropionate
Methandrostenolone	Testosterone cypionate
Ethylestrenol	Testosterone enanthate
Stanozolol	Testosterone propionate
Fluoxymesterone	Methenolone enanthate
Norethandrolone	Boldenone undecyclenate
Methenolone acetate	Trenbolone acetate
Mesterolone	Trenbolone
Testosterone undecanoate	Stanozolol

The Drug Enforcement Administration (2020) reported the following synthetic derivatives of testosterone are among the most commonly encountered by law enforcement: Testosterone, Trenbolone, Oxymetholone, Nandrolone, Methandro-Stenolone, Stanozolol, Boldenone, and Oxandrolone. DEA (Ibid.) does not mention a number of steroids primarily favored by competitive bodybuilders, such as: Anavar (often used with Winstrol and Testosterone), Deca Durabolin, Dianabol, and a number of non-steroidal drugs, such as HGH, Clenbuterol, Proviron, and Arimidex, each with a specific function, taken for a particular reason to either increase the effect (strength, muscle size) or to combat adverse effects of the cycle, such as gynecomastia and bloating. Some of these drugs are also freely available from doctors who advertise them as an "anti-aging treatments" (e.g., HGH, Anadrol, Rapamycin, Metformin, etc.).

The table above was provided for reference by Maravelias et al. (2005) who also noted that *stacking* AAS, in order to increase their efficiency (an many athletes do) causes commensurate increases in their side effects. AAS do have justifiable medical uses and even among athletes, some uses can be justified, such as improving recovery from an injury. The key positive effects of steroids are as follows:

- Increase in nitrogen retention (Ibid.).
- Increase in protein synthesis in skeletal muscle cells.
- Increase in muscle mass and strength.
- Promoting anti-catabolism by blocking the gluco-corticosteroid effects of depressed protein synthesis during stressful training (Haupt & Rovere, 1984).
- Promoting the healing of injuries.
- Decreased recovery time.
- Increase in aggression (arguably a positive effect), as athletes "often experience a state of euphoria" (Maravelias et al., 2005, p. 169).

Common knowledge of AAS and their effects are such that, more than fifty years ago, Ariel and Saville (1972) were able to establish that a significant physiological effect of placebo existed among female college athletes who *thought* they were taking Dianabol. Placebo effect is also well known among those who deal in black market steroids and regularly dilute or even completely substitute the drug with oil and other ineffective (though sometimes extremely dangerous and harmful) substances (such as vegetable oil, baking soda, etc.).

Even pure AAS may have serious side effects, which the likes of Mike Matarazzo, Momo Benaziza, Andreas

Münzer, Nasser El Sonbaty, Rich Piana, Greg Kovacs, Dallas McCarver, George Peterson, Anthony D'Arezzo, and many others lived to regret. The most frequent deaths occur because of heart failure, cardiovascular insufficiency (cardiomyopathy), enlarged and diseased liver and kidneys (nephrosclerosis), thyroid carcinoma, internal (stomach) bleeding.

Steroids are used in treating autoimmune diseases because they suppress the natural immune system of the body which in turn means that those who take steroids are "not only more susceptible to infections" but more likely "to have severe or unusual infections" (Zoorob & Cender, 1998, p. 443). What is more, extended use of steroids suppresses the natural production of Cortisol. One of its functions[149] is the regulation of blood pressure. Adrenal suppression during steroid use may cause a subsequent drop in blood pressure (adding to the complications of an enlarged heart, as well as an extreme stress upon the heart due to the increase in the body mass). The heart is then unable to supply oxygenated blood to the body, causing cramps, shallow or labored breathing, and possibly resulting even in death. Other significant effects upon the hypothalamic-pituitary-adrenal (HPA) axis have been noted even with single application of AAS, not to mention repeated, chronic use of steroids of varied kinds, such as the now popular "low T replacement therapy" (Younes & Younes, 2017, p. 270).

---

[149] Other functions of Cortisol include: the regulation of stress response (fight or flight reaction), control of metabolism, suppression of inflammation, regulation of blood sugar, control of the sleep-wake cycle.

Neurological Effects

Special attention should be paid to the neurological effects of AAS. Individuals who suffer from MD are also more likely to suffer from depression, and from ED associated comorbidities. The likelihood of these negative effects increases with the use of AAS. Hildebrandt et al. (2014) found that steroids increase beta-endorphin levels, decrease cortisol levels, and increase ACTH levels[150] – leading to positive associations with exercise as well as dependency and abuse. Tests on rodents showed that the dependency may be so strong that the individuals will continue to self-administer the drug "even to the point of death" (p. 88).

Piacentino et al. (2015) warned against AAS abuse and dependence because they are frequently linked to psychiatric symptoms, such as mood swings and schizophrenia-related disorders. However, it is not clear whether AAS abuse causes such disorders by "determining neuroadaptive changes in the reward neural circuit" or whether the AAS users have had "premorbid abnormal personalities" or a "history of psychiatric disorders" which attracted them to the AAS abuse in the first place (p. 101). For example, Pope et al. (2005) found that 86% of men with MD had an additional history of non-muscle-related BDD. Concerns with appearance (hair, skin) lead to appearance-fixing behaviors which are mitigated by exercise and the use of AAS. BDD need not be related to MD, but the two may overlap, in which case the diagnosis would focus on dieting and frequency of exercise (Ibid.). The same study also reported a higher number of suicide attempts, poorer quality of life, and non-AAS related substance abuse among the sub-group of individuals who suffer from BDD and MD.

---

[150] Adrenocorticotropic hormone, produced by the pituitary gland, often in response to stress. It increases the production of cortisol and is related to the circadian rhythm.

Many readers are familiar with the term *roid rage*. A very simplistic way to explain roid rage is that anabolic steroids stimulate the production of dopamine, which increases aggression and contributes to the executive function in the medial prefrontal cortex. However, unlike what is commonly assumed, Wood et al. (2013) found that the aggressive impulse is not altered by testosterone. Thus, long-term exposure to AAS does not increase motivation for aggression and does not enhance impulsive behavior (Ibid.).

Therefore, contrary to the established byword, long-term use of AAS causes destabilizing effects, primarily through depression, particularly marked during withdrawal ("off-cycle" in athletes). AAS are also linked to psychotic behavior, anxiety, and suicidal ideation, likely associated with the changes in hormonal and neurotransmitter levels (serotonin, GABA). In the long term, AAS also decrease motivation (Cafri et al., 2008; Griffiths, Murray, et al., 2016; Palamar, Kiang, & Halkitis, 2011).

Conclusion

In conclusion, MD can be an extremely debilitating disorder because it may cause serious impairments in various psychosocial domains. Individuals with MD are highly avoidant, "particularly in contexts where their bodies are believed to be scrutinized" (Cunningham et al., 2017, p. 260). They tend to be withdrawn, housebound, absent from various social functions and roles, and – specifically men suffering from MD – find it "difficult to maintain interpersonal relationships" (Ibid.). Pope et al., 2005 found that 50% of men with MD have attempted suicide at least once (C. Pope et al., 2005). The lethality of these attempts is in direct proportion to the number of comorbidities associated with MD (Lecrubier, 2001). Preexisting DSM III R diagnoses are a strong predictor of lethality.

Unfortunately, many MD conditions go unnoticed or are interpreted as healthy. Steroid discontinuation is critical to both physical and mental health, and should be the first step in MD treatment. Related BDD and eating disorders should also be addressed, especially as they are expected to exacerbate with the cessation of steroid use, simply because the artificial supply of exogenous hormones suppresses their endogenous production.

Finally, everyone who is suffering from MD would be well advised to limit their social media exposure to muscle-oriented communities, wherein the urge to rigid diets and exercise practices is fostered, triggering the feelings of guilt, insufficiency, and inferiority which feed in to the cycles of ED and depression. These media sites present objectified muscular bodies and propagate eating disorders while often appealing to the basic needs for belongingness, appreciation, and love.

Changing the Body Image

Status Quo

Mainly under the influence of mass and social media, Beauty and the focus on self-improvement have become the burning issues of every modern individual. Globalism and computerization have made this a world-wide phenomenon, turning Beauty into a business. However, Beauty is not a fungible experience – it is a form of experience which is unique, and uniquely personal. As such, it is fluid, consisting of many impressions, and fluidly absorbed. It moves with the individual as he or she proceeds on their daily journey, projecting, and perceiving body images within and around them.

The perception of body image is invariably an aesthetic experience. This fact has several implications: first, what is and is not "aesthetic" is a matter of individual judgment; second, this judgment is primarily subjective; third, if the observer surrenders this judgment to the objective domain, he thereby surrenders an important part of selfhood. Therefore, if there is no absolute, universal, and objective aesthetic judgment, then Beauty is subjectively determined, and includes predispositions which are both cultural and environmental, unique to each individual. Aesthetic judgment is then a matter of degree. No such judgment can be deemed "wrong" or "right."

Therefore, there is also no absolutely beautiful body image, and the body images experienced by everyone in their everyday lives are relative to environment, and functionally related to the self-identity of each individual: when one dresses up for a rendezvous, when one goes to the gym, has a formal dinner, retires for the day to the privacy of his or her bedroom... one assumes different personas, dresses differently, and perceives a gamut of diverse, often seemingly disparate, emotions and feelings about the self vis-à-vis the other – sometimes filled with apprehension, sometimes with excitement, sometimes relaxed, sometimes indifferent. What is key to happiness in each such body-instance is being true to one's self on the given occasion. This requires that the individual be constantly engaged in the microsphere of their habitat, able to communicate and understand human desires and needs – in other words, empathy is the primary prerequisite of aesthetic judgment and a necessary component of a healthy mind in a healthy body. Only then can a healthy body image take form.

Body image mediation (its inter-personal transfer and understanding) is ever so much more difficult because of the pervasiveness of internet and social media that often substitute personal contact, providing few clues and opportunities to read one another's gestures, to "see" the "real *Me Myself*" behind the image which is but a snapshot-in-time of the ever-changing *I*. The need for social media presence requires that the individual create a stable image, a stamp-in-time of a perfect self, in full bloom, beauty, achievement, and success, asking to be merited in the imaginary computer-screen or I-phone screen mirror. Alas, that stamp-in-time image becomes no more than an artificial face, an avatar, not unlike the perfect death mask uniting the image and the body. It may be gratifying, and may even motivate the alien observer sitting miles and miles away browsing his account – but it invariably distorts reality, and therefore fails to bring true gratification in the long run.

As has been indicated above, different cultures hold diverse aesthetic judgments and diverge in traditional concepts of Beauty. Some (non-Western) societies regard plumpness as a sign of higher status, good health, beauty, and fertility (Jung & Lee, 2006). Asian women are predominantly concerned with their faces, undergoing eyelid and nose surgeries, in order to approach the Western ideal of beauty (Kawamura, 2004, p. 245). Hispanic women (both in the U.S. and in Latin American countries) have a higher body weight dissatisfaction than Black American women, and even White European women (Altabe & O'Garo, 2004, p. 251). Local cultures and traditions often collide with global media influences and the "mammoth power" of the diet, fashion, beauty, and cosmetic industries that profit from the "enormity of the body insecurity" that they "allege to ameliorate" even as they are reinforcing and amplifying it (Orbach, 1993, p. 52).

Surveys indicate that body image dissatisfaction with "overall appearance" is not only universal among various human races and cultures, but also almost equally common among men as it is among women. Surveys from three different years conducted by the popular psychology magazine *Psychology Today* concluded that 56 percent of women and 43 percent of men were dissatisfied with their "overall appearance" (Wykes & Gunter, 2005, p. 156). Equal dissatisfaction was perceived with the mid-section and weight. However, body image dissatisfaction has been found to cause depression only in women, not in men (Davis & Katzman, 1997). Further surveys also indicated that more than 4 in 10 women were actively pursuing some diet in order to lose weight (Wykes & Gunter, Ibid.), a finding not paralleled among men. Body image dissatisfaction and associated eating disorders have been found in countries as dissimilar as Norway (Wichstrøm, 1995), China (Davis & Katzman, 1997), Italy (Santonastaso et al., 1995), and Argentina (Martinez & Spinetti, 1997).

It would therefore appear reasonable to conclude that body image dissatisfaction is a universal phenomenon, part and parcel of the human condition – and so is the desire to change it, either by altering the body, or by changing the image. Some readers may conclude that, far from finding it wrong and unhealthy, concern with how one looks a sign of cultural and social adaptation, as well as a healthy sign of the desire for self-improvement.

One may also hypothesize that there are the "image people," who insist on making a good image of themselves by all kinds of natural and artificial means (such as make-up, costume, presentation); and the "body people" who are focused on altering their bodies (by the means of exercise and dieting, but also via tattooing and piercing the skin, medication, as well as surgery). Of course, these two groups may intersect and even be a subset of each other but, philosophically speaking, there are people who believe in the givenness[151] of the material part of the I, and people who believe in its changeability and malleableness. Neither exists to the exclusion of the other. Neither is right or wrong. It is a matter of personal approach.

---

[151] In its facticity, thrownness, and finitude.

Assessment, Research, and Evaluation Tools

In order to address body image issues of various kinds, that preoccupy and often undermine individual self-development, all causal and related factors must be explored. First, some form of assessment is necessary, in order to ascertain these factors. For this purpose, various body image-measuring tests have been developed that assess body image disturbances (BID), and examine how they affect cognitive and behavioral functioning. Figural scales and questionnaires are among the most common assessment techniques. There are also projective techniques, such as the Human Figure Drawings (HFDs), Thematic Apperception Test (TAT), and various association techniques, such as Rorschach, intended to determine the strength and stability of the body barrier, and feelings about the prominence of body-parts (the Barrier Score, the Body Prominence Score), from which various body image criteria can be derived.

All of these tests can summarily be divided into those that focus on Affective Components (how the body image and its aspects affect the individual), and Behavioral Components (how the individual behaves as a result of such affects). Thompson and Van Den Berg (2004) also included Cognitive Measures, which focus on "the degree of dysfunctional cognitive schema regarding one's appearance" (p. 150).

Nevertheless, Cognitive and Affective components can hardly be separated because one's thoughts and feelings about oneself cannot be separated. Some feelings may be pure affects (such as feeling someone's touch), others may be cognitive (such as feeling "under the weather") but to what degree, if at all, are such feelings exclusively affective versus cognitive is debatable. Moreover, behavior follows the aspect – one will dress up or dress down not only in accordance with custom and social occasion but also, perhaps above all, depending on how one feels on a given

338

occasion. Such feelings are often temporary, and may have nothing to do with any body image dissonance. To generalize them might then lead the assessing professional to a body dysphoria diagnosis where there is none – which is why there are precise protocols psychiatrists and psychologists have to follow in the diagnosis and treatment of BDD, and related comorbidities.

Diagnosis and treatment of BDD often consists primarily of observation, assessment testing, and cognitive-behavioral therapy (CBT), sometimes in synergy with selective serotonin reuptake inhibitors (SSRIs). SSRIs inhibit the reabsorption of serotonin in the brain, thus lowering anxiety and making the body use its own serotonin more efficiently. Randomized controlled trials (RCTs) revealed that BDD is frequently diagnosed "10 years after first presentation" and, even then, is often treated "inappropriately" with antipsychotic medication, addressing serotonin reuptake, not BDD (Veale, 2001, p. 125). Therefore, mere lengthy observation and continual assessments do not cure BDD and, arguably, do not even contribute to the treatment of BDD.

Figural Drawings

Figural drawings consist of a set of schematic figures which represent the frontal view of either male (for men) or female (for women) figures. The participants then select one figure for their "perceived current size" and one for their "ideal size" (Gardner et al., 2009, p. 114). The difference between the perceived and the ideal size is said to represent body size dissatisfaction.

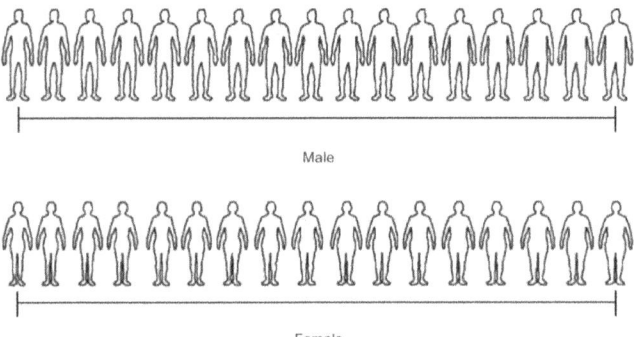

The latest 17-figural drawing scale (Gardner et al., 2009).

The drawings increase in size by five percents from 40 to 160% of average BMI. While guiding as to obesity and future health complications, there are several problems with this measurement.

First, the BMI does not take into account factors such as bone density or muscle mass. It also accommodates neither race nor age of the tested individual. In fact, the BMI had been developed in the 1830 by a Belgian mathematician and sociologist with a special fondness for statistics, Adolphe Quetelet (1796–1874). Quetelet collected data on men's heights and weights, and concluded that there is a definite relationship between the individual's weight and their height. The so-called Quetelet's Formula (today known as the BMI) is calculated "by dividing an individual's weight in kilograms by their height in meters squared" (Humphreys, 2010, p. 696). However, Quetelet made his findings in Belgium of his day, measuring these values only in Belgian men. Thus, the BMI analysis can be misleading for an average American today, not to mention for members of various non-white races and cultures.

Second, the anthropomorphic Body Image Assessment Scale–Body Dimensions (BIAS-BD) does not take into consideration person-specific characteristics and dimensions: some women will never have wide hips and greatly feminine curves, just as some men will never be skinny or build V-tapered latissimus triangle with broad shoulders – yet, they may be perfectly happy with how they are built. While the figure drawings printed here minimize such distortions, other scales can be found in clinical practice that do not do so. What is more, in figural drawings, the length of the limbs and the proportions between the head and the torso are almost always universalized, which may lead to distortions in self-image perception and even exacerbate the existing BDD already present (though as yet undiagnosed) in the tested individuals.

Criticism may also be raised that no figural scales portray distortions specific to sports. Athletes may be shaped in a way specific to their discipline or event, and such a shape does not say anything about their body image self-perception, or self-esteem. Indeed, it would be altogether amiss to use these generic figure drawings with athletic population (about as much amiss as using generic ED surveys with these groups). If such scales are to be used, they ought to be sport-specific, and modified accordingly.

Gardner (1996) found that when the figure scales are drawn and presented in a descending, as opposed to an ascending fashion, the same individuals produced different results. If the first figure is the smallest and thinnest one, then the tested person is more likely to select a thinner ideal version of one's body image. This has been confirmed using the video size-estimation methodology: If the initial image presented to the individual is a much thinner version of their actual self, the individual will tend to adjust the ideal self to portray a thinner version of one's true self, and vice versa (Ibid.). Not surprisingly, Nicholls et al., (2006) found that "overall satisfaction was higher for the original descending scale than for the ascending scale" (p. 1027).

Two significant findings have been made using the figural drawings: First, the smaller the actual body size of the person is, the greater their over-estimation of their actual body size will be (Sepulveda et al., 2002). This corresponds to the findings by Nicholls et al. (2006), cited above. Second, the greater the body dissatisfaction, the more likely the individual is to suffer from eating disorders and body image problems, such as BDD. The latter is evaluated using the Body Perception Index (BPI) as proposed by Slade & Russell (1973), which relates size estimated by the subject to real size: perceived size/real size.

What is also interesting is that primarily cognitive (as opposed to perceptually affective) estimation of one's body image yields a greater BPI. This conclusion can be made from a study conducted by Sansone et al. (2010) on 126 women in an inpatient psychiatric unit using 5 measures for body image and 2 measures for Borderline Personality Disorder (BPD). Participants with BPD demonstrated more self-consciousness about one's appearance and a more negative evaluation thereof, indicating "less comfort and trust in their own bodies" (p. 579). In general, Sansone et al. concluded that body image measures that were "more perceptually grounded" were "more likely to be similar to non-BPD participants," whereas body image measures that were "more cognitively grounded" were "more likely to be statistically significantly different in comparison with non-BPD participants" (Ibid.).

This conclusion underscores the importance of actual sensual awareness and self-perception. In conjunction with conclusions of research founded on figural drawings, it also shows that outside influence (mass/social media, criticism, bullying, etc.) competes for body image formation with perceptual findings (self-perception), but that the latter must remain guiding, key, and crucial if the individual is to develop healthy body image. In plain English, over-thinking it and over-imagining the ideal (or "model") body image is ultimately self-destructive and undermines one's true self.

Techniques affiliated to the figural drawing include depictive techniques, and metric methods (Sadibolova et al., 2019). So called *depictive techniques* include the following: measuring the width of certain parts of the body, such as the face, the hips, or the waist, in order to establish a Body Image Index (akin to BPI); comparing the experience of one's own body with its image in a distorting mirror (Traub & Orbach, 1964); the distorted photograph technique (Glucksman & Hirsch, 1969[152]); video distortion (Probst, Vandereycken, Van Coppenolle, & Pieters, 1998); and template matching (Gandevia & Phegan, 1999).

The *metric methods* involve: comparing the experienced size of one's own body to a physical length (Slade & Russell, 1973); image marking or "patterning" of the body image "related to the localization of somatic complaints" (Askevold, 1975, p. 71); and the Adjustable

---

[152] Glucksman and Hirsch (1969) made an interesting finding during their study. They conducted a survey of obese subjects following weight loss during a period of weight maintenance and found that the subjects overestimated their own body size despite the weight loss. They concluded that these subjects manifested a *phantom body size* phenomenon, perceiving themselves "as if they had lost almost no weight" and consistently overestimating "the size of other stimuli external to themselves before, during, and following weight loss" (p. 1). It can therefore be concluded that body modification does not immediately alter body image. A period of habituation to the new body is necessary in order to form, apprehend and accept the new body image.

Light Beam Apparatus[153] (Thompson & Spana, 1988). These methods are one-dimensional and primarily focus on one dimension at a time, such as length, width, or circumference.

Researchers have demonstrated that body image self-perception can be manipulated through exposure to either thinner or larger body images (Brooks et al., 2016). In as little as one minute of exposure, the return to a "normal" body image is perceived as distorted because it has been manipulated by the ideal. These findings have significant implications for media exposure, especially with respect to young, susceptible individuals. Even as little as two 30-second commercials on television can distort the self-perception of a suggestive person, especially if she already suffers from preexisting comorbidities, such as ED.

Surveys

Various surveys and questionnaires are used to assess the individual's feelings about his or her body and body image. These surveys reflect constitutional, attitudinal, and cognitive variables which should be taken into account in the evaluation. Some surveys focus solely on body weight, others on eating disorders and attitudes to food, still others are more socially-constructed, i.e., "what others think of me" and "how am I perceived in public."

Garner and Garfinkel (1979) developed an Eating Attitudes Test (EAT), which measures symptoms in Anorexia Nervosa (AN). The EAT scale is presented in a 6-

---

[153] The Adjustable Light Beam Apparatus is used to measure an individual's accuracy in estimating one's own body size. An overhead projector, with the apparatus attached, is placed at 1.5 meters (4 ft 11 inches) from a blank wall. Participants "adjust rods on the apparatus to beam rays of light on to the wall" using each beam of light to "approximate the width of four body parts in turn (cheeks, waist, hips and thighs)" thereby creating an adjustable silhouette of one's body image (Waldman et al., 2013, p. 8).

point, forced choice, self-report format of 40 questions. It is easy to administer and score. This test does not directly measure body image but focuses on AN. Compared to normal population, anorectics score statistically significantly higher. The test is also sensitive to clinical remission, with recovered anorectics scoring in the normal range. It can therefore be used as a clinical device in monitoring recovery progress among affected subjects.

A measure of cognitive body image disturbance is provided by the Beck Depression Inventory (BDI), and Beck Anxiety Inventory (BAI), often applied in conjunction with anthropometric measurements, such as the body mass index (BMI), and percentual determination of subcutaneous body fat (e.g. by means of the skinfold caliper). These tests show that BDD is directly linked to the symptoms of anxiety, and depression. Not surprisingly, EAT and BDI scores in tested subjects were found to be similar, which means predictive of each other (Lee et al., 2018).

As an aside, for the diet-minded and nutrition-conscious readers, it should be noted here that student cohorts who were trained in nutrition and dietetics scored higher on these tests and were more prone to eating disorders than population not educated in nutrition (Negriz-Unal, 2014). The same relationship was observed in sports population practicing endurance and aesthetic sports, such as long-distance running, bodybuilding, ballet, gymnastics, or figure skating (Matusik et al., 2022). Young women (under 18) were found to be ten times more susceptible to eating disorders and depression than young men (Ibid.).

More specific questionnaires, such as the Body Shape Questionnaire, focus on the body image perception among those who are suffering from body image related problems, such as anorexia nervosa and bulimia (Cooper, Taylor, Cooper & Fairburn, 1987). The BSQ questions are phrased so as to detect insecurity, and feelings of inferiority related to a particular body part or body area, for example:

"Have you thought that your thighs, hips or bottom are too large for the rest of you?" or "Have you worried about your flesh being not firm enough?" or "Have you worried about your thighs spreading out when sitting down?" (Evans, 2023). The BSQ (see Appendix C) is a self-report measure taken during an interview, intended to provide further topics for discussion and raise issues related to one's shape and body image. It can be a useful device for breaking ice and starting conversation with subjects who are ashamed and unwilling to confide about their problems. These questions go to various factors that measure a general concern with one's body image/shape, body image/shape self-consciousness, and behavioral characteristics clinically correlated with eating disorders.

It should be noted that a specific questionnaire for women versus men is desirable, because different body-parts are of different concern to each, and that the researcher or psychologist evaluating the test should take into account the momentary disposition of the person, because periods of illness, grief, work-related problems, menstrual cycle, etc. can significantly skew the results. Limbert (2004) found that if other factors are not included, the results of eating disorder questionnaires may be faulty. Leaving out any of the five subscales – "drive for thinness, perfectionism, bulimia, interpersonal distrust, or maturity fears" – can cast significant doubts on the results (p. 165).

Scales and Inventories

The number of body image measuring scales and inventories has been constantly increasing in recent years. Some of these measuring instruments are focused specifically on subjects already suffering from body image disturbances, others concentrate on minorities, as well as sundry non-western cultures, still others take into account specifically classified psychiatric conditions. Apart from Body Shape Questionnaires (BSQs), and the inventories listed in the previous chapters, there exists a plethora of symptom-intensive scales. It should be noted that many different scales bear the same name (i.e., "Body Image Scale"), but may contain different, sometimes overlapping, items which were adapted by researchers for a particular subset of population.

From among several Body Image Scales, the Body Image States Scale (BISS) is among the most advanced instruments because it evaluates both positive and negative aspects of body image experience, as well as the context in which it is taken. The BISS measures the following factors: 1) satisfaction and/or dissatisfaction with one's appearance, 2) satisfaction and/or dissatisfaction with one's body size and body shape, 3) satisfaction and/or dissatisfaction with one's weight, 4) feelings of physical attractiveness and/or unattractiveness, 5) current feelings about one's looks "relative to how one usually feels," and 6) the evolution of one's appearance "relative to how the average person looks" (Cash, 2004, p. 166). BISS is a useful tool in determining dysfunctional investment in one's appearance which, in turn, is a reliable predictor of negative body image.

The Drive for Muscularity Scale (DMS) is also among the most favorite investigative devices focused on the investigation of the correlation between the excessive investment in one's appearance and body image dissonances. The DMS has been tested on men, including minority and gender non-conforming individuals (DeBlaere & Brewster, 2017). It considers attitudinal and behavioral components among men who have internalized "societal expectations of a muscular mesomorphic body shape," which implies lean yet highly muscular men, even where the individuals lack natural predispositions to conform with the muscular standard, that is men who are endomorphs or ectomorphs (Ryan & Morrison, 2014).

The Adolescent Body Image Satisfaction Scale (ABISS) was developed in addition to other measures focused on body image, and body image related behaviors (Eating Disorders Inventory, Body Image Satisfaction Scale, Eating Attitudes Test, Rosenberg Self-Esteem Scale, Body Esteem Scale), in order to address specific pathologies present in adolescent males predominantly likely to focus on muscularity, self-esteem, and body-pride or, conversely, body-shame. The pilot version of ABISS contained 16 items, positive versus negative statements, such as: "My body makes me feel proud," versus: "I am ashamed of my body" (Leone et al., 2014, p. 2663). The final 32-item ABISS is scored using a Likert 1-4 scale to assess body image satisfaction of the cohorts. Higher scores show a higher level of body image dissatisfaction. Researchers often incorporate other scales, as well as interviews, in order to accurately measure intrapersonal, interpersonal, and social factors that contribute to the adolescent male body image.

The Body Image Coping Strategies Inventory (BICSI) is a 29-item measure focused on the body image coping factors, such as avoidance, appearance fixing, and a positive rational acceptance. Cash et al. (2005) found that the BICSI "significantly converged" with other "pertinent measures of body image evaluation, affect, and investment, and with psychosocial functioning," such as self-esteem, social support, and possible eating disorders (p. 191). Coping strategies were also found to be predictive of quality of life, and attitudes to eating and exercise. Compared with men, women used all coping strategies more frequently, especially "appearance-fixing strategies" (Ibid.).

The Multidimensional Body-Self Relations Questionnaire-Appearance Scales (MBSRQ-AS) have been developed to address different factors and aspects of the body image/body-self-perception, such as the mental body schema, the subjective components of body image, including one's thoughts, beliefs, feelings about and satisfaction with one's body, the degree of satisfaction with one's own body, as well as behavioral components, including specific behaviors that people "perform regarding the consideration of the shape of the body and the degree of satisfaction with it," such as exercising, dieting, covering imperfections, or emphasizing positive features (Lizana-Calderón, 2023, p. 628).

The Multidimensional Body-Self Relations Questionnaire (MBSRQ) and Body-Self Relations Questionnaire-Appearance Scales (MBSRQ-AS) are multidimensional constructs that focus on the evaluation of appearance, body area satisfaction, preoccupation with one's weight, and the shape of one's body. The MBSRQ includes five subscales, related to: appearance evaluation, appearance orientation, overweight preoccupation, self-classified weight, and body areas satisfaction scale. Both scales yield solid reliability, and convergent and discriminant validity coefficients, and have been translated into other languages (Vossbeck-Elsebusch, 2014). They are recommended for a multidimensional assessment of appearance-related aspects of body image in both research and clinical practice (Cash, 2000).

The Assessment of Body Image Cognitive Distortions (ABCD) is a clinically-favored measure of cognitive body image distortions. It focuses on cognitive-behavioral techniques to target individuals with some degree of body image dysphoria. Jakatdar, Cash, & Engle (2006) found that the ABCD "uniquely predicted body image quality of life and disturbed eating attitudes above and beyond other body image predictors" (p. 325). The researchers found that "heavier women" and White women were "more prone to body image cognitive distortions" than thinner women and Black women (Ibid.).

The Appearance Schemas Inventory (ASI) is a scale designed to "assess core beliefs or assumptions about the importance, meaning, and effects of appearance in one's life" (Cash & Labarge, 1996, p. 37). The ASI scales body image vulnerability, self-investment, and appearance stereotyping. It correlates to and confirms other measures of body image and psychosocial functioning. Researchers noted that women who sought treatment for a negative body image scored higher on the ASI than their peers (Ibid.).

The Appearance Schemas Inventory-Revised (ASI-R) is a revision of the original Appearance Schemas Inventory. It assesses the individual's psychological investment in her appearance (Cash, Jakatdar, & Williams, 2004; Cash, 2009; Cash, Maikkula, & Yamamiya, 2004; Cash, Melnyk, & Hrabosky, 2004; Cash, Morrow, Hrabosky, & Perry, 2004; Cash, Phillips, Santos, & Hrabosky, 2004). This revised measure contains 20 items and two subscales examining the tested individuals' beliefs about "how their appearance influences their personal or social worth and sense of self," as well as the extent to which they "attend to or seek to manage" their appearance and perceived appearance-related issues (Thompson et al., 2019).

There also exists a plethora of tests measuring self-esteem and body image in relation to and during sexual activities.[154] Virtually all of these studies, tests, and measures found that body image dysphoric feelings should be considered in the treatment of individuals with sexual dysfunction. In fact, arguably the most well-known and guiding book on the treatment of body image related problems, T. F. Cash's *Body Image Workbook*, starts with a survey of dissatisfaction of sexual life and lack of orgasm in women caused by dysfunctional body image perceptions.

The Body Exposure during Sexual Activities Questionnaire (BESAQ) is a measure of "body image experiences in the specific, situational context of sexual

---

[154] Many of these forms and assessment tools are available from Dr. Thomas Cash, for a nominal fee, for personal use and research. *See* http://www.body_images.com/assessments/order.html

relations" (Cash, 2012, par. 1). This 28-item tool focuses on preoccupation and avoidance of exposure of certain body-parts or nakedness in general during intimate contact[155] (Cash et al., 2004; Cash, Jakatdar et al., 2004; Cash, Maikkula et al., 2004; Cash, Melnyk et al., 2004; Cash, Morrow et al., 2004; Faith & Schare, 1993; Yamamiya, Cash, & Thompson, 2006). Faith and Schare (1993) termed this phenomenon *spectatoring*.[156] They found that it strongly correlates with body satisfaction and investment in appearance. Conversely, body image scores "significantly predicted frequency of sexual behaviors" for both genders (Ibid., p. 345). General sexual knowledge and psychological adjustment bore no causal relationship to spectatoring. The BESAQ was wound to be a strong predictor of pleasure and desire, as well as sexual satisfaction.

Yet another measure which can be used in evaluation of sexual satisfaction and body image is the Multi-dimensional Body-Self Relations Questionnaire (MBSRQ). Brown, Cash, and Mikulka (1990) conducted an analysis of the BSRQ on a random stratified sample of 1,064 females and 988 males, and found this questionnaire to be highly reliable for the following factors: appearance evaluation and orientation, fitness evaluation and orientation, health and sickness evaluation and orientation. Females demonstrated a "somewhat greater differentiation of body image attitudes" than did the males in this study (p. 135), especially with

---

[155] For example: "I don't like my partner to see me completely naked during sexual activity." "During sexual activity I try to hide certain areas of my body." "I am self-conscious about my body during sexual activity." Respondents rate each item on a 5-point frequency scale (0 = "Never" to 4 = "Almost Always") – higher scores reflect more self-conscious focus and avoidance.

[156] *Spectatoring* refers to a "cognitive self-absorption, wherein individuals fixate on and carefully monitor personal body parts and/or the adequacy of personal sexual functioning" (Faith & Schare, 1993, p. 345).

regard to specific physical areas (face, lower torso), and body image attributes (weight, height).

Appearance Schemas Inventory (ASI) is a 14-item assessment scale (including items such as: "I should do whatever I can to always look my best." Or: "My appearance is responsible for much of what has happened to me in my life."). The ASI evaluates the degree of psychological investment in the tested individual's appearance (Cash & Labarge, 1996). It has been found to have a high internal consistency (.84 for men and .85 for women).

The Sexual Self-Schema Scale (SSSS) is an inventory that measures one's self-concept as a "sexual person" (Cash, Maikkula et al., 2004, Ibid.). It consists of 50 items for women and 45 items for men, comprising three dimensions: passionate versus romantic, open versus direct, and not embarrassed versus conservative, for women; and passionate versus loving, powerful versus aggressive, and open-minded versus liberal, for men. The goal is to explore the intrapersonal and interpersonal aspects of sexuality, and examine the impact and degree to which sexual self-concept is caused by body dysmorphic feelings. The SSSS ranks responses as either: positive, co-schematic, a-schematic, or negative (Andersen & Cyranowski, 1994; Andersen et al., 1999).

The Changes in Sexual Functioning Questionnaire (CSFQ): is a 14-item measure which compares the experiences and sensations to sexual functioning. Like SSSS, CSFQ is different for men and women, with subscales for: 1) sexual pleasure (1 item), 2) desire/frequency (2 items), 3) desire/interest (3 items), 4) arousal (3 items), and 5) orgasm (3 items) (Clayton, McGarvey, & Clavet, 1997). Clayton, McGarvey, Clavet, and Piazza (1997) found that psychiatric patients diagnosed with "a mood disorder" had "significantly lower sexual functioning" in comparison to nonpsychiatric outpatients, medical students, and psychiatry residents combined (p. 747). As a consequence of this research, the CSFQ is recommended as an efficient tool for psychologists and psychiatrists in treating sexual dysfunction in patients with various mood disorders.[157]

A vast majority of these instruments assess and evaluate various dimensions of self-concept and body image, and try to capture attitudes and behaviors, satisfaction, and coping strategies and mechanisms. Some are confined to the measurement of only specific components of the individual's body image, such as body dissatisfaction related to certain body-parts. Experts constantly try to update these questionnaires and tools, in order to develop a more comprehensive tool which would cover all aspects and dimensions of body image. Since there is a strong association between body image disturbances and culture, such a tool would have to contain variances related to a particular society and culture. As noted above, however, the more specific the tool, the better the results will be during its application. As apparent from the sundry tools used to assess the relationship between body image and sexual dysfunction, more specificity, rather than more comprehensiveness, is desirable (for example, an eating disorder measure developed specifically for South Korean women will have more utility in the field than a generic eating disorder questionnaire used in the United States). Generic and generalized advice must be offered with caution, at least until the individual is examined with specificity as to their particular disorder.

---

[157] The level of self-consciousness in various body areas during sex (chest, breasts, hips, buttocks, thighs, scalp hair, etc.) was also examined by Cash, Maikkula et al. (2004).

Somatoperception

Anyone who has ever attempted to draw a portrait of themselves, or even of another human being, has immediately found out how difficult it is to gauge and copy the proportions of different body parts in relation to one another, and to the whole. This is one of the reasons why Human Figure Drawing tests have been found "questionable" (Radika & Hayslip, 2004, p. 155). Other reasons include finding a reliable scoring system, and interpreting the drawing in individualized context (Ibid.).

Linkenauger et al. (2015) conducted an experiment in which the researchers asked the participants to judge the length of different body parts in units of length versus a noncorporeal object: for example, how many "units" would fit in a size of a body-part (e.g., one's own hand). A pattern of length misestimation emerged, suggesting that the sizes of different parts of the body were misinterpreted more often than others (e.g., torso and arms versus legs and the head). What is more, visual perception positively relates to tactile sensitivity and physical size.

Somatoperception is an activity necessary for body image mapping in the somatosensory cortex. While tactile spatial acuity is "routinely tested in neurology" and it consistently follows the "proximal–distal gradients" and body innervation density (Mancini et al., 2014, p. 917), it is rarely, if ever, tested in conjunction with questionnaires and assessments that inquire about how the individual at question perceives his or her body image.

Indirectly, however, Penfield and Rasmussen (1950) showed that a compensatory distortion of subject's body image exists, indicating that body-parts of particular concern to the individual are distorted in somatosensory mapping, in order to compensate for a perceived deficiency. Arguably, therefore, for reasons that may be interoceptive (including valid biases, even of genetic origins), rather than proprioceptive (tactile, sensual), or exteroceptive (i.e., triggered by the ecosystem, microsphere, media impact, etc.), the individual is driven to compensatory behaviors (such as extreme dieting or exercise).

In other words, visceral organs signal to the brain their states, and such signaling contributes to the formation of the body image. Since these interoceptive data are three dimensional, intangible, and invisible, they may interfere with the conscious two-dimensional concept of the self (what one sees in the mirror or perceives by touch) in seemingly inexplicable ways.

For example, Keizer et al. (2011) found that higher levels of body dissatisfaction in anorexia nervosa (AN) affected subjects were related to more severe inaccuracies in the visual mental image of the body, and "overestimation of tactile distances" (p. 115). In their further research, Keizer et al. (2012) discovered that this overestimation in AN subjects was directly related to their overestimation of the size of their bodies, thus bearing a direct witness to BDD in both, visual and somatosensory areas, which means involving "both bottom-up and top-down processes" (p. 530). In connecting the visceral inability to feel hunger (repeated suppression of hunger in AN subjects), Pollatos et al. (2008) highlighted the "importance of investigating interoceptive sensitivity in the pathogenesis of eating disorders" (p. 381), thus also highlighting the potential importance of interoceptive sensitivity in the pathogenesis of eating disorders. In lay terms, pragmatically interpreted, this means that if an individual repeatedly omits to eat regularly, consequent desensitization to hunger may trigger AN, with consequent related comorbidities (e.g., BN).

The modal verb "may" in the previous sentence is in order here, because both AN and BN are multifactorial disorders with a "strong genetic component" (Paolacci et al., 2020, p. e1244). Siblings and consanguineous relatives are similarly affected (Ibid.). Zipfel et al. (2015) found that there is a "fourfold increase in susceptibility to AN among family members," and that the risk among female relatives of AN is eleven (11) times greater compared to the "normal population" (as cited in Paolacci et al., Ibid.). Eating disorders are clearly heritable diseases, although it is not exactly known yet what specific genes are their carriers.[158]

However, this does not mean that non-susceptible individuals should experiment with various yoyo diets and borderline AN "tactics" – simply because self-perceived "top-down" control and manipulation may provoke unexpected "bottom-up" reactions from the body. Therefore, somatosensory investigations of body image can contribute not only to diagnosing and treating BDD, AN, and other body image disturbances and related disorders and comorbidities but they may also play an invaluable role in body image assessments in the non-BDD suffering population. Reduced interoceptive awareness may indicate visceral changes or conditions that would otherwise be left to fester until discovered in a direct examination of the blood, or disease-specific tests. Last but not least, they may also serve as a useful predictor of susceptibility to body image dysphoria.

---

[158] According to the Anorexia Nervosa Genetic Initiative (ANGI), the Genetic Consortium for Anorexia Nervosa (GCAN), and the Welcome Trust Case Control Consortium-3 (WTCCC-3), along with UK Biobank, the investigation of 16,992 cases as well as 55,525 controls from 17 European countries identified the following genetic loci that potentially carry the ED: NCKIPSD (OMIM *606671), CADM1 (OMIM *605686), ERLEC1 (OMIM *611229), MGMT (OMIM *156569), FOXP1 (OMIM *605515), CDH10 (OMIM *604555), PTBP2 (OMIM *608449), and NSUN3 (OMIM *617491) (Watson et al., 2019).

Practice and Practical Implications

Each measure of assessment, every test, survey, scale etc., contributes to human knowledge about body image dysfunctions, but each such measure is also limited because: 1) the body image is fluid and complex, and (by the same token) it 2) takes only a snapshot in time (someone momentarily dissatisfied with an aspect of their body image does not necessarily suffer from BDD or ED); further, more often than not, it also 3) focuses on the negative aspects, neglecting when and where the individual is satisfied with their body image; 4) it is often oriented on a particular area, body-part, aspect or trait (such as anxiety); and 5) many measures fail to capture the context, thus can only be averaged out over time; and, furthermore, 6) an identified "disturbance" or dysphoria may actually be true (a person may really be fat or have a "perceived" deformity) but it may not necessarily be the cause of any body image problems to the individual because he or she likes and has fully accepted their body image. This is often the case with various subcultures, (sub)categories of gender identity, and even with many obese people. What all assessments and body image measures do, however, is that they offer the opportunity for the all-important self-reflection.

Krueger (2004) underscored the importance of such self-reflection in changing one's body image – the individual may rationally understand the processes and even the causes that have led to her current body image feelings and perceptions, yet, because such an understanding is self-referential but not self-reflective, she is impotent to address BD issues with any measurable long-term success in real life.

It is apparent that a "false body self" (p. 463) makes it difficult to operate in real world because – if the individual finds it difficult to be her "real self," how can they adequately and honestly communicate with others? The inability to communicate results in perceived ostracism and self-hatred. Stronger individuals may become obsessed with dieting, exercising, and various forms of body-self-flagellation; while the individuals who are less strong are at risk of becoming attached to purging, and guilt-contrition ritualistic behaviors; while the truly weak individuals resort to self-harm, often harming others in the process.[159] An individual suffering from BDD may even move among the three states up and down within a short period of time, all to no apparent effect or solution.

The fact that psychological and physiological aspects of body image are intertwined may appear detrimental at first, but it can be seen as beneficial once it is understood, absorbed, and applied to solve body image related conditions – simply because psychological crutches lift the body and vice versa. Every such crutch creates a point of reference to one – and, in turn, points at another – undifferentiated, unrecognized body image issue. Returning to when the first abuse, scorn, moment of deprecation, or other hurtful episode took place, reviewing it and analyzing it, creates not only a referential point but also a modus operandi to address the issue, e.g., "My mother beat me because she had been beaten herself when she was a little girl" (logical rationale). "She slammed the door as if to lock me in. It felt like a slap in the face" (psychological rationale, naming the feeling). "[Hence] every time someone slams the door, I feel like vomiting, and running away…" (physiological rationale, naming the feelings). The feelings of vomiting and confinement have become physiological requirements, potentially manifested in the present ED. They need to be addressed in words that distinguish them as somatic "body-issues" – as opposed to image issues. Once distinguished and named, they can be addressed and dealt with (see below).

---

[159] Morbidity among the ED patients is significantly higher than among "normal" population (Genis-Mendoza et al., 2019).

This is exceedingly difficult for someone who feels totally alone or is afraid and unwilling to confide in anyone. Such an individual often turns to self-help, in order to change the body – because he finds it impossible to change the mind. Frankly, even experts at "changing the mind" are sometimes at a loss and relegated to changing the body because there are simply too many factors at play in body image formation, including hereditary and environmental components; and it may very well be that the *cortical mapping* in the case-at-hand has become irreversible. Although neuroscientists continue to investigate how neurogenesis can "learn representations of sequential, complex events" and contribute to cortical mapping, such investigations have yet to yield practical recommendations for body image experts (Finnegan et al., 2017, p. 443).

Changing Your Body image

The good news is that the human being is a living, self-renewing organism, as is one's body image. In fact, as explained in previous chapters, it would be amiss to speak of a singular body image one is trying to achieve. Each Human Being contains multitudes. Thus, returning to the episodes of hurt and abuse in the past, in order to analyze them, and to determine the steps that need be taken, in order to cope with the current situation, and to prevent future moments of despair and frustration, is an example of only a partial path to renewal and return to the healthy self. In order to take practical steps to improve one's body image, one need not take half a dozen tests and visit a host of psychiatrists. One must only learn to know and appreciate oneself, determine what causes any given body image disturbance, feelings that flow from it, and try to prevent them, focusing on the path which led to it.

The advice provided here is offered to an average, inquisitive reader, someone who is not in any psychiatric treatment, and does not have a history of any serious psychiatric condition. There are situations where medical intervention is necessary, be it on the side of the psyche/image, or the body, or both. The self-treatment tips, and succinctly presented advice in the following chapters, are not intended to contradict or counteract any professional intervention.

Find a Friend

First, find a friend, a real friend, not a social media follower, but someone who knows you personally, in whom you can confide. You can also speak with someone you trust, such as a parent, sibling, teacher, spouse, or your mentor. Investing trust, time, and energy into a relationship is never a bad idea. Research shows that individuals suffering from various forms of PTSD, as well as victims of bullying and harassment, overcome their trauma without slumping to suicidal ideation, if they have at least one trusted friend (Condor-Fisher, 2021). The same is true with ED and BDD, where serious (even fatal) comorbidities are always a potentiality. You may be surprised how supportive and positive the reaction of a person who knows and in whom you decided to deposit your trust will be.

Evaluate Your Body

Second, realistically evaluate your body, including the body-parts you are uncomfortable with. Would changing the body (or the problem body part) improve your self-esteem? Would it lead to a better concept of the self, a more comfortable body image? The first question always will be: Why do I feel this way? The very next questions should be: On what occasions, and what triggers my feelings? Is it important that I change? Why?

One cannot avoid social contact and avoidance is not a solution. Positive thought matters. Never use slurs to describe yourself. Never address yourself in self-deprecating words and phrases, not even in your thoughts! Learn to love yourself. You have a beautiful soul, which is a gift from God. You had better believe it.

Analyze Your Body Image Story

Third, your body image has a story behind it. The story is composed of many components which come from your DNA, interpersonal experiences, culture, and the media. Most of these experiences and influences cannot be altered. What can be altered is your attitude and acceptance of the self. Cash (2004) recommends that one start a "body image diary" in which one should write down the following (p. 167):

- Activators: events that trigger body image discomfort and distress.

- Beliefs: activator-associated beliefs and thoughts about one's body image.

- Consequences: emotional and behavioral reactions that follow the Activators and Beliefs.

Think of the journal approach like an athlete having a training log. Professional trainers and nutritional analysts, not to mention serious athletes and their coaches, require such a journal as a necessary precondition to success. It has been stated that feelings about one's body are always self-reflective but, in order to achieve progress and improve how one feels about oneself, such feelings must be *self-referential* (Krueger, 2004). This means that they must contain facts that present a point in time describing the self in the given environment – because, after all, one's body image is fluid and tends to escape a static moment of "capture," a snapshot in time. The feelings of being good and doing good (e.g., after an episode of binge eating), eludes and escapes just as easily as it came on, and – unless one determines what triggered the BN, how one felt, and why –

362

the individual will never snap out of the vicious cycle. Similarly, a feeling of disgust or disappointment with one's body was likely triggered by a particular event – perhaps a T.V. commercial, perhaps a comparison with one's peer, or a disparaging comment from a close family member. One cannot deal with the feeling and eradicate it, unless one first ascertains what triggered it.

What is more, negative feelings about the self may be caused by some lower unfulfilled need on the "hierarchy of needs" (Maslow, 1970, p. 38). The BN hunger (desire to purge) is likely not for food but for an inner fulfilment, for love, for belongingness. One might also argue that the binge eating-purging episode is an attempt at mental purification through the body, an attempt to get rid of a burden one feels but cannot define (such as childhood abuse). Establishing a written journal will facilitate understanding and assist in arriving at the original need (or trigger) which led to the moment of body image dissonance.

Accept Your Experiences

The feeling of acceptance is fully within your domain and power. Consider this: If I will not accept myself, how can I expect others to accept me? Further, if one has a significant body image concern, it impacts one's self-worth, and shows in his or her conduct.

In the now well-known experiment conducted by Kleck and Strenta (1980), individuals were "led to believe that they were perceived as physically deviant" in one-on-one interaction, even where no such actual perception of deviance took place (p. 861). Subjects (all female) were given a set of written instructions that randomly assigned them to one of three conditions: 1) allergy, 2) epilepsy, or 3) a facial scar. The instructions informed them that they would be "involved in a discussion with another female" to test whether the other's behavior was affected by their condition. In the case of the scar sample, they were given a small hand mirror to confirm that an "authentic-looking scar had been placed on her face" by the make-up artist (p. 863). As the subject put the mirror down, the experimenter informed the individual that he was "putting a moisturizer over the scar" to keep it from "cracking and peeling off" (Ibid.). In the process of "moisturizing" the scar, however, the experimenter removed it – without telling anything to the subject.

In the subsequent interaction, the interactant "did not, in fact, perceive them as deviant," even though persons who thought that they possessed a "negatively valued" physical trait, found a "strong reactivity to the deviance in the behavior of their interactant," whereas those with a "more neutrally valued characteristic" (epilepsy, allergy) did not (p. 861). In addition, those who observed the behavior of the interactants on a videotape subsequent to the experiment also perceived a "greater reactivity to an imputed negative form of deviance" than to a neutral one (Ibid.). Consequently, the researchers showed that an expectancy-perceptual bias mechanism exists but also that there is a "self-fulfilling prophecy dynamic," that is: one who thinks they are "scarred" will not only perceive the perceiver as biased, but will "fulfill the prophecy" of such perception and will, in fact, be perceived as "scarred" (p. 868).

Acceptance consists of recognizing that feelings about one's body image are inner experiences that will remain invisible to others. Unless you find such experiences intolerable and begin to outwardly project anxiety, shame, and overt self-consciousness on others, the realization of the inner experiences is always to your benefit. Cash (2008) speaks of "mindful self-monitoring" (p. 72). According to Cash (Id.), appearance assumptions are the greatest culprit in the creation of BD. Assumptions about the body image and that everything in life revolves around it – happiness, success, love,... – results in poor quality of everyday life, as well as in personal body image distress and dissatisfaction. Those who doubt such assumptions (i.e., those who impute less importance to body image) are on average at 5% likelihood of developing body image distress while those called "assumers" (who are constantly concerned about their body image) are 92% likely to develop body image distress (p. 82).

How to avoid being an "assumer?" Stop focusing on how others view what you look like – because, the fact is, they could not care less. Focus on your actions and seek friends among those who think likewise. Further, if you fix an appearance problem and it does not fix how you feel, the problem is not in your appearance. Hence, in the journal (see above), pay attention to the voice which asks you: How do I feel when I focus on the uncomfortable body-part? What thoughts run through my head?

There will be a pro and a con voice, one speaking for the image, one for the body. The first voice may, for example, say: "I feel really bad about my big fat nose." "I keep thinking about it all the time, feeling as if everyone is staring at my nose when they talk to me." The Body Voice will rebut: "It's just your imagination. Even if it were so, there are so many people with big noses. I was born this way and I like it. It goes well with my mouth and my cheeks. Moreover, it is not bad to have a big nose, it makes the face interesting."

Correct Your Mental Distortions

Mental distortions are prejudicial errors in thinking about body image. They originate in the assumptions (discussed above) that everything in life is founded on how you look. Cash (2008) characterizes such assumptions as "mental distortions" (p. 110). As in other spheres of life, prejudices in the form of mental distortions come from seeing the world as black-and-white: either I am fat or I am skinny, either I am beautiful or I am ugly, either others think that I am successful or they think I am a failure.

If you think this way, you will think this way not just about yourself but also about others, perceiving them primarily in terms of their size, weight, prominent body-parts, beauty, and visible success (possessions). That leads to misery. What is more, it is completely distorted, because the world is not black-or-white. It contains all shades and colors in between. So do you. You can see the world objectively, which leads to being less judgmental and critical – primarily about yourself – which, in turn, will lead you to being less judgmental about others. Assuming less, reframing the world in positive terms, that is the road to happiness.

In *The Nature of Prejudice,* Gordon Allport (1958) identified the origins of prejudice in conformity to custom and *"the need to... maintain the cultural pattern"* (p. 272) [italics original]. The cultural pattern which focuses on images (and their symbolic value, e.g. as status symbols) is the pattern which creates prejudice. Paradoxically, prejudice is isolating, and ultimately always self-destructive. It may stem from the desire to conform, but because it lacks personal judgment (which is subjected to the pressure of the majority, be it the master race ideology, or the prevailing views about women and men propagated through mass media), it removes the individual thought and substitutes it with superimposed image.

In practical terms, this means that one should spend about equal time pondering the positives as one spends dwelling on the negatives. Accept criticism the way you accept flattery – both may have a grain of truth in them, but neither is evidence. Opinion is not evidence. The fact that someone (or even you yourself) espouses an opinion about a fact (such as the shape and size of your nose) is not evidence. Cash (2008) made an interesting point: "Replace 'I am" thoughts with 'I feel" thoughts" (p. 131). How you feel is easier to change than who (you think) you are!

Finally, do not compare yourself to an ideal out there. NEDC[160] (2023) recommended that such comparisons be avoided at all times. Each person has many dimensions and there is no ideal. Accepting this reality undistorted means being comfortable as yourself, in your own skin.

Create a New Body Image Voice

Create a new body image voice, which will always be mindful of your positives, who you are deep within, will always flatter you, and will always respond: "Don't be judgmental! Be tolerant! Love yourself!" Write a positive statement in this regard on a sheet of paper, and pin it to your bathroom mirror. For example: "I feel good. I look good. I am goooood!" Every time you shave or use makeup, you will see it. It will stick with you. Make yourself feel gooood!

Body Image Warrior

Hiding, avoiding certain people or places, putting on tons of makeup, covering up your perceived "deformities" – those are not actions of a brave Body Image Warrior. Such actions originate in, and lead back to, being judgmental about body image.

Recall the encounter between the Prime Minister Winston Churchill and Bessie Braddock, MP, late one night in 1946, as Churchill was leaving the House of Commons (Langworth, 2011):

---

[160] National Eating Disorders Collaboration, an Australian association of organizations and people within the purview of the Department of Health and Ageing.

"Winston, you are drunk, and what's more you are disgustingly drunk!" Ms. Braddock stated.

Here is what the Prime Minister said in response:

"Bessie, my dear, you are ugly, and what's more, you are disgustingly ugly. But, tomorrow, I shall be sober and you will still be disgustingly ugly."

The rumor has it that he was tired and not drunk, hence the response (Ibid.). However, there is more to this conversation than meets the eye: Being drunk says nothing about the person's body image – or does it? No doubt, it was meant as a remark upbraiding Mr. Churchill about his manners. One may argue that if he was not drunk, and Ms. Braddock knew it, then she may have been criticizing something else. But what if Churchill did interpret it as a disparaging body image statement? After all, are not drunks usually dirty, smelly outcasts? Hence, perhaps self-righteously, he responded with his own body image counter-salve.

Both actors present to this spat were highly educated, savvy, and even wise and witty people. Therefore, their remarks should be interpreted not as shallow statements about looks but as deeper insights into human nature: being ugly and acting ugly are as inseparable as being drunk and acting drunk. Even in reverse, acting drunk projects the body image of a drunk, whether one is drunk or not. Conversely, a beautiful lady would likely not call a gentleman of Winston Churchill's prowess and caliber a disgusting drunk. Being judgmental leads to being treated in a judgmental fashion. It is the shortest path to a mutually assured self-destruction.

At least, one might suggest, they did not try to avoid each other (which would probably have been easier, but certainly less entertaining, leaving not a bit of wisdom to us, their wisdom-hungry "posteriors"). Indeed, it should be noted that evasive actions lead to destructive ends – simply because one covers up the true body image, and projects onto another something made-up which cannot be adequately

368

mediated – the evader then receives a retort which is likewise not based in fact. Should Mr. Churchill have responded: "Dear Ms. Braddock, I am not drunk, I am terribly tired?" But how could he have? Politicians, after all, live in the world of images.

Eradicate Negative Rituals

Negative rituals are rituals that lead to negative body image feelings. Body image rituals can include anything from staring in the mirror, dressing and undressing oneself, checking and re-checking some blemish or imperfection on one's face, to preparing for a binge episode by accumulating food, making certain no-one will be at home at the time. These rituals are not difficult to delay, but the affected individuals find them nearly impossible to eradicate. The reason is that the opportunity arises and the desire becomes irresistible.

Once again, it must be stated that the desire is not for the ritual itself but, rather, for the satisfaction obtained through it. In this regard, the ritual is tantamount to the image. Getting rid of the bathroom scales, buying healthy food, calling on a friend to come over or meet you for dinner, evading moments of loneliness at all costs, even supplanting existing negative rituals with positive ones (e.g., a moment of yoga or mediation, a moment reserved for a new diary entry, or socialization with one's loved one) is the right way forward.

Many people who have overcome eating disorders did so by treating their body somewhat like a car which needs to be refueled. A car is also a means to the end – it gets you somewhere. It is not the end in itself. It should not be.

Sometimes, it helps to talk to your body as if the body were your best friend: "I know we have not always had a good relationship, but you are my best friend, and I am sorry

I mistreated you. You are not bad looking at all, especially compared to some of the bodies out there... Let's do something which will make us both happy in the long run."

Rituals are problematic because they become a habit. A habit, as they say, is an iron shirt – nearly impossible to take off. It is therefore critical that any ritual you may wish to introduce into your life have a positive impact on your body image *in the long run*. For example, ten minutes of yoga or stretching in the morning, a walk with the dog, a moment saved for pruning the roses, cleaning the room, or exercising – all in order to have fun and enjoy the freedom of your body – are all great rituals. People who want to exercise, but hate it, should set up regular times, let us say three times a week, always at the exact same time, and establish a positive routine (ritual) during which they will refuse to answer the phone or talk to anyone. Your favorite music may do the trick. Just being with your own self alone, enjoying your body, relaxing your mind should be the goal.

Whenever you lapse or relapse, stagnate or succumb to despair, ask yourself why. Define the original moment, why it happened, how it happened, and analyze your feelings. Write it down, state what you will do differently next, and do so. Choose a *long-term* positive path for yourself and your body image whenever you are at the crossroads. Often, such a path lies in the fulfilment of the need for belongingness, be it in going out with a friend or watching a good movie with someone near and dear to your heart.

Changing the Body Image – Medical Context

Trauma

There is probably not a single human being who has escaped some form of trauma in life. Trauma is usually understood as a deeply disturbing experience (psychological trauma) or a serious injury (physical trauma). Physical trauma often leaves psychological scars, and vice versa. Although medicine is primarily concerned with physical trauma, such trauma is often treated only superficially when not considered with its psychological implications, which invariably either precede it or follow in its wake. Therefore, trauma has a significant, lasting impact on human interactions, the impact often caused by a change in the perceived body image.[161]

Traumatology as a sub-branch of medicine deals with both physical and psychological trauma. Since trauma is a complex phenomenon, which involves abstract rationale and has its invisible components, it cannot be approached and dealt with solely on concrete terms. The good news is that it need not be. Traumatic events are "encoded and processed at a subcortical level" at which past, present, and future are "not differentiated" – which is why the past constantly emerges, seemingly out of nowhere, to bother the individual and detract from the enjoyment of the present moment (Ogden et al., 2006, p. 165). Traumatic events of the past may thus cause cognitive distortions of the events presently experienced. This often manifests in depression,

---

[161] Even in the context of the body image of a nation, trauma (such as Civil War) will leave indelible wounds, turning into mental scars – not unlike the scars applied on experimental subjects in Kleck and Strenta's 1980 experiment (p. 126 above) – which the nation will perceive more than the outsiders, and, consequently, will strive their best to conceal, in order to present its best "body image" on the world stage. Meanwhile, the soul may fester and the nation self-flagellate to destruction.

despair, self-loathing, suicidal ideation, emotional maladaptation, and various forms of autonomic dysregulation. The cycle of stigmatization and self-distortion is triggered by the traumatic thought or feeling (e.g. "I feel worthless") and is completed by it ("I look worthless. I am worthless").

Focusing on repairing the body image will prove ineffectual, unless the root cause of the distortion is found. That is why most therapists seek to make the patient "stable" first. This means achieving a state of safety and mental equilibrium ("I am no longer threatened. I am safe."). This is equivalent to addressing physical trauma by stabilizing the body and bodily functions. Akin to the trauma medicine approach, when dealing with psychological trauma, the image and its functions need to be stabilized prior to further intervention.

Top-Down/Bottom-Up Interventions

The difference between Top-Down intervention and Bottom-Up intervention is similar to that between inductive and deductive reasoning. Top-Down interventions focus on cognitive regulation of affect. They consist of creating a narrative and understanding of the traumatic experience. Bottom-Up interventions follow the sensations coming from the body and changes in sensorimotor experience, from which the understanding is gradually derived. While these approaches are used in professional therapy, they can be similarly applied either in the form of self-intervention or intervention by a close friend who will listen to the symptoms and observations of the individual and help connect the proverbial dots, to understand where and how the trauma-related feelings originated, and what the responses are, how to approach and regulate them, how to understand them.

Lanius et al. (2010) showed that there are two specific types of responses to trauma, a dissociative subtype, and a non-dissociative subtype. Dissociation means fragmentation "of the usually integrated functions of consciousness, memory, identity, body awareness, and perception of the self and the environment" (p. 641). Focus on a particular body-part may be symptomatic of the dissociative disorder, commonly caused by trauma.[162]

Emotional content may prevent the individual from accessing and understanding the context of the traumatic experience, or the context may be altogether absent from memory – because trauma (such as severe bullying – which may even be self-bullying, as in the case of Erin's story, *see* below) alters memory encoding, which leads to "fragmentation and compartmentalization" of memory, as well as impaired retrieval. Body image fragmentation and the discontinuity of body images (inability to integrate them into one whole and healthy Self), are the direct consequence of dissociation. Desensitization to pain, or inappropriate awareness of pain (which does not fit the situation) have also been found (Ibid.).

Ogden at al. (2008) recommended the use of a "mindful exploration" of "present-moment experience" in order to break free from the process of numbness and stultified cognitive processing, such as what is witnessed in patients suffering from eating disorders or BDD. For example, a friend might invite a resisting bulimic to a restaurant, in order to "explore" what will be happening to her body when she eats "normally." This would take place as a top-down intervention, and self-intervention. He might then want to slowly and gently suggest certain physical actions and ask about her feelings, including feelings of harm, danger, denudement, guilt, or even disintegration, the

---

[162] For example, *see* the story of Sarah and her earlobe tear, in *Changing the Body – Actual Stories* (p. 405, below).

tension and freezing in response to communication, all of which would be gathered bottom-up, in order to integrate the body image.

The greatest obstacle to treatment appears to be the fact that "re-experiencing trauma symptoms is an involuntary process" (Zepinic, 2017, p. 2061), which may involve any or all of the following: 1) lack of self-awareness, 2) affect without recollection (impulse drive), 3) memory fragmentation, and 4) occurrence of "spontaneously intrusive memories" which the individual is interpreting and to which the individual is attributing meanings (Ibid.). The occurrence of hyperstimulation through the senses (smell, color, sound) is something which takes the affected individual by surprise and revives the trauma. Intentional recall is therefore difficult because unintentional, fragmented imagery may appear. This leads to rumination, thought suppression, dissociation, and various safety-seeking behaviors, with which professionals dealing with chronic PTSD are wholly familiar.

Trauma-focused therapies involve associative learning and perceptual priming, triggering memories and matching cues, in order to: 1) explain behaviors and emotions, 2) prevent avoidance and reappraisals (e.g. hypervigilance to threat, belief that trauma is inevitable), 3) increase in direct symptoms (feelings of insecurity), and 4) avert needlessly dwelling on the traumatic event (e.g. grief, rumination).

Body Image and Pain

Trauma is invariably associated with pain. Pain may be psychological as well as physical. In fact, studies show that both psychological and physical pain leave the same imprint in the human brain (Condor-Fisher, 2021; MacDonald & Leary, 2005; Mee et al., 2007; Weinstein, 2009); although pain is perceived differently, depending on its type, and the individual appraisal of its duration and intensity (Rainville, 2002). Neuroimaging studies in chronic pain patients show that brain activity, "especially in cortical and mesolimbic regions," is different from "activity observed during acute pain" (Becker et al., 2018). Further, the pattern of activity within the anterior cingulate cortex and other classical limbic structures is similar in all human beings. This means that the body-schema and body image may undergo permanent deformation as a result of chronic pain, whether psychological or physical. Neuroimaging further evidenced that endogenous mechanisms[163] modulate pain. This finding may be key to dealing with trauma (see below).

The affective and sensory components of pain often function independently of each other. Thus, a painful event, such as a surgery or auto accident, may have a delayed onset of mental pain or, conversely, the mental pain may come in anticipation of a traumatic event or events (e.g., cancer treatment, loss of a loved one). Thresholds for pain are also highly individual: some people perceive ostracism and bullying as extremely painful and traumatic, while others will seamlessly shrug it off. For the same reason, even a partial body image fragmentation or dissonance may cause great affect in some individuals, while leaving others

---

[163] Mechanisms which exist in the organism, as opposed to mechanisms existing outside the body (exogenous). Endogenous mechanisms of self-protection and self-repair block pathophysiological processes that lead to neurodegeneration.

unscarred. It should be emphasized that even a small pain, but of long duration, especially where there is no resolution in sight, may become unbearable. It little matters whether such pain is mental (grief, BDD, gender dysphoria, etc.) or physical (e.g., MS, cancer, chronic injury).

Mee et al. (2007) noted that "I can't stand the pain any longer" is among the most frequent explanations found in suicide notes. The "torment of psychological pain" may make it seem that suicide is the only solution (p. 681). Body image dysmorphic disorders, depressive disorders, physical, as well as psychological pain and severe trauma are closely related (Ibid.). Pain intensity and body integrity correlate and are causally related to depression, and to subsequent body image dissatisfaction.

Animal studies revealed that ascending nociceptive (pain perception related) and descending modulatory pathways "play a critical role in the modulation of pain" (Rainville, 2002, p. 195). This means that the motivation to deal with pain caused by trauma, whether physical or mental, is key to its resolution. Somewhat paradoxically, this requires an increased focus on the pain, thus also on the painful body part which causes or significantly contributes to negative body image. This is paradoxical at first because, in the short run, it increases the preoccupation with pain, thus increasing the pain itself. However, the focus must be positive, i.e., the pain is a sign of healing (the body speaks to the soul), not negative, i.e., taking the pain as a (perhaps necessary) evil.

In the long run, what is needed is to achieve mastery and self-regulation. Hence the so-called *mind-body therapies* have taken center stage in recent years (Astin, 2004; Daubenmier, 2005; Gard et al., 2019; Oswald et al., 2017; Todd et al., 2019). Gard et al. (2019) listed the following positive effects of the Basic Body Awareness Therapy (BBAT) used in the Nordic European countries: increased overall health, and improved self-efficacy, increased use of functional coping strategies, reduction in musculoskeletal symptoms, reduction in posttraumatic stress disorders, anxiety, depression, eating disorders, and mitigation of the comorbid mental illness. It should be noted that mind-body awareness is applied across the board in virtually all sports, in order to improve efficiency, movement awareness and quality, and to improve contact with the body. In non-athletes, mere focus on the correct posture, balance, breathing, and coordination by performing "simple movements and exercises during stillness and action" have been noted to significantly improve body image dissonance associated with pain (p. 3). Exercises are performed without weights, using gravity, in order to ground the body and establish body ownership, which is key to a healthy body image and self-mastery.

In conjunction with body-mind awareness exercises, psychologists use *journalling,* which basically means writing down confidential statements, messages, and narratives about one's pain. Researchers found that expressing trauma in writing strengthens the body's immune functions and improves overall health (Rakel, 2007). In fact, there is an entire branch of literary canon which originated not in fantasy and amusement, but from dealing with personal trauma. Not all such literature is bad, as fans of Eugene O'Neil and Tennessee Williams may attest to, but all of it is weighty, emotional, interlaced with rumination, and pregnant with thought, literally *embodying* the suffering of the author. Needless to say, all writing purifies and organizes one's thoughts, and it may even bring about the much-needed closure to a distressing psychological event, which may have been the cause of extreme physical pain, leading to body image disintegration. Hence, many gurus in treating pain suggest that the individual commence by confiding the malaise of the moment into a personal journal.

Exhibitionism and Gymnophobia

Exhibitionism and gymnophobia are manifestations of body dysmorphia. While trauma need not always be their source, fragmented body image, and disintegrated self-concept are often either part of etiology or solely responsible for the associated display of paraphilias which invariably affect feelings about one's naked body. Non-exhaustively, these paraphilias[164] include: *actirasty* (excitement from the exposure to sunrays), *alloerasty* (using nudity of another person to arouse one's partner), *nudomania* and *omolagnia* (arousal from nudity).

Exhibitionism is an "uncontrollable urge to exhibit one's genitals to an unsuspecting stranger" (Aggrawal, 2015, p. 1). The urge must be recurrent, long-lasting, and marked by a form of personal distress or "interpersonal difficulty" (DSM-IV-TR 302.4.B). Exhibitionism is a form of obsessive compulsive disorder, also belonging to the class of paraphilias listed above.

While *gymnophobia*, which is the fear or anxiety of being seen naked, "even in situations where it is socially acceptable" (Ibid.) is commonly cited as the opposite of exhibitionism, the etiology of both disorders reflects deficicncics in the body image acceptance and formation often stemming from trauma. The differences lie in outward manifestations of the inner disorder. However, the disorders themselves may overlap, or even appear to be identical.

Both gymnophobia and exhibitionism arise from feelings of inadequacy, often in comparison to the images idealized in the media, and in the community of one's peers. Marginalized communities, such as LGBTQIA+ may be affected by these disorders more than population in general, simply because of their need for belongingness, and

---

[164] The word *paraphilia* is derived from Greek παρά [para] "beside" and φιλία [philia] 'friendship, love."

association with various sub- and counter-cultures, some of whom may extol these disorders as forms of cultural counter-protests (e.g., naked bike-ride parades in the first case, and various forms of body disguise in the painted productions of unholy "Sisters of Indulgence" in the latter[165]). What these disorders have in common is an unhealthy relationship with the self (frequently including acts of self-deprecation, self-denigration, and self-hatred), hence the use of the naked body as a purportedly soulless tool of revenge and instrument of inflicting fear in others.

The etiology of these two disorders is likewise not unconnected. Attempts to contact a partner or being mentally "stuck in" the precontact mating stage of courtship has been cited as one of the key causal factors (Morin & Levenson, 2008; Tichý, P., 1996). Body-self disturbances projected in these paraphiliac behaviors may also be associated with monoamine receptor malfunction,[166] and Huntington's disease,[167] which points at disturbances in the brain-stem nuclei, as well as at the cerebral cortex, consequently affecting the "feeling of knowing" one's self, and the formation of integrative maps of the self (Damasio, 2010, p. 205).

---

[165] Satanism is a cult which inverts Christian norms, thus also the foundations of Western civilization. It represents the "alienated, anxious, and powerless" who hope to obtain some "magical power and control over their destiny" (Ivey, 1993, p. 180).

[166] Quinn et al. (1983) noted that patients suffering from Parkinson's disease who were treated with Sinemet (levodopa, metabolic precursor of dopamine), and bromocriptine or pergolide (dopamine receptor agonists), experienced an uncontrollable urge to undress in public as well as masochistic tendencies.

[167] Huntington's disease (HD) is an "autosomal-dominant, progressive neurodegenerative disorder with a distinct phenotype, including chorea and dystonia, incoordination, cognitive decline, and behavioural [sic] difficulties" (Walker, 2007, p. 218). Why exactly HD patients display pathological exhibitionistic tendencies is unknown, but the body image dissociation and fragmentation is marked here as clearly comorbid.

Psychoanalysts have hypothesized that castration anxiety may be the primal cause of paraphiliac behavior, whether it be exhibitionism, gymnophobia, or other abnormal forms of obtaining arousal. Arguably, this would explain the disorders in the male only. However, when the impetus is seen as that of the need to belong, coupled with self-affirmation (i.e., "Here are my sexual organs! I am what you can see!"), then the original anxiety may be imputed to body image disturbance in both males and females.[168] Exhibitionists do not always achieve arousal by displaying their sexual organs. For example, a transsexual female displaying her breasts in public as an apparent form of social protest is, in fact, displaying her most vulnerable identity, which had been hidden from social acceptance for most of her life. Conversely, in gymnophobia, an argument can be advanced that the individual is hiding his or her identity and body image for the same reasons, i.e., either the fear of castration, or fear of the naked display of it – because it is the most vulnerable part of the body.

Perhaps a more acceptable psychological analysis of the underlying etiology is the one which argues that some individuals who were abused and traumatized as children tend to re-enact the acts of traumatization and sexual violence which, in exhibitionism, takes place in public, whereby the individual seeks to overcome the feelings of low self-esteem, shame, and inadequacy. Exposing genitals "thus becomes a sexualized form of *countershame*" intended to display power and to create control over the observer

---

[168] An even more Freudian explanation would be that by publicly displaying their "mutilated" genitalia, the females are threatening the males with the same fate (Aggrawal, 2015). Before completely dismissing this hypothesis, one should recall Sheela-na-Gigs (Sheelas), the figures of naked women "displaying an exaggerated vulva, found on churches, castles, and other buildings, particularly in Ireland and Britain dating from 12th century" (p. 1). These are said to impart a religious warning against the "sins of the flesh." Any distinction between a "warning" and a "threat" is that of degree, not intent.

(Aggrawal, Id.) [emphasis added]. In the same light, gymnophobia, interpreted as an attempt to hide the body from the potential trauma, may appear to be more natural – but many historians and kinanthropologists would argue otherwise, i.e., that the shame of nakedness is the result of the Christian dogma, not a natural state of being.

Homoeroticism and homosexual tendencies have also been cited as causal factors here. If one neither has nor craves a partner of the opposite sex, being relegated to masturbation and the pleasures of one's own body, it is not inconceivable that the homoerotic tendencies would then occur as an extension of self-love, i.e., love of the same body, whether projected outward in public or actually practiced in private. Aggrawal (Ibid.) noted that both homosexual men and exhibitionists often display *automonosexualism*, a phenomenon in which the individual is sexually excited by his own body (often simply by being nude). There appears to be no reason to make a different conclusion in cases of female homosexuality.

McGuire et al. (1964) suggested that sexually deviant behavior is a conditioned behavior and may thus be induced. Individuals with overlapping body dysmorphic disorders or paraphilias may behave similarly when part of the same subculture and conditioned to do so by the dominant elements of that subculture. This would imply that conditioning and behavioral therapy could be used to disengage the systems that lead to such behavior. However, it should be noted that not all such behavior is pathological or contains an underlying sexual motive.

Obesity and Fitness Enhancement

Obesity is a worldwide problem, related primarily to poor diet habits and inadequate exercise. Obesity is also correlated with dieting, psychiatric morbidity, and eating disorders (Patton et al., 1999). It is the main cause of chronic diseases, such as diabetes, hypertension, cardiac disease, and cancer. Obese individuals, irrespective of age and gender, also consistently report negative self-esteem, and body image dissatisfaction (Goldfield et al., 2010). There is, however, a significant difference in gender with respect to weight estimation. Chang and Christakis (2003) found that 27.5% of women and 29.8% of men "misclassified their own weight status by medical standards" (p. 332). The difference was in the opposite directions: while the women of normal weight (factoring in age and height) tended to overestimate their weight, men who were medically overweight thought they were "about the right weight" or "underweight" (Ibid.).

There also exists a documented comorbidity between obesity and body image dissatisfaction, in particular among women. Weinberger at al. (2017) found this relationship to be "complex," dependent on many individual factors (p. 424), including "age, marital status, race, income, and education" (Chang & Christakis, 2003, Ibid.). It is the self-perception of obesity (or lack thereof) that dictates long-term psychological success, manifested by congruence of the body and the image. Needless to say, such congruence is not always present, not even where there has been a marked physical improvement. In other words, many obese individuals will not achieve long-term body image satisfaction even when they have achieved a lasting weight loss.

Conversely, Martin and Lichtenberger (2004) documented significant appearance related positive changes associated with exercise and "improved fitness" (p. 405). These changes take place regardless of actual body image changes. In other words, exercise and fitness contribute to mental well-being even in people who go to the gym every day, lack instruction or exercise structure, often do not know how to work the machines but, rather than educate themselves or hire a personal trainer, move around haphazardly imitating others – even in such seemingly ludicrously acting individuals, whose body has not changed over years of regular gym attendance, important secondary appearance-related positive changes will take place, improving their body image. Improvement in physical fitness, such as stamina and endurance, are not always tangible in muscle mass, mainly because they utilize red muscle fiber; nevertheless, overall conditioning significantly enhances self-efficacy, and thus self-esteem, which is then reflected in a more positive body image. What is more, such improvement is achieved whether "real or imagined," as long as it is *perceived* by the individual as *"personally meaningful"* (p. 416) [italics original].

This corresponds to the finding that women overestimated their attractiveness "in the cosmetics-present condition" (with makeup on), and underestimated it when without makeup (Cash, 1990, p. 69). What is more, the more makeup women wore, the better they felt about themselves which, Cash postulated, shows that "cosmetics make a positive difference on self-image as well as on social-image" (Ibid.). At the same time, contrary to the male perceivers, female perceivers did not grade women's appearance differently whether with or without makeup. Research also showed that it was the women concerned with attentional self-focus and body image focus, women who were "more feminine on a particular measure of sex-role identity" – a measure reflecting histrionic emotionality and the need for social approval and attention – that engaged in "aesthetic self-management with cosmetics" to a greater degree than their peers (p. 70).

The gym is a place of social cohabitation where many people show up, in order to boost their self-image, and find commonality of purpose, as well as a sense of safety (belongingness). Notice the chest and arms revealing shirts, make-up, tights, manicured nails, etc. Even the conduct of these self-professed "gym rats" is manifest in self-assurance and self-esteem: men bubble with muscle power, women pass from machine to machine in catwalk fashion, eyeing themselves in the mirror walls. From the accoutrements and clothing, to the mood and muscle-enhancing substances, everything revolves around body image. Interestingly, the same placebo effect one achieves from merely entering and cohabiting in this environment, and dressing in the like fashion, has been found to exist from the use (or non-use, rather) of performance enhancing substances. What is more, studies have shown that even a placebo effect (perceived effect from getting better, dressing in a certain way, going to the gym – while the body remains the same) may not only lead to the perception enhancement, but may be actually performance enhancing. Maganaris et al. (1999) showed such effect with powerlifters, Foster et al. (2004) with cyclists, and Jackson (1995) proved that the state of *flow*[169] is a controllable state dependent on self-confidence, motivation, and arousal level, as well as on measurable factors, such as preparation and training.

Paradoxically, therefore, physical exercise *for body image* should focus not on improving one's body image (imitating a bodybuilding ideal, measuring the circumference of one's arms or waist, or taking weight at regular times, marking these data in a journal, as bodybuilders frequently do) but, rather, physical exercise

---

[169] *Flow* is a state of absolute abandonment in the activity, total focus and complete concentration. Athletes are familiar with it also under the term or phrase of being *in the Zone*. The term was coined by the cofounder of Positive Psychology, Mihalyi Csikszentmihalyi (1990, 2002, 2014).

should focus on improving strength and endurance, which leads to the improvement in self-esteem and, therefore, one's body image. This means that short workouts, focused on *perceived* ability to perform, execute movements with weight, as well as high intensity training for cardio purposes, will have a more marked and meaningful effect on the body image than any form of exercise which focuses primarily on what the body looks like.[170]

---

[170] HIT, High Intensity Training, also known as HIIT, High Intensity Interval Training, consists of short bouts of high intensity performance (90% heartbeat rate), usually not more than five minutes, and an equal period of rest (50-60% heartbeat rate), for the overall length 20-60 minutes. The HIIT workouts burn more calories than traditional aerobic workouts because of the extended post-exercise period, referred to as EPOC, which stands for Excess Postexercise Oxygen Consumption: for about 2-3 hours after the HIIT workout, the body consumes more oxygen and up to 15% more calories at rest.

Body Image Workout

Following the analysis and conclusions above, it is clear that both sarcoplasmic and myofibrillar sets are needed for overall body image improvement. Powerlifters focus on *myofibrillar hypertrophy*, which means multiplying the number of myofibrils in the muscle by training hard, heavy, in the low rep range. Endurance athletes focus on multiple sets and reps, in order to increase endurance and, arguably, *sarcoplasmic hypertrophy*. Bodybuilders do both, in order to achieve mass, vascularity, and eliminate excessive fat. The latter, sarcoplasmic hypertrophy, is somewhat of a misnomer because the muscle does not really increase in volume long-term, only temporarily. Bodybuilders understand that it is in the process of temporary sarcoplasmic oxygenation and absorption of fast carbs when the muscle gets pumped backstage, immediately before the contest.

In order to better understand the composition of the workout, some fundamental terms describing the human muscle must be explained: individual bundles of muscle fibers are referred to as *fascicles*. The cell membrane surrounding the muscle cell is called the *sarcolemma*, and beneath the sarcolemma lies the *sarcoplasm*, which contains the cellular proteins, organelles, and myofibrils.

Myofibrils are composed of two major types of protein filaments: the thinner *actin* filament, and the thicker *myosin* filament. The arrangement of these two protein filaments gives skeletal muscle its striated appearance. For practical purposes, whatever is not myofibrillar in the muscle, is sarcoplasmic (see below).

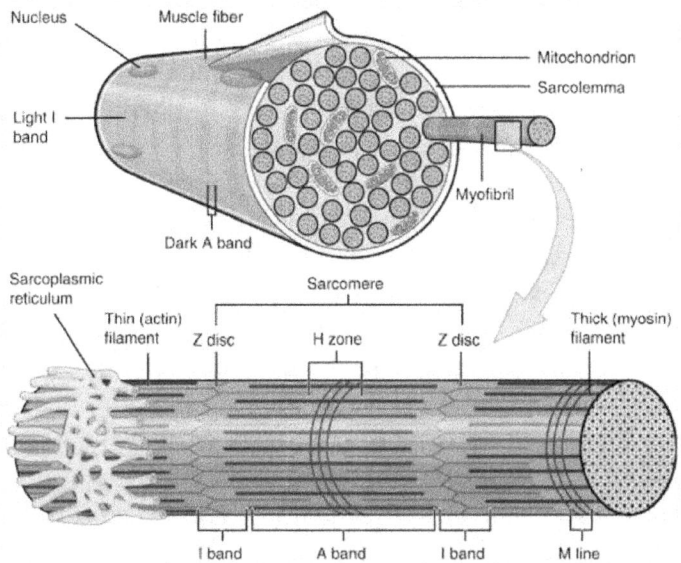

All human beings are born with a certain proportion of red and white muscle fibers. What is more, the proportion of these fibers differs from muscle to muscle in every single individual. Red muscle has a greater concentration of the pigment myoglobin (which is why it is red), while being lower in soluble protein content and glycogen. Red fibers are smaller in size than white fibers, are "better supplied with capillaries, and contain more mitochondria" (Cassens & Cooper, 1971, p. 2).

On the other hand, white fibers are better equipped for glycolytic metabolism, have a greater calcium-binding ability, and a higher ATPase activity.[171] White muscle fibers have faster twitch (reaction) but get quickly tired. They are

---

[171] ATPases are large macromolecular biological catalyst enzymes that catalyze the hydrolysis from ATP to ADP. As the enzyme hydrolyzes ATP, it yields a free phosphate ion, ADP, and energy. The reaction proceeds slowly (if at all) in the absence of enzyme, but proceeds well in the presence of the ATPase.

referred to as FT, fast-twitch fibers. Red fibers are referred to as ST, slow-twitch fibers. They are high in oxidative enzymes, such as SDH,[172] but low in glycolytic enzymes, such as phosphorylase, as well as low in ATPase, while "the opposite is the case for the white fibers.

Studies revealed not only that competitive endurance athletes have more ST than FT fibers and sprinters more FT than ST fibers, but also that the proportion of these fibers can be altered by exercise (Costill et al. 1976; Saltin et al. 1977). This alteration can be significant, although inborn proportion of FT:ST ratio is also undeniable, which is why some people appear to have a "talent" for long-distance events and others seem to be born for sprint. It is much easier to foster and increase the inborn ratio than reverse it, that is to make a sprinter out of a natural long-distance runner, versus vice versa. This proportion exists regardless of sex (i.e., there are "born" female sprinters and "born" female long-distance runners, just as there are male ones). Any body image-oriented exercise plan should take this into account. Mastery and ultimate body image satisfaction will be achieved faster if the natural propensities of the individual are followed.

Therefore, while it can be generically stated that a positive body image change will be easier to achieve in men when myofibrillar growth is stimulated, it may not always be so. Men who are born "long-distance" ectomorphs, may acquire mastery and improve self-esteem in workouts that preference sarcoplasmic growth. Generally, however, rapid gains in muscle mass through myofibrillar growth will be

---

[172] Succinate dehydrogenase (SDH) is part of both the citric acid cycle and respiratory electron transfer chain. Within the citric acid cycle, SDH oxidizes succinate (a salt or ester of succinic acid) to fumarate. Fumarate is an intermediate in the citric acid cycle used by cells to produce energy in the form of adenosine triphosphate (ATP). It is formed by the oxidation of succinate by the enzyme succinate dehydrogenase. Fumarate is then converted by the enzyme fumarase to malate.

more suitable for women than men. Since over 3,000 genes have been "identified as being differentially expressed between male and female skeletal muscle," it is safe to assume that there are inborn differences which should be reflected in the approach to training by personal trainers (Haizlip et al., 2015, p. 30). Consequently, gym workouts for body image enhancement in men should incorporate at least one pyramid set for a major muscle group per workout, which will follow the warm-up set. The pyramid set should look as follows. Let us take the squat as an example:

15 reps with 25% bodyweight
12 reps with 50% bodyweight
9 reps with 75% bodyweight
6 reps with 100% bodyweight
3 reps with 125% bodyweight
1-2 reps with 150% bodyweight
6 reps with 100% bodyweight
MAX reps with 50% bodyweight

The first two sets, and the last one can be characterized as sarcoplasmic, while the remainder is primarily myofibrillar. This exercise should be preceded by a warm-up exercise, such as leg extensions, and followed by a muscle-group specific exercise, such as narrow hack squats or lunges for the outer quads. The number of sets depends mainly on the fitness level of the individual. Obviously, other factors, such as age, and the potential for injury should also be considered.

Myofibrillar sets are not as crucial in female development as in the male muscle development, although it should be emphasized to them that muscle mass increases basal metabolism (burning of fat), and that it is virtually impossible for an average woman to acquire the muscle mass of an average man, unless the woman specifically trains with this end in mind (e.g., powerlifting) and possibly also uses performance enhancing drugs. While female muscle has the same structure as the male muscle, the female muscle has fewer myofibrils and is more prone to sarcoplasmic growth (relative to body weight and size), given the same conditions and workouts. This means that in women, self-mastery is achieved faster by multiple sets and reps, thereby leading to enhanced endurance and improved perceptions of self-competence and self-reliance, the key assets in addressing BD and related conditions. An average female workout will thus contain more exercises per muscle group, and each exercise will be composed of multiple sets with no more than the individual's bodyweight.

Mastery and body image improvement in females is not induced when the female athlete compares against a male athlete in workout. It follows that females should have a female spotter and males a male spotter, and if the trainer is of the opposite gender, he or she should approach the workout on a highly individualized basis, with the trainee's sex, age, ability, experience, and FT:ST ratio in mind.

For females, the sets cited above should be limited to bodyweight and although the pyramid is also useful, stimulating myofibrillar growth, it should be flat on top, consisting of 3 sets of bodyweight to failure.

For both men and women, each individual workout should not exceed one hour and the number of exercises should not be more than 6 per large body-part (e.g., latissimus) and 3 per small one (e.g., biceps). Stretching and yoga are crucial because individuals with body image issues always need to improve their body-mind connection which is achieved primarily during contractions in the actual workout (the peak contraction) and in extensions during warm-ups, warm-downs, and stretching. Off days should always contain stretching and some activity which does not involve the gym.

Body Image Diet

Assuming that most body image concerned people are either extremely conscious of what they eat, or follow some diet plan that they researched online, or studied nutrition and feel fairly competent in the area, the following advice is tailored for those less knowledgeable. The former are advised to think of food as an enjoyable, social activity, not a drudge or command under the whip of some invisible blond-haired, gray eyed sadomasochistic chef. Try to experiment with ingredients and when you use "forbidden ones" (such as butter or cream), simply factor in the extra calories when you eat, and lower the portions accordingly. Never avoid meals, seek them. One meal out of order in a week does not throw even the best of the best off balance. To the contrary, the body is satiated and feels no need to expect another week of starvation and suffering. It is a complex mechanism but works on some very fundamental principles which are not difficult to grasp.

Eating for body image means eating with discretion, confusing the body, not denying it supply of healthy nutrients but, rather, eating with measure and moderation. One who eats healthy is looking forward to every meal, but does not need to think about it all the time. Eat to live, do not live to eat. Even those who are busy in their occupations can stick to the principles of Body Image Diet, described below:

1) Never allow yourself to starve. Always have something, even when you are at work or on the road. One apple or banana will do. Find a snack which is rich in complex carbohydrates, or make one.
2) Purposeful fasting is not starvation. This is usually applied in conjunction with the Keto Diet which means diet rich in fats, wherein fewer meals are consumed which contain a sufficient supply of calories in fats, such as MCT and CLA oils.

391

3) Unless you stick with the Keto Diet (wherein up to 60 percent of calories are consumed in the form of fatty acids), think of the macronutrients as 40-40, carbohydrates to protein ratio, in which case fat takes care of itself. Do not consciously combine carbs and fat, and minimize simple carbs. It is also not a good idea to combine starchy and fibrous carbs (as they do when they serve you raisins on the salad when you are eating out). The reasons are beyond the scope of this book to explain but have to do with digestion and enzymatic processes.
4) Take 15 calories per pound of bodyweight when you are working out, 12 when you are not working out.
5) Eat 6 times a day (a small snack is a meal).
6) Never consume more than 50% of your calorie intake in some artificial form, be it protein shakes or bars.
7) Never limit your carbs to zero, because then you would be consuming your muscle tissue for energy. Muscle burns fat, you need muscle.
8) Learn all about the glycemic index and know the glycemic index of the carbs you consume, so that you understand how long they will last for energy, how much they will weigh down your system, potentially causing insulin spikes.
9) Do not weigh yourself more than once a week under the same conditions (empty, in the morning). In fact, even once a week is too often as you can only effectively lose or gain 1-2 pounds a week – any more than that is either water (bloating) or added fat, or, when losing weight, muscle tissue and water.
10) Avoid social media exposure to unhealthy models, unproductive discussions, and unachievable beauty or muscle standards. Stay natural. Stay yourself. Love yourself.
11) Avoid the use of diuretics at all times. They kill your kidneys.

Ketogenic Diet

The ketogenic diet has become increasingly popular in recent years, hence it deserves a few words here. This diet, commonly referred to as Keto, was created by Russell Wilder in 1921 as a treatment for epilepsy. After about ten years of use, it was replaced by anti-epileptic drugs and not widely used or known until its recent rediscovery by nutritionists and bodybuilders. The keto diet consists primarily of fat and protein, typically 60% fat, 35% protein, and 10% carbohydrates (Ayele et al., 2023). This diet works by creating a state called "physiologic ketosis" and, although its "exact effect on the body is unclear," what is well-known is that when the natural glucose production from carbohydrates is not met, the body resorts to manufacturing glucose endogenously (Ibid.). During ketosis, acetoacetate is produced as a result of the metabolism of fatty acids. Acetoacetate is broken down into acetone and beta-hydroxybutyrate, increasing the level of ketone bodies which are then used for energy. Ketone bodies are generated normally but in low amounts, without changing the pH levels of the blood – as opposed to ketoacidosis, in which a significant increase in ketone body production causes high acidic shift in the blood's pH levels (Masood et al., 2022). This diet has been found effective by many, but should definitely not be followed long-term (over 4-6 weeks).

For example, Ayele et al. (2023) cited a case of a 36-year-old female, hospitalized for "persistent nausea and vomiting, along with fatigue and malaise." She was on a ketogenic diet and lost over 30 pounds in 2 months (which in itself is extreme and strongly indicates that ED and BDD were present). Her diet consisted of eggs, beef, avocado, chicken, and peanuts. She had no history of hypertension, diabetes, or kidney disease. As a result of the keto diet, she suffered an acute kidney injury and cholelithiasis.[173] She was given IV fluids and supportive care, and recovered in less than a week to normal.

Some researchers have alleged that the keto diet leads to hyperlipidemia, vitamin and mineral deficiencies, fatigue, and kidney damage, among other complications (Joshi et al., 2019). The rationale is that the increased acid production triggers metabolic acidosis and weakens bone health (Masood et al., Id.). Combined with high protein diet, some studies have reported that increased fatty acids result in a high phosphate content, gut microbiome dysbiosis, and inflammation. Experimental rat studies showed that "increasing the protein dose increased the expression of proinflammatory genes" and, in pig models, "consuming a high-protein diet over a long period resulted in 55% more renal fibrosis and 30% more glomerulosclerosis" (Ayele et al., Ibid.). When used in the pediatric epilepsy community, ketogenic diet caused nephrolithiasis.[174]

On the other hand, Torres et al. (2019) found that ketosis ameliorates polycystic kidney disease (PKD) and causes regression of renal cysts. In the experiments Torres et al. conducted rats were given unrestricted access to a high-fat, very-low-carbohydrate (caloric ratio of 91% fat, 2% carbohydrates, and 5% protein), and compared to animals with the same access to non-keto diet (caloric ratio of 62% carbohydrates, 25% protein, and 13% fat). The keto group marked a "remarkable reduction in the 2-kidney to body weight," as well as a reduction in the cystic area (cysts literally shrank and burst), decreased blood glucose, and

---

[173] Cholelithiasis or gallstones are hardened deposits of digestive fluid that can form in the gallbladder.

[174] Nephrolithiasis is the medical term for kidney stones (also known as *renal calculi*).

increased BHB levels (p. 1013). They initially attributed these results to the almost complete decrease in protein intake. However, further experiments showed that the results were mainly due to time restricted food intake (TRF). Fasting 12-15 hours a day induces ketosis, which increases the output of BHB, consequently reducing kidney and heart disease. Even supplementation with artificial BHB has produced similar results (Quigley, 2020). Animals treated with BHB for five weeks had the PKD significantly reduced, there was a commensurate reduction in the 2-kidney to body weight ratio, the cystic area, and kidney fibrosis (almost complete elimination of myofibroblasts, improved kidney function, and inhibition of proliferation).

In conclusion, ketosis causes a radical shift of fuel source: 1) decrease in glucose, 2) increase in fatty acids, and (3) increase in ketones. In particular, in PKD patients, the cystic cells flourish on glucose. Once glucose is eliminated, they shrink, burst, and die away. Keto diet of five weeks has shown an altered cellular metabolism, beneficial to the whole body (decrease in blood sugar levels, heart pressure, cardiovascular health, and kidney disease). However, researchers cautioned that the studies on which these conclusions were made were conducted in rats, not in humans (Bae et al., 2016; Newman & Verdin, 2017; Rojas-Morales et al., 2016; Torres et al., 2019). The studies in rats experimented with diets extremely high in fats and low in protein, which is not the case when the keto diet is utilized by humans. Therefore, a word of caution is still in order here: the ketogenic diet ought to be implemented in conjunction with regular blood testing, limited to 5 weeks, upon which a period of low protein diet should follow, in order to prevent potential chronic liver and kidney damage.

Body Image and Eating Disorders

A recent worldwide survey revealed that the incidence of eating disorders (ED) has risen by about 5% in the last ten years. Stice et al. (2013) noted that 13% of women suffer from ED. Lifetime prevalence estimates of DSM-IV anorexia nervosa, bulimia nervosa, and binge eating disorder are .9%, 1.5%, and 3.5% among women, and .3% .5%, and 2.0% among men. All 3 eating disorders are comorbid (associated with each other, and with other disorders). Further, lifetime anorexia nervosa (AN) correlates to low weight (body-mass index <18.5), while lifetime binge eating disorder (BD) is associated with "severe obesity," defined as BMI over 40 (Hudson et al., 2007, p. 348). Evidence further indicates that disordered eating behavior is associated with Obsessive-Compulsive Disorder (OCD) and that both bear similar pathologies: an intense preoccupation with a particular stimulus, a particular food, weight, or shape, and contamination (in OCD); all elicit "negative affects followed by compensatory behavior" (e.g., purging in BD or washing hands in OCD), in order to reduce the negative affect (Altman and Shankman, 2009).

Kaye et al. (2004) found that the rates of most anxiety disorders were similar in all three subtypes of eating disorders, with two-thirds of the ED individuals suffering from one or more lifetime anxiety disorders. The most common were "obsessive-compulsive disorder (OCD) (41%) and social phobia (20%)" (p. 2215). Significantly, anxiety disorders invariably preceded the onset of eating disorders. They were found to also follow the ED diagnosis, making the subjects more prone to succumb to ED again. It can therefore be concluded not only that OCD, social phobia, specific phobia, and generalized anxiety disorder in childhood predict the development of ED in future, but also that a history of an eating disorder makes the individual more "anxious, perfectionistic, and harm avoidant" (Ibid.).

Phobic, fearful, and anxious individuals should therefore be cognizant of the fact that they are more susceptible to eating disorders than the general population (as should their parents and loved ones). Low self-esteem is also correlated to ED, such as low esteem during childhood predicts a development of ED in adulthood (Doris et al., 2014). As everywhere, an ounce of prevention is worth a pound of cure here too. Prevention in individuals prone to ED should consist of a stable daily routine, including regular measured meals, and exercise. Acquiring good habits also boosts self-esteem and personal security in a fearful individual who may be prone to phobias. Loose, unstable, or partially fragmented body image makes these individuals susceptible to internalizing negative outside influences and criticism, coming from their peers, social circles, mass, and social media. It is therefore crucial that the individual be instructed to avoid negative exposure to such stimuli, consciously evading social media platforms that expose them to dieting, body perfectionism, as well as targeted commercials that use various forms of skinny (or excessively muscular) body images.

Where the body image input is primarily cognitive (as is the case in the individuals afflicted with various forms of ED), not perceptual or sensual, the most effective treatment requires gradual restructuring of the cognitive matrix by redefining what the "body" means, what it means to be the "right weight" versus "thin" or "obese," and accepting the fact that no human possesses only one body image at all times (as well as the fact that a "perfect" body image is truly unachievable). The individual must consciously start avoiding self-defeating practices, such as weighing, looking in the mirror, compulsively exercising, and engaging in artful masking of their perceived defects (Garner, 2004). This will not happen overnight but only step-by-step, akin to stretching or exercising with weights during which the muscle and tendons and ligaments gradually accommodate and acquire a new "muscle memory."

Individuals prone to ED should also avoid dieting.[175] Dieting is a predictor of AN and BD, causes an increase in BD, and predicts the onset of depression (Stice, 2004). The negative affect associated with ED then feeds into the negative body image, thus creating a vicious circle. Patton et al. (1999) found that women who adhered to a strict diet "were 18 times more likely to develop an eating disorder" than those who did not diet, while those who dieted "at a moderate level" were 5 times more likely to develop an eating disorder than those who did not diet (p. 765). Psychiatric morbidity[176] predicted the onset of ED "independently of dieting status," with subjects suffering from a psychiatric disorder being seven times as likely to develop ED (Ibid.). Batista et al. (2018) further found that a "general psychological maladjustment" is the best predictor of ED, followed by "females with higher thin-ideal internalization" (p. 399).

This internalization can be prevented by intervention. Posavac et al. (2001) documented that even a brief targeted intervention prior to media exposure to the "thin ideal" achieved the desired effect of de-internalization of the ideal. Posavac et al. (Id.) used three experimental targeted interventions, each "with the goal of leading women to define media images of female beauty as dissimilar to others, and therefore inappropriate comparison targets" (p.

---

[175] ED studies consider dieting as either or combination of the following: counting calories, reducing food quantities at meals, skipping meals. eating healthy, avoiding excessive fats, and excessive calories per se is not dieting. However, eating "healthy" to the point of orthorexia (viz.), when one is limited in social contact and cohabitation by food, is.

[176] Psychiatric morbidity is a mental illness, characterized by a behavioral or intellectual impairment in functioning which causes some distress or impairment in the life of the individual. It may arise from a single traumatic episode, but may also occur continually, or on a relapsing and remitting basis.

328). Each intervention consisted of a videotape of a psychologist speaking about the specific topic of the intervention. The experimental interventions consisted of "Artificial Beauty," "Genetic Realties," and "Combination" messages (Ibid.). The researchers found that, compared with participants who did not receive an experimental intervention before media exposure, participants who received an experimental intervention were less likely to: engage in social comparison, be concerned about their weight, make a "Negative-Self statement or Drive for Thinness statement" (p. 337).

Since all eating disorders are multifactorial in nature, they have to be approached with multiple factors in mind and an eye keen on comorbid conditions. Apart from the avoidance of external factors, such as media pressure and social media exposure, and the treatment of a potential related psychiatric comorbidity, such as OED, the treatment should focus on empathy because individuals with ED (in particular AN patients) have been found lacking in cognitive empathy (ability to recognize and understand mental states of others). This, in turn, affects their emotional regulation and social relations (Davies et al., 2013).[177] Meanwhile, their affective empathy (ability to share feelings) remains untouched, and may even surpass the norm, which makes them particularly susceptible to uncontrolled emotional flow without understanding what and why is happening. In other words, they are not in touch with their bodies. Negative affect is further associated with negative information bias, resulting in a negatively skewed body image and susceptibility to outside influences – which can, sometimes, be for their general betterment but, more often than not, are misdirected and harm them. Directed therapies, involving

---

[177] Empathy is the ability to recognize the feelings in others, the ability to relate to others and to partake in their emotional experience. Cognitive empathy means the cognitive comprehension of feelings. Affective empathy means the observer's emotional response to affect in others.

meditation, yoga, dance, focus on body sensations, exploring various forms of artistic expression… should all be used with all ED individuals.

Finally, Yager et al. (2006) emphasized the importance of "core attitudes regarding weight, shape, and eating" in the family, including alcohol and substance abuse, family history of obesity, and interactions which may perpetuate and undermine potentially all clinical efforts to cure the ED (p. 12). On the other hand, where removal from the environment is not possible, the intervenor should avoid casting blame on other family members, as this may also be detrimental to the patient's care and recovery. The stressors may affect the whole family or microsphere that the individual inhabits which may require careful monitoring prior to intervention. Positive involvement of the entire family in a "blame-free atmosphere" appears to be necessary to achieve ultimate success (p. 16). Behavioral therapy, psychosocial programs, and engagement in creative activities, such as a variety of nonverbal therapeutic methods, such as painting, writing, music, but also movement therapy (mentioned above) have proven successful in long-term treatment and prevention of relapse.

Body Image in Dermatology

The skin is the largest organ of the body (comprising about 15% of adult bodyweight), and it is also the most obvious barrier with the world (Pohanka, 2001). It serves as a protective shield but it also communicates information about the individual, including their physical and psychological "problems and processes" (Tomas-Arragones & Marron, 2016, p. 48). The latter issues have been raised and discussed in the subchapter entitled *The Skin the Skin and Social Discourse* in relation to various cultural and ethnic aspects of body image. Acne, psoriasis, and vitiligo are the most visible skin conditions that do not necessarily communicate anything about the internal state of the individual. However, there can appear self-inflicted physical damage (e.g., cutting, tattoo) which may point at some deep-seeded psychological issues. Still other conditions may appear as side-effects of a bodily disease projected outward (such as cancer or liver damage). All these conditions may lead to depression, anxiety, feelings of stigmatization, and even suicidal ideation.

Gupta and Gupta (2013) concluded that a specific term, Cutaneous Body Image (CBI), is appropriate, especially in cases of individuals who are at high risk for depression and social avoidance behaviors because of social stigmatization. The CBI is defined as "the individual's mental representation of his or her skin, hair, and nails" (p. 48). It is an important clinical factor in dermatological disorders and is often "the primary consideration in deciding whether to proceed with cosmetic procedures" or treatment (Ibid.). Since CBI is a subjective construct, it must be approached on a highly individual basis; akin to what has been stated about coordination between cosmetic/plastic surgeons and psychiatrists, dermatologists are advised to correlate the physical and psychological symptoms, taking into account cultural, psychosocial, and psychiatric factors

401

and, where necessary, referring the patient to a mental health expert.

There are also dermatological conditions that result from trauma, PTSD, and stress, sometimes in conjunction with endocrine and neural factors. Among the most prominent and well known are alopecia areata[178] (AA), and atopic dermatitis (AD). Many patients with AA or AD also suffer from psychiatric diseases (Ibid.). However, psychiatric conditions are not their sole factors of causation. AA and AD may be caused by various environmental stressors. Such stressors trigger perfectly natural defensive mechanisms, activating a host of neuroendocrine mediators, such as adrenocorticotropin, β-endorphin, catecholamines and cortisol – all of which are produced in response to stress. The resulting increase in endogenous glucocorticoids may then disrupt the chief function of the skin as a shield and protector of the body, leaving the individual "vulnerable to inflammatory disorders" like AD and AA (Senra & Wollenberg, 2014, p. 38).

Jafferany (2007) divided psychodermatologic disorders into the following four broad categories: (1) psychophysiologic, (2) psychiatric with dermatologic symptoms, (3) dermatologic with psychiatric symptoms, and (4) miscellaneous. A non-exhaustive list of these disorders includes:

1. Psychodermatologic:
   - psoriasis
   - atopic dermatitis
   - acne
   - herpes simplex
   - rosacea
   - pruritus
2. Psychiatric with dermatologic symptoms:

---

[178] AA is defined as a "nonscarring hair loss" which affects the scalp, eyebrow eyelashes, and inguinal regions (Kara & Topkarci, 2018, p. 131).

- eating disorders
- delusions of parasitosis
- obsessive-compulsive disorder
- phobic states
- dysmorphophobia
- neurotic excoriations

3. Dermatologic with psychiatric symptoms:
   - alopecia areata
   - vitiligo
   - generalized psoriasis
   - chronic eczema
   - albinism
   - rhiophyma
   - neurofibroma

4. Miscellaneous:
   - chronic itching in scalp
   - psychogenic purpura syndrome
   - suicide in dermatology patients
   - pseudopsychodermatologic disease

Almost all of these skin conditions cause some degree of social stigmatization, withdrawal, anxiety, and even depression. The psychological symptoms may exacerbate the somatic ones, which then results in a lifelong struggle with the condition, with no apparent way out (Jafferany, 2007). Since inherited factors, environmental influences, and psychosocial issues often collide, and the individual struggles with significant emotional distress, a multidisciplinary approach is necessary. Many individuals resort to self-help, purchasing various crèmes, undergoing laser therapy, as well as various forms of homeopathic procedures without any long-term improvement.

Consequently, it is important to realize that only certain skin conditions can be treated with success by dermatologists. The division above is instructive in which these are, and where mental professional should be consulted. While some conditions may also require cosmetic surgery or intervention (physical removal), others will benefit from a multifaceted approach, including Cognitive-Behavioral Therapy (CBT) and psychoeducation.

CBT is a treatment of psychological problems grounded in how individuals think and behave. It assumes that psychological problems are acquired through learning processes and can thus be unlearned or altered. Patients are assisted in identifying and modifying their behavior patterns, in order to eradicate dysmorphic feelings and symptoms. Yoga, meditation, hypnosis-induced relaxation, symptom-control imagery training, exercise, but also antidepressants are included in the treatment (Shenefelt, 2003). *Mindfulness-based cognitive hypnotherapy* is a term which embraces cognitive-behavioral therapy and hypnotherapy, to address emotional aspects of dermatological conditions (Shenefelt, 2018). Research showed that this form of therapy produces "specific improvements in skin disorders through psycho-neuro-endocrine-immunologic mechanisms" (p. 34).

Psychoeducation is focused on providing individuals (patients) with information about their disease or condition, etiology, therapeutic options, and prognosis. Educating patients about the links between their physical condition and their feelings helps them understand how, for example, what appears to be a simple case of acne or dermatitis may result in unanticipated emotional trauma and even BDD. Such understanding can be helpful in reducing the feelings of depression, isolation, and social stigmatization.

There are also dermatological conditions that one cannot eradicate because they are not curable, such as vitiligo. Group therapy leading to body image acceptance is advisable in these cases.[179] Technically, there is a difference

---

[179] Group therapy was first introduced by Joseph Hersey Pratt (1872-1956) in 1905. Dr. Pratt invited eight patients with pulmonary tuberculosis, for whom no place could be found in the sanatoria, to participate in group sessions in his clinic at the Massachusetts General

between *group therapy* and *group work*. The latter takes place in a non-clinical setting and addresses primary affects. By contrast, group therapy is a psychosocial treatment practiced in a clinical setting by qualified mental health professionals such as psychiatrists, clinical psychologists, psychiatric nurses, psychiatric social workers, and occupational therapists specialized in mental health (Ezhumalai et al., 2018). What is key for group sessions of either kind is the definition of purpose, setting, time, frequency, and members' condition. Homogeneousness, cohesiveness, and trust are also important. Group work and group therapy can be recommended not only for diverse addictions and psychiatric disorders, but across the board in body image dysfunction, which is also why many people find their kindred in groups with similarly afflicted members, such as bodybuilders or swimmers, among whom body-image related conditions and comorbidities are often found.[180]

Hospital in Boston. Pratt reported very positive results and the rest, as they say, is history; history which, however, should not be forgotten, despite the fact that Pratt's achievements were overshadowed by the rise of behavioral psychotherapy in the 1960s.

[180] While many in the "lay populace" may have been surprised when Michael Phelps came out as a recovering addict, those familiar with the swimming world certainly were not. Fighting alcohol and drug addiction, in 2015, Phelps said he was "in a dark place" and "did not want to be alive anymore" (Kunst, 2023). Much like Princess Diana's admission of eating disorders, Phelps shed light on a social taboo, in order to help others. It would not surprise the reader to learn that body image dysphoria is a significant component of these clandestine issues.

Body Image and Cancer

Cancer is one of the most serious diagnoses one may receive. Treatment of the body leaves lasting psychological scars which may appear as body image dysfunctional disorders. Research into this field has shown that the need for body image treatment and care is the greatest not during the treatment but upon discharge from the hospital, and that its need is directly correlated to the length of the treatment, not necessarily its intensity (Konradsen, 2012). Negative affect is further exacerbated by the constant presence of the stigma associated with confiding details about one's body image, as well as the social taboo regarding any communication about cancer and private medical details in general (Rasmussen et al., 2010). Consequently, even physicians administering adjuvant therapy and palliative care should consider the psychosocial impact of the disease on the individual and ascertain the stability of the patient's body image before, during, and after the treatment.[181]

For practical purposes, White (2004) divided body image concerns in oncology into concerns related to appearance, and sensory-related concerns. Some patients have to undergo a radical surgical reconstruction or an immediate irreversible change (e.g., mastectomy), others are treated gradually and body image changes occur as the treatment progresses (e.g., colon cancer); some suffer detrimental sensory reactions, while others are concerned primarily with social impact of the treatment. Adverse chemotherapy reactions may include hair loss, dermatitis, pustules, sensory deficiency, even auditory changes, as well as changes in speech (e.g., in laryngeal cancer). Appearance

---

[181] Adjuvant therapy is defined as "additional cancer treatment" which is provided after the primary treatment, in order to lower the risk of comeback; adjuvant therapy may include chemotherapy, radiation therapy, hormone therapy, targeted therapy, or biological therapy (National Cancer Institute, 2023, par. 1).

related changes resulting from treatment "are often ranked as more severe" than side effects (p. 381). Nausea, fatigue, insomnia, lack of appetite and other side effects are generally much less traumatizing than associated lack of self-confidence, inability to perform the activities one has been used to all his life, dependency on others, and overall well-being. For many, the looming threat of impending death may also skew the perception of reality in assuming that the body, not to mention its image, simply do not matter. Here, Dylan Thomas' "Do not go gentle into that good night, / Old age should burn and rave at close of day," acquires a whole new meaning. Positively directed anger can be productive.

Consequently, it is recommended that the valuation each individual places on their body image play an appreciable role in treatment. Some people will fear cancer-related appearance changes (image-impact) more than actual changes in the body, such as amputation (body-impact). For some patients, lumpectomy will be a more acceptable form of treatment than mastectomy, although it may not be medically as effective. Sometimes, the need for psychological peace and social habit outweighs the advantages of a radical approach to treatment. To what degree a surgical intervention should be applied may also depend on the individual's family history, occupation, and personal wishes, related to their family background and social standing.

Even tolerance for pain could be a decisive factor. Teo et al. (2015) found that "higher levels of pain led to higher states of body image dissatisfaction" (p. 1377). Pain disrupts bodily integrity and may erode, partially disintegrate, or even completely fragment the body image. Since initial greater body integrity beliefs were shown to lead to higher dissatisfaction with one's body upon diagnosis and treatment (resulting in depression and BDD-related symptoms), screening for body image integrity is advisable both prior to treatment, during treatment, and upon discharge (Ibid.).

Although research in this area is far from satisfactory, it shows that all cancer patients will benefit from some degree of intervention – which may be psychodynamic, or static (in the form of psychoeducation). Psychodynamic approaches include embodied experiences, body-based transferences and counter-transferences referred to as "felt experience" (Krueger, 2004, p. 464). Emptiness, fullness, paralysis, sensory experiences of certain parts of the body, such as relaxing and clenching the muscles, creating awareness of the body-part which has been altered by treatment, in order to achieve a sense of control over it may be helpful. The first step should be from the external to the internal point of reference, to *embody* the experience. Once the internal point of reference is achieved, the somatic and emotional components distinguished, the patient can formulate his or her feelings, which is the first step toward the mastery of body image. As with other spheres of human existence, it is necessary to transform extrinsic motivation to the intrinsic impetus that not all is lost and that, indeed, the most important things in life cannot be ever lost, unless they be willfully discarded. Of course, physicians cannot give the patients false hopes; on the other hand, research has shown that abandonment of hope leads to a spiral of depression which exacerbates the physical condition of the suffering individual.

This is not merely a philosophical or psychological contention. Utilizing correlative behavioral and neuronal studies, Dubner and Ke (1999) demonstrated that (p. S45): (1) behavioral context modulates neuronal activity in nociceptive[182] and non-nociceptive somatosensory

---

[182] Nociception refers to the central nervous system (CNS) and peripheral nervous system (PNS) processing of pain, including its depth, frequency, and sensitivity, which is a highly subjective criterion (Kendroud et al., 2022).

pathways, (2) descending modulation influences behavior and neuronal activity at spinal cord levels after inflammation and persistent pain, and (3) there are descending facilitatory as well as inhibitory influences on behavior and spinal cord neuronal activity that may impact persistent pain particularly of deep muscle and visceral origin, thus "supporting the hypothesis that responses in these pathways are not immutable" and that cortical and subcortical pathways "can be modulated by attentional, motivational and cognitive factors" (Ibid.). In other words, it appears that the human brain uses the same mechanisms it habitually uses for learning as it uses when there is a threat of tissue damage, persistent pain, inflammation, or noxious stimuli such as disease. Therefore, survival in critical situations, including cancer, can be greatly advanced and facilitated via learned response.

Relatives, friends, and loved ones of the afflicted individual should likewise be acquainted and familiarized with this research, in order to provide the individual with a constructive body image support through responsive body-language, and behavior. Their observation is often crucial because "gestures predate affect" and often divulge more about body image dysfunction than the diagnosis or description of symptoms (Krueger, 2004, p. 466). The unity of movement and affect, position of limbs in relation to the torso, coordination in time, gestures, symbolic content, and reenactments of movements that display a primary attachment can all be observed and explored to mirror the body image and create self-awareness, cohesiveness, increase body-self integration, and self-mastery in these difficult circumstances. The sense of loss of control and an inevitable downward spiral must be avoided at all costs.

As a logical extension of the focus on sensory affect and body image awareness, recent studies have shown that social activities such as dance and yoga therapy have a positive effect on cancer patients (Costa et al., 2022;

Dibbell-Hope, 2000; Mahmout, 2023; Rao et al., 2017). Cancer-related fatigue, and sleep disorders, as well as the pain triggered by the effects of endogenous opioids, increase negative body image while decreasing self-esteem and stress, thereby causing mental imbalance (Costa et al., Ibid.). Physically active individuals have shown a significant reduction in these symptoms. In particular, dance therapy has been used to promote body-mind integration. Physical performance with music is particularly motivating and captivating (Hohmann et al., 2017). It is for the same reason that people with BDD tend to find refuge in body image sports, such as bodybuilding. Some associations, such as the INBA even celebrate and give special awards to those who have undergone cancer and cancer treatment, as well as the individuals with radical "body transformation."

Exercise may reduce not only physical but also mental pain, activating the noradrenergic system,[183] modulating the nociceptive pathways, and lowering pain thresholds (Costa et al., 2022). Regular physical exercise has also been shown to reduce oncologic fatigue and improve sleep quality by regulating inflammatory cytokines[184] (Zimmer et al., 2018). Where exercise is in the form of spontaneous movements, such as in dancing, it allows for the

---

[183] The noradrenergic system has been implicated in the pathogenesis of neuropsychiatric disorders and has become a "pharmacological target" in various psychiatric, neurologic, and cardiopulmonary disorders (Hussain et at., 2023). Norepinephrine, also known as noradrenaline, was first identified in the 1940s by Swedish physiologist Ulf von Euler. It plays an essential role in the regulation of arousal, attention, cognitive function, and stress reactions.

[184] Exercise influences inflammation by lowering the release of proinflammatory cytokines such as TNF-α and "promoting the production of mediators with anti-inflammatory effects, especially myokines, such as interleukin-6 (IL-6)" (Ferioli et al., 2018, p. 14015). IL-6 stimulates skeletal muscle oxidative metabolism, improves insulin sensitivity and increases the concentration of anti-inflammatory cytokines IL-1ra (interleukin-1 receptor antagonist) and IL-10.

410

externalization of depressive symptoms, promotes the release of beta-endorphins, vascular endothelial growth factor, brain-derived neurotrophic factor, and serotonin, thus stimulating hippocampal rejuvenation (Ferioli et al., 2018).

Changing the Body Image – Actual Stories

This chapter is intended to provide the reader with a selection of stories recounted or reported by those who struggled with their body image, and eventually overcame the BDD and related psychopathologies. Some have grown beyond them, and are now providing others with advice founded on the benefits of their experiences, others learned to live with them, still others have faced relapses and continue fighting.

Sarah

Sarah is a brunette with a beautiful smile, to whom other girls come for advice. She says that others tell her with admiration how "comfortable" she seems in her own skin, how "totally accepting" of who she is (female), what she looks like ("skinny," she says), and that she is "always encouraging and optimistic," which projects a "high level of self-esteem" (Laviajera, 2019, par. 8).

Still, Sarah says she used to be defensive about her looks, questioned compliments, and was extremely bothered by her acne, her "crooked teeth," unwanted facial and body hair, as well as scars. For many years, she was not able to "look past" her "physical flaws and imperfections" (par. 12). Since she could not compete with other girls in "looks," she focused on educational progress and engaged in the pursuit to acquire "the most beautiful mind" (Ibid.). Since she hated her "crooked teeth" so much, she learned how to write and communicate primarily in writing. Her acne made her unsure of herself in human interaction, insecure in speaking in public, and made it virtually impossible for her to engage in any job interviews. What is more, her obvious body hair made her feel like an invalid on the beach and prevented her from enjoying swimming. She also alluded to her physical scars which turned into long-term mental scars. The scars were caused by an infection following an earlobe injury she had suffered on a vacation in rural Nebraska (where she slept with dangling earrings and, apparently, tore her earlobe). The surgery was not performed on her ear until years later.

Based on her experience, she passes on to others the following points:

1) If you "focus only on your looks," you are "missing out big time" (Id., par. 24).
2) You can hide to heal your wounds, but not "your beautiful self" from those who love you.
3) Accept the things you cannot change, accept your flaws and scars. They are who you are.
4) Love someone who has flaws and imperfections, healing yourself in the process.

Today, Sarah lives in Spain, works as an English teacher and tourist guide in Madrid. She is happy with herself, unconcerned on the beach, swims, and has recently fallen in love.

Sarah's story can be called a success not only because she has successfully treated her body image disorders, but also because she did not slump into the cycle of ED and depression. Rather, she was able to look outside herself and seek happiness in activities not directly related to her body image, such as education and discovering new horizons. Her very realization as a junior high student that she "could not compete" in her looks with others, but could strive to have "the most beautiful mind" was the one step needed to recover from what might have become a downward spiral to the vicious ED cycle and suicidal ideation.

Erin

Erin calls herself a "body image bully" (Kerry, 2023, par. 1). At the age of eight, she called herself "fat, ugly, disgusting," and, "the worst – unlovable" (Ibid.). In the fifth grade, she had an epiphany that, perhaps, having a boyfriend would solve all her problems. This is a frequent assumption, not uncommon even among many insecure adults who often believe that marriage will magically solve their insecurities. Her "cycle" of self-love and self-rejection began; the cycle which coincided with her first having, and then losing, a boyfriend: "[A]s soon as I won over my male," she says, the "feelings of shame would quickly overshadow my victory." Her feelings of guilt were directly related to the fact that she knew she was "using someone" for what she defined as "personal gain." The feelings of guilt were even stronger in her than they would have been had she not also suffered compunctions on account of her strict Catholic upbringing.

Before long, in high school, she began to struggle with depression, and cyclical suicidal ideation. Her self-bullying continued, to the point when she began to hear voices, which led to psychiatric treatment. She gained 30 pounds in two years, for which she blamed the antidepressants. At that point, she says she "knew for certain" that she was "not only unlovable" but "CRAZY and unlovable" (Ibid.) [emphasis original]. She rejected the guidelines of her upbringing, her family, "gave up on God" and hit "rock bottom."

It was not until she became pregnant, nursing a new life in her womb, that she was "restored" because – her body had "a purpose." She looked in the mirror with pleasure, and "embraced her belly" with pride and self-satisfaction. After giving birth, she lost twenty-five pounds, and finally fell in equitable, reciprocal love.

Her ultimate message she wishes to pass on to others is that "body image issues" do not come from what others think about our bodies, but what we think about ourselves. Today, Erin enjoys reading the Bible again, and is proud to see and absorb a clear parallel between the temple of the Lord and the human body:

> Do you not know that your body is a temple of the Holy Spirit, who is in you, whom you have received from God? You are not your own; you were bought at a price. Therefore, honor God with your body. (Corinthians 6:19)

Clearly, there is a lot that Erin leaves undisclosed, but her suffering and the arduous journey to self-love is apparent from her final words: "Now, when I look in the mirror, I will choose not to listen to the bully. I will choose to embrace the way I look... I will choose not to step on a scale and be defined by the number there. I will choose not to compare the old me."

These words penetrate the core of BDD, which lies in cognitive comparison: either you are a beauty, or you are a beast; either you are admired and loved, or rejected and unlovable; either you are worthy, or not. Such a worldview leads to others: observing imperfections through the magnifying glass, comparing yourself with an incomparable ideal, blaming your body for your misfortunes in life, and seeing distortions where there are none. In brief, as Erin pointedly stated, failing to see the "Truth."

Kaelin

Kaelin remembers when she was eight years old and "refused to wear pants at all" because she was worried about "showing everyone how chubby" her thighs were (Guillaume, 2015, par. 1). She was bullied for having baby fat, hence the word "fat" was always on her mind. As a 15-year-old, she remained unnoticed by boys and began to feel that there was something "inherently wrong" with her. She even saw a psychiatrist who specialized in eating disorders, but even he failed to persuade her that she was not fat and did not need to diet. She started counting calories, obsessively using the treadmill, and only considered her day successful if she ate less than 1000. Before long, boys started being interested in her which pleased her but did not satisfy her.

Even as boys started "paying attention" to her, she tortured herself by constantly comparing herself to everyone around her. She began to "pick out" her "problem areas" – her arms, butt, stomach… almost every part of her body turned into a "problem area" (Ibid.). In her confession, she intentionally omits to describe in detail the "two eating disorders" that "engrained themselves" into her psyche "as old friends," creating a "comfort zone" (par. 3).

By way of commentary, it should be noted that the "comfort zone" (which could also be called a "safe zone" or "zone of stability" or equilibrium) is always lacking in the lives of people who suffer from eating disorders. It can only be provided by self-confidence which stems from true love, love for oneself, and one for others. Internal suffering undermines such feelings.

In Kaelin's case, there existed love for music, but the "safe zone" of ED gave her more comfort than music. Not until she was 21 years old, did she realize that her eating disorders were damaging her voice and that if she continued "being unkind" to her body, she would completely destroy it. She began therapy again, this time with a renewed endeavor and serious purpose. "Through music, through therapy, through friends," she learned that her "most important job" was to take care of herself (Ibid.).

Kaelin's story is typical of many teenage girls who are uncertain of themselves, insecure, feel unloved, even unlovable, and seek a purpose in the world. Many, like Kaetlin, realize the purpose as they grow older. However, this does not eradicate the ED and related comorbidities. Those must be addressed with more acumen and detail, as this book suggests and instructs. Although socioeconomic factors are at play, genetics have been shown to be an important factor in ED acquisition and predisposition (Berrettini, 2004). Those who have suffered from ED once, will face periods of potential reoccurrence, triggered by stress, uncertainty, grief, and other slings and arrows life may throw their way. Information, awareness, and preparedness go a long way to achieve long-lasting, permanent happiness with oneself.

Jenna

Jenna has never been athletic. Her body is average, slightly on the pudgy side. As a teenager, she considered herself fat and constantly compared herself to her "skinny friends" (Guillaume, 2015). She claims her "teenage insecurity" was triggered by witnessing other "beautiful women" on television agonize over slightest imperfections.

She joined the gym and lost 10 pounds, to which her friends responded with flattery, evoking a sense of personal pride in her. Before long, however, she started on weight loss pills, laziness took over, and depression followed suit. Her hard-won sense of pride and self-worth was nothing but a flash-in-the-pan, it seemed.

Interestingly, Jenna grew up in a "fat-phobic" home and "fat-hating society" thus, she says, she became "the thing that everyone hates" (Ibid.). Her hate was not just self-hate herself but also multiplied by the hate of the hate itself. The feeling of shame and unworthiness consumed her. Shame is a sister of guilt, and self-guilt is among the most common conditions that ED patients suffer from.

As is the case with so many anorectics and bulimics, food – once a source of nourishment and delight – became a tool of self-harm for Jenna, even though it also was a means of revolt against the world. At the same time, physical exercise turned into a fearful reminder of how far she fell from what she used to be. Regretfully, she concluded: "The more of me there was, the less of me I felt."

Today, she is looking back at her tortured past, trying to love her body and be kinder to herself but, she says, "It's a daily struggle." What gives her hope is that she is not alone in this struggle.

Jenna's story underscores the importance of reframing the struggle with one's body image as an interpersonal disadvantage in life which requires an interpersonal solution. This does not mean a uniform, universal life-changing turnaround but a gradual progression to self-acceptance. The first step is to avoid self-defeating habits, such as taking one's weight every day, staring in the mirror, photographing certain body-parts, avoiding compulsive exercise routines, etc.

Next, the afflicted individual must be led to realize that food is a form of compensation for something else which is lacking in her life – more often than not, it is love and friendship, but also self-fulfillment and gratification. Finding a hobby, focusing on something else which also creates social connection to others is key. Conversely, dieting and focusing on food is a sign of psychosocial problems. It predicts the onset of depression and "subsequent increases in bulimic pathology" (Stice, 2004, p. 307). What is more, dieting is a science and directly affects bodily functions. Therefore, one should always consult with a licensed nutritionist or professional trainer.

With eating disorders, the solutions focus on autosuggestion methods, meditation, self-talk, and self-appreciation (NEDC,[185] 2023). Interestingly, as Jenna realized, the path to success consists not so much in turning away from one's self but, rather, reframing and reshaping the understanding of the self, in order to achieve self-respect and self-love through self-appreciation, not self-denigration and self-hatred. This implies making conscious decisions about what to emphasize, look at, intellectually absorb (social media, advertising), and being realistic about one's social image.

---

[185] National Eating Disorders Collaboration, an Australian association of organizations and people within the purview of the Department of Health and Ageing.

Gena

Gena was a professional dancer for 5 years. She toured across the globe several times, "training vigorously six out of seven days a week" (Hamshaw, 2011, par. 4). She ate almost exclusively meat and white rice, not thinking much about it or studying nutrition at all. Everything seemed to work fine for her until the team was assigned a new dancing instructor from Asia who was stricter and harder than any of their previous instructors, and calculated instantly how much each dancer had to shed to remain competitive, instructing them on what to eat and what not to eat. The calculation was based solely on the competitor's height. For Gena, it was 11 pounds.

Consequently, she began to starve herself while working out harder than ever – what could possibly go wrong? What was even worse, this Asian teacher knew very little about nutrition herself, hence Gena ended up eating "low in calories and high in protein" beef jerky and only items that contained less than 100 calories. Her period stopped but so did others' – which was generally considered a "good sign" (Ibid.). Everyone on the team became "increasingly obsessive" about their "weight and numbers." She notes that nothing mattered to them "more than the blinking number that showed up after the beep on that little plastic black scale" (par. 8).

The teacher was watching them, everything they ate, made them feel proud when they lost weight and, conversely, shamed them when they ate something tasty which was deemed to be "off limits" for them. Before long, Gena developed diet-related stress, cried during rehearsals, became incapable of controlling her emotions, and felt like a different person. After an episode of food poisoning during a tour, Gena finally reached her stated weight goal. Still, no matter how skinny she was, she still was able to "pinch bits of fat" on her body, which made her feel too fat. Step by step, her old cheerful self was gone; she became a different person: glum, depressed, without any enjoyment for life and activities she used to love.

During summer break, she found out about a book on veganism from her vegan friend, and became captivated by the philosophy founded on care for others, namely well-being of animals. She stopped dancing, gained healthy weight, and became engaged in pro-animal welfare causes. The turning point was her realization that "the people in our lives are not going to love us any more or less based on how much we weigh" (par. 13). Compassion for others taught her to be compassionate and forgiving toward herself.

Gena's story is interesting because it shows how dance, a combination of art and physique, can be turned into an exercise in self-destruction. This is even more apparent in events in which the body is a means of achievement, judged by comparative means (including sports, such as bodybuilding, professional dancing, figure skating, etc.). Individuals with BDD tend to compare themselves with others, in order to "validate the perceived flaw" which they then try to fix by any means necessary (Mahmood, 2023, p. 2). Note that the obsession with sports and results is a form of perfectionism which makes such people more vulnerable to ED. Misdirected obsession is as destructive as misdirected anger.

On the other hand, under proper guidance, these sports can help body image issues where defects are real, and the goal are realistic. Dance is actually recommended as one of modern experimental body image therapies (which embrace visual, auditory, and kinesthetic methods) in the treatment of breast cancer patients (Dibbell-Hope, 2000). In these instances, dance is a means of social communication, creating empathy, reinforcing hope, self-confidence and self-expression. It also helps conquer depression, isolation, anger, fear and other negative emotions (Karaferi et al., 2022).

Hannah

The case of Hannah Carpenter is unusual in that she enjoyed the support of her family, was outwardly successful, in a loving relationship, and seemingly happy. Yet, there were telltale signs.

Hannah had suffered from eating disorders since she was 13. Her parents took her to a general practitioner in 2010 with a malnutrition complaint, stating that she was refusing to eat. She was referred to an anorexia specialist, and from 2010 to 2011, she gained 9 kilograms (20 pounds). She went from 36kg (79 pounds) to 45kg (99 pounds). At this point (March 2011), the specialist decided to end her appointments and declare her "cured." Consequently, her family believed that she was "in recovery" and became less concerned – until – five years later, when she was found dead in the woods nearby her home.

Her parents discovered that Hannah had been using laxatives, secretly binging and purging, hiding all this, thus providing them with no visible sign or indication that there was anything wrong with her. It was not until they found her dead that her phone revealed thousands of pictures of different parts of her body. In giving the verdict of suicide, the coroner stated: "This was a case where Hannah was concealing the way she was feeling from virtually everybody" (par. 20).

Vandereycken and Van Humbeeck (2008) carried out a retrospective survey of (ex-)patients with eating disorders. All respondents (401) reported a variety of methods to conceal their eating disorder, which ranged from sundry excuses to avoid eating together, giving a false impression of having eaten, to eating with gusto then secretly purging, hoarding food in secret, and falsifying weight. Many of these methods were described as a deliberate strategy to achieve their psychological goal. The denial of the seriousness of this illness, and self-denial, coupled with concealment, made it even more difficult to treat.

Sometimes, the eating disorder is unspecified, falling within a generic category for ED but not so serious that it would be immediately destructive of the individual's social life. It is then referred to as Other Specified Feeding and Eating Disorder (OSFED). For example, in BN, the binging and purging is less frequent, or, in AN, the individual has normal weight. There is also an OSFED called Purging Disorder (when the individual purges without binge eating), and NES (Night Eating Syndrome), characterized by a strong urge to eat at night (at least 25% of daily calorie intake takes place at night), anorexia in the morning, insomnia, and depression (Allison et al., 2010). OSFEDs are common among athletes like Hannah, and professionals in stressful fields with little or no time to eat during the daytime. They should never be ignored or disregarded by the individual as something they have "under control." Treatments are highly individualized, employing various forms of CBT, light therapy, progressive muscle relaxation techniques, education about nutrition, logging of sleeping and eating habits, encouragement of coping skills, regulating sleep patterns, and weight management (Allison et al., 2010; McCuen-Wurst, 2018).

Chris

Many men silently suffer from eating disorders. For example, bulimia nervosa (BN) is reported in 4.8% of women and 4% of men (Striegel-Moore et al., 2009). Eating disorders (ED) in men are even more insidious than in women because the beauty culture is focused on women and ED among women has become a frequent topic of research, surveys, and media conversations. Men, on the other hand, are expected to be tough and resilient, silent where emotions are concerned, and obsessed with women, not with their own bodies. Furthermore, being overweight is often better socially and individually tolerated in men than in women.

Chris is a case in point. He was brought up to eat as much as he wanted and when he wanted, although, most of the time, he did not want to eat, but his Italian mother and grandmother made him eat (Tognotti, 2017). His eating disorder battle started "with a single slice of white bread" (par. 4). Chris grew up in the carefree "upper-crust, outdoorsy liberal bastion of Marin County, California" but soon found himself insecure, unable to "weather" his "chubby adolescence." This led to depression, especially as he inevitably began to compare himself with "sinewy, fit male bodies" that surrounded him (or seemed to surround him) at every corner.

Being overweight at 12 was not the same as being overweight at 18 when the sexual impulse kicked in. He grew increasingly lonely, and slumped into a "passive… tired, apathetic inner-dialogue on repeat" during which he reminded himself how "slow, comparatively unattractive, and comparatively unhappy" he was (par. 10).

Compared to what? Compared to the ideal of the macho culture, his inner voice replied, in which men do not even talk about such issues. It was this culture of the macho ideal that forced him to pretend that he was well adjusted, "even-keeled, dry-humored, and emotionally bulletproof" because, he assumed, that was what the society wanted him to be (Ibid.).

When Chris was 21, he joined two of his friends in an aggressive exercise plan. At this time, his weight was 238 pounds. Without a plan but, keeping a promise to his friends, Chris went to 172 pounds in one year, achieving an above-average male physique. He began receiving compliments on his looks, which only reminded him of how much other people focused on his weight. This brought to the spotlight his body image and the emphasis others placed on it. it was a heavy thought, especially as he realized that his lack of self-confidence and self-worth had nothing to do with his body but, rather, that it was all about his "state of mind" (par. 20).

He worked as a front desk receptionist at the same gym where he would work out which seemed to be an ideal arrangement. However, before long, he began to loathe the job, dislike the gym, and started to indiscriminately devour protein bars and other treats, in complete disregard to the needs of his body. Why? Because it was his mind that mattered, not his body, he told himself.

He gained weight again, and his body image struggle continues. As of the writing of this story in 2017, he embarked on another bout of dieting and exercise.

While unsuccessful in his endeavor, Chris had made a great deal of progress toward learning about society and himself. Although it would appear to be so to a disinterested observer, his current diet is not the same as any of his previous diets – it is not in response to a socially normalizing impetus or muscle-bound inspiration. Today, he is on a new diet, in order to be healthy. The goal of his diet is to make himself happy, not suffer for some ideal perceived by others.

Chris' story is the epitome of stories of many other men who have shown an outwardly tough, thick skin for many years, only just to realize that the image does not really protect them but that it stands as a barrier between their real selves. This realization is key to recovery. Although Chris did not report any ED, current or past, obesity shares comorbidities with ED. Thus, attaining weight appropriate to one's age, height, and sex is crucial in preventing future ED issues, even though Chris has not reported he had suffered from any ED.

It should be noted that 55-77% of people with other specified feeding or eating disorder, and 67% of people with of avoidant/restrictive food intake disorder are men (Eddy et al., 2015; Hay et al., 2015), and that men have traditionally been underrepresented in ED surveys. Due to the general awareness of ED existence among women, men who suffer from an ED may also feel unmanly and subject to greater stigmatization should they "come out." Such fears may lead to depression, anger against oneself, and others.

Nik

Nik is a musician, writer, and advocate for gay and transgender rights. The latter because he grew up as a lonely man without any social support. He had come out as gay fairly early in his life and was referred to not by his name but as "that gay kid" (Mitchell, 2022, par. 7). He sought refuge among the pop culture crowd but found himself an outsider. His loneliness and rejection persuaded him that he needed to change his body, in order to "experience love, sex, or even friendship" (par. 10). That was when his struggle with body image and ED began.

Nik developed "really unhealthy restrictive habits around food" and was prone to exercising impulsively and "overexercising" (par. 11). A typical AN behavior ensued, represented by the avoidance of social occasions where food was served, skipping meals, stepping on the bathroom scales every morning and evening… As a young adult in the gay community, he soon discovered that "[e]verything was geared towards praising people with 'perfect bodies' and tearing others down," which only encouraged him to pursue his AN and ED as a means to fit in (par. 13).

At some point, he gave up on this struggle to conform. Instead, he began advocating against body-bullying among the gay community. Today, he feels well-adjusted and is able to celebrate his own body and his sexual identity. Still, he perceives the "toxic side" of this community and continues to fight against it.

Research examining men with eating disorders revealed that gay men are one of the two critical groups susceptible to ED, the other being athletes (Fawkner & McMurray, 2002). As Nik's story confirms, gay men are at risk of ED because of the increased pressures on appearance and physical attractiveness. Athletes, "especially those who compete in weight-prescribed sports" are also at risk (p. 138). Comparison works in reverse here, compared with the females, which is why it was described as *reverse anorexia* or muscle dysmorphia (Pope et al., 1993). Steroid use has been associated with ED in athletes (Pope et al., 1997, 2000). Again, however, the individual's primary purpose is indicative of a possible ED or BDD: men who exercised for the enjoyment of exercise, as opposed to the men who worked out to show off or improve their appearance, were less likely to suffer from eating disorders. What has been mentioned in the section on *Workout for Body Image* above, should be referenced here: a regular exercise routine positively influences the mood and self-esteem (Fawkner & Murray, 2002). Impulsive, compulsive, and excessive exercise does the opposite.

What Nik encountered when he started to work out was the realization that there is a difference between exercising for health, and exercising for body image. Although they overlap to some degree, it is the primary intent that matters. What is more, exercising for health improves one's body image, but not vice versa. A further complication arises because exercise and increased masculinity in men are often associated with the narcissistic stereotype, which involves constant comparisons of body images among men.

What is more, the ostentatious visibility of male bodies that Nik described is not pertinent solely to the gay subculture. Since the 1980s, men's bodies "have become increasingly visible in popular culture," mainly through marketing and advertising (Fawkner & Murray, 2002, p. 139; citing Mort, 1988). It is no wonder that the pressure among men to look more masculine, and to conform to the advertised ideal has increased over the last several decades.

Ben

Ben's story is instructive in spreading awareness about how insidiously ED can creep up on a busy professional, especially one who is unaware of their genetic predispositions to ED, and the subtle, insidious nature in which the disorder creeps in upon the individual.

Ben is a 30-year-old professional who has been suffering from AN for the past 3 years. He has always been overweight and has what he calls a "problem" with his body image, always dreaming about and thinking of how to be more "fit, toned, muscular, and attractive" (Eating disorders.org, 2023, par. 3). As a teenager, he had made an effort to go on a diet and exercise but it was not systematic and he was insufficiently motivated. At some point, he became bulimic. Although he was in a relationship, and had a steady professional job, he was not happy with himself. His diet was irregular and poor, which led to his gaining weight.

In a short span of time, Ben lost his grandfather, his mother attempted to commit suicide, and his girlfriend told him that she was not interested in him because of his weight. On top of all other misadventures, his house was burglarized and his car vandalized in a parking lot. What spurred the onset of AN was the combination of stress and irregular diet, although these were not the root causes.

As is the case with most ED patients, Ben bought a brand new set of bathroom scales and started weighing himself daily. He exercised compulsively and his life "degenerated extremely rapidly" from this point on: "Food started dominating my thoughts and feelings," he says (par. 11-12). He became obsessed with losing weight, severely restricted his food intake and started weighing himself several times a day. Although he claims that his life became a "set routine" because he planned his exercise and meals, it was governed by his hunt after some body image ideal, not by being healthy or living happily. He became a slave to the eating disorder and, before long, his life was "falling apart" (par. 15).

Certain characteristics of ON are apparent in Ben's conduct: he carefully selected his meals, he was always thinking about healthy or low-calorie food, and he was averse to eating with others, in particular as he would schedule his workouts after meals. As a consequence, he was "chronically fatigued" and hamstrung at work, frequently sick due to stress and suppressed immune system. Hypoglycemia also made him less tolerant of other people and their problems. His social life dissipated, and his friends "drifted away" (par. 20). He even went so far as to take the phone off the hook, in order to avoid conversations, something bulimics do when they need to be alone with their ED.

After several months of living with the ED, Ben was caught unprepared when, all of a sudden, he began hyperventilating in a parking lot, feeling as if his heart was giving out. Since then, panic attacks became a frequent occurrence and fear a part of his life. After three years of AN and BD, his body was literally becoming starved to death and needed help from a professional. He says he has been depressed, tired, confused, gaining no joy out of life, terrified both of losing, as much as gaining, weight.

His path to recovery began gradually, out of dire need for help. He did not trust his own thoughts and feelings and, most of all, distrusted his body. In order to recover, he had to trust someone which, at first, was his physician and his psychiatrist. As he was instructed to socialize again, he caught up with friends. His productivity and enjoyment of work soon improved. Today, he does not consider himself "recovered" yet but on the road to recovery.

The advice he provides to others is: "Please arm yourself with a strong support network of health professionals, family, and close friends" (par. 38). Not by coincidence, this is also the first advice offered in the chapter entitled *Changing Your Body Image* (above). Ben's story clearly shows that men are just as much prone to ED as women, given the same adverse constellation of stressors and circumstances beyond one's control, such as a combination of personal grief, professional stress, and frustration.

The influence of feminism, equality at work, women taking over traditionally male professions, debasement of male power and dominance in both professional and personal spheres, propagation of the term "toxic masculinity" and prejudice to the traditionally straight male with the appertaining implications (traditional family values), the rise and idolatry of the gay, trans, and queer movements, as well as the objectification of the (naked) male body by the media and commercial machinery, have all contributed to the increase vulnerability of the modern man to ED and BDD. Fawkner and McMurray (2002) further noted that there has been a marked rise in the incidence of heart disease, diabetes, stroke, and Alzheimer's disease among men (as opposed to infectious diseases), and the increased emphasis "placed on the self-management of one's health" (p. 3).

Striegel-Moore et al. (2009) suggested sex and gender differences in data for ED may also be the result of varied questionnaires, surveys, and expectations. Women are expected to suffer from ED more than men, but when the researchers looked into details, they found that the incidence of binge eating is about the same (4.9% vs. 4.0%), and with respect to both anorexia and bulimia, it is the definition that matters (p. 472). Thus, women were found to be purging themselves even where they were not "binging" on food, while men were more likely to binge without purging, thus facilely gaining weight, and becoming obese (one must also note: with the absence of the compunctions common among women). Compare the following data collected by Striegel-Moore et al. (Ibid.):

431

	Women	Men
Overeating	18%	26%
Binge eating 2/wk.	7.8%	5.8%
Fasting	6.3%	4.0%
Laxatives	3.1%	3.0%
Exercise	6.0%	5.6%

This research showed that almost all values were roughly similar in both sexes, except for overeating and vomiting (women were significantly more likely to use vomiting in purging: 3.7% versus 1.5%). Striegel-Moore et al. (2009) also documented gender differences in body checking, and body avoidant behavior: one in five women versus one in ten men acknowledged engaging in such behavior, women being also "significantly more likely than men" to be "consciously avoiding checking body weight or shape" (p. 473). Therefore, body avoidant behavior should also be considered among the BDD criteria (which is currently not the case).[186]

---

[186] *See* Substance Abuse and Mental Health Services Administration. DSM-5 Changes: Implications for Child Serious Emotional Disturbance [Internet]. Rockville (MD): Substance Abuse and Mental Health Services Administration (US); 2016 Jun. Table 23, DSM-IV to DSM-5 Body Dysmorphic Disorder Comparison. Available from: https://www.ncbi.nlm.nih.gov/books/NBK519712/table/ch3.t19/

Jason

Jason is a short, muscular male with curly black hair. He wears glasses and teaches economics at a prestigious university. His story is that of a lifelong struggle with body image, eating disorders, and steroid abuse.

Jason was born as Jane, but felt "different" ever since his mother tried to make him wear skirts and dresses. Before long, he began to hate everything female in himself and his own body. Unfortunately, he lived in a religious, highly conformist family, and was not allowed to express his real feelings. He always liked girls and hated his own body, but every attempt to be himself was swiftly dismissed as "ridiculous" by his parents. Eventually, he began to hate school, play truant, and his grades went down as his depression increased.

When he was 16, he started going to the gym but, by then, he had developed breasts, and was long past menarche which he was suppressing by underground hormonal treatment. No amount of bandaging "the top" could help and the masculine body appeared ever so elusive to him… Restrictive eating and excessive exercise were a means to rid himself of fat, lose the periods, and "become himself." After nearly a year of dieting and torturing himself in the gym, he met a competitive bodybuilder called Paul, who was using a gamut of performance enhancing drugs, virtually indiscriminately.

Paul seemed to like Jason (who, at the time, was still officially Jane) and they began to date. Jason told Paul all about himself when, to his great surprise and amazement, he learned that Paul was struggling with similar issues "in reverse." Thus it was that Jason lived vicariously through Paul's body, and Paul enjoyed the attention Jason paid to him the way no other man could. This went on for some time. They thought they were a perfect couple but, after less than a year, their relationship seemed to deteriorate. They realized

433

that each of them loved and envied the other's body "as his/her own." All this time, Paul had been using heavy doses of steroids, and hated himself for it. Jason also hated to daily witness how Paul was destroying his body.

About a year passed. By then, Jason had become addicted to orthorexia and compulsive exercise, visualizing himself as in Paul's body. Meanwhile, Paul competed in bodybuilding and received some degree of notoriety. Only Jason knew what a heavy toll it took on Paul, how it destroyed his body and mind, and how it "wasn't the right thing to do" for him. In the end, it was Jason who obtained the contact, made an appointment, and forced Paul to go to a specialist in gender dysphoria – even as he himself continued to "fight it." By then, Paul had nearly destroyed his liver and kidneys with steroid abuse which, Jason says, was Paul's ultimate goal.

Today, after much suffering, many sleepless nights, several radical cosmetic surgeries, with the help of steroids and hormone suppressors, Jason is finally satisfied where he is in life. He is in a relationship with a woman who understands and loves him for "who he is." What about Paul? He lost track of Paul. Last time, he remembers seeing him on the stepper, sweating off the hard-gained muscles. "Paula," he said, "good luck!" "Paula" beamed with joy.

The story of Jason and Paul is a true story which incorporates both FtM and MtF transgender BDD and exemplifies the associated symptomatology. Murray (2017) posited that the female gender and "feminine gender role endorsement" are accompanied by the drive for thinness, and "thinness-oriented disordered eating psychopathology" and, conversely, the "masculine gender role endorsement" is linked to the reverse AN and "muscularity-oriented disordered eating psychopathology" (p. 1). While the truly transgender individuals often strive to live in the role of the assigned sex for many years (there is commonly 10-15 years' difference between the realization of one's true gender between MtF and FtM transgender individuals, favoring the FtM, who usually make the decision earlier), the moment they do realize their gender identity is a permanent "burden" (for lack of a better word), they are subject to the ED psychopathologies associated with their gender identity, not their birth-assigned gender, and that even to a greater extent than their cisgender peers, simply because these psychopathologies affirm their gender identity.

Murray et al. (2012) examined the case of two MtF transsexuals and concluded that a highly individualized approach is needed because the body image psychopathology is impacted by both gender role orientations (i.e., cis- and trans-) during the process of acceptance of the individual's gender identity. This process is exemplified here by the case of Jason and Paul, who suffered from alternating symptomatology, even during their transition, with Paul/Paula being more likely to suffer from AN and BN than Jason, who was more aligned with the typically male OSFED. Guss et al. (2017) researched the associations of gender identity with disordered weight management behaviors, nonprescription steroid use, and weight perception, comparing these psychopathologies among trans- versus cis-gendered high-school students in Massachusetts, and found that "specifically," compared with their cisgender counterparts, transgender youth had "significantly higher odds of fasting greater than 24 hours" and "using diet pills and laxatives in the past 30 days," in order to lose or maintain their weight" (p. 18). Compared to cisgender males, transgender males had a higher incidence of using non-prescription steroids where and if available, similar to the transgender females seeking the female hormonal therapy, often by any means necessary. Interestingly, compared to cisgender females, transgender females had "higher odds of perceiving themselves as healthy weight/underweight when they were overweight" or even obese (Ibid.).

Although no peer-reviewed research has been performed in this area, it would appear that a dyadic relationship of the same gender identity in a cis-woman–trans-woman scenario is more likely to be supportive than the cis-male–trans-male relationship, simply because of the sociological nature of the typically female, versus male genders. In the females, their struggle with BDD and ED is unifying, and the relationship is that of concern and care. Given the heightened emphasis on the acceptance of body image, transsexual women also suffer from the typically female concerns that other women can well understand. On the other hand, the hierarchy in the male world does not revolve around the image of the body as much as in the female world. Male desirability is founded on virtues of heroism, perseverance, trust, faithfulness, kindness, moral integrity, and charisma – which have nothing to do with body image.

Fatima

Fatima is a Pakistani native who was born as Ahmed. In her early twenties, she revealed to her parents that she "had a female soul" and "wanted to live like a female" (Yousafzai, 2022, p. 375). She realized that this revelation was "catastrophic" because her parents raised her as an "archetypal man" (p. 376). Her parents were "deeply shocked" and completely rejected her.

Relegated to her resources, Fatima visited many different psychiatrists and physicians, but encountered only scorn, dismissive attitude, and apathy. She was "continuously judged and stigmatized" and either diagnosed as either a homosexual, or "Hijra" (Ibid.).[187] She turned to the transgender community for help and support, but she found them patronizing, without much empathy. She became depressed, thinking of suicide nearly every day. She tried to seek help from plastic surgeons but did not find "any positive response and reassurance" (Ibid.). Over the five years of this struggle, she faced "nothing but labels, sarcasm and mordacity" (Ibid.).

At tether's end, she made an appointment at Shifa International Hospital, where the physician was well acquainted with the transgender concept and sex reassignment surgery (SRS). The reception and information Fatima was given made her ecstatic – for the first time, she

---

[187] *Hijra* is a derogatory term for non-binary people. They are recognized as a "third gender" in various countries across Asia, their history going back to pre-antiquity. Non-binary individuals had been criminalized under Section 377 of the Indian Penal Code (1860), and labelled as a "criminal tribe in 1871" (Hinchy, 2019, p. 96). It was not until April 2014 that the Supreme Court of India recognized the transgender status and decreed that it is legal and can be listed as the "third gender" (Mahapatra, 2014). This law is now accepted in India, Nepal, Pakistan, and Bangladesh. It application includes greater freedoms in education, employment, and offering transgendered individuals the option to state "third gender" in passports and other official documents.

was treated in an unbiased, unprejudiced fashion, and provided with realistic options. A meeting was set up with plastic surgeons and endocrinologists, opinions from various sources, not all of whom approved the diagnosis. Endocrinologists "refused to go for hormonal therapy" and plastic surgeons likewise did not accept the gender dysphoria diagnosis. She was repeatedly told about adverse consequences of such actions and refused treatment. In the end, they told her that she must obtain the permission from Supreme Court of Pakistan for SRS.

She requested an official report from her psychiatrist, left the country and, within six months, underwent her much-desired SRS abroad. One year later, she returned to the same psychiatrist at Shifa International Hospital as a "fully developed female" with "noticeable breasts, long hair, soft and tender voice" and a "very composed demeanor" (Ibid.).

Today, Fatima lives a very happy life, has a husband, coveted position of a professional in a prestigious international company, and is fully content and satisfied. Yousafzai (Id.) noted that she is "not only a successful leader," but that she, "won the battle between her physical self and intuitive self" (p. 376); in other words, the battle between the body and the image.

Alex

Alex is in his late twenties, an average looking man, with a professional standing, and much going for him in his life. At 5'7", he is slightly below average in height. That is to say, he was – until recently.

When Alex was a teenager, he was often teased about his height but did not think much of it, until he grew older and, he claims, began to "get routinely spoken down to" because of his height (Ede-Osifo & Wilson, 2023, par. 2). Consequently, he began to *perceive* himself as extremely short, and therefore inadequate.

He did some research and found Dr. Shahab Mahboubian, a surgeon at the Height Lengthening Institute in Burbank, California. He became one of his patients and, withing months, Mr. Mahboubian performed a "leg-lengthening surgery" on him for $75,000, which Alex gladly paid. The total cost came up to $100,000. The insurance company compensated him $10,000 during the recovery phase.

Understandably, this surgery is extremely painful. It consists of sawing the thigh bones and inserting rods inside, which are then lengthened by 1 millimeter (0.04 inches) per day, via an external remote control. Meanwhile, new bone grows over the rods, which are eventually removed. Physical therapy is lengthy and Alex still requires a cane to walk.

"My goal was never to be tall," he claims. "It's to be in a place where no one comments on my height" (par. 4).

Rather than judging Alex too harshly, one may want to reflect on the consequences of social maladjustment, bullying, and body image ideals in society. While many readers may dismiss this type of cosmetic surgery as "insane" (Alex admitted as much), and even unethical, Alex expressed his unreserved gratitude to Dr. Mahboubian, and said the procedure was worth all the pain and money.

Alex's diagnosis of BDD is specifically termed *Short Stature Dysphoria* (SSD). This means a deep dissatisfaction with one's height. Consider that, before the surgery, Alex was so depressed and distressed that he would "walk around the neighborhood and cry" (par. 17). He had attended therapy, but to no avail. He perceived every remark about his height as "body-shaming" and even references to "short kings" (a term which is apparently used as a slang for dating charming men of short stature who are charismatic, confident, and attractive) seemed "mocking and backhanded" to him which, indeed, they were (par. 21). Alex still blames social pressure and prejudice for his BDD.

Today, he stands 5'10", slightly above the average height for a man in the United States.

Expounding about the SSD, Dr. Mahboubian remarked that he expected to perform fifty "stature-lengthening operations this year" (2023), which was "more than double the 20 he did three years ago" (par. 13). The most significant risks involve nerve injury and potential loss of the range of motion (Ibid.).

Facts are no doubt stacked against short men: 58% of the men on the Fortune 500 list are taller than 6 feet, even though only 14% of American men are that tall (Ibid.). Judge and Cable (2004) found that taller men earn more and have significant advantages in workplace as well as in private lives (dating).[188] Undurraga et al. (2012) conducted research of height preference in non-industrialized contexts and found a positive height correlation only among children and young adults. The research qualified four values: strength, dominance, social concern, and knowledge. The cohorts deemed all four values to be greater in taller children, but not necessarily in taller adults. Only greater strength was attributed to taller men and women, but not greater dominance, social concern, and knowledge. This research is

---

[188] *Cf. The Napoleonic Complex*, p. 197.

contrary to the data collected from industrialized nations where taller people are invariably "attributed positive socioeconomic and character traits, such as intelligence, employability, and leadership" (Ibid.). Height is also positively associated with greater self-esteem and self-consciousness (Booth, 1990), as well as wages, overall prosperity, and other socioeconomic indicators (Perisco et al., 2004).

On the other hand, Samaras and Storms (1992) documented men <175.3 cm (69 inches) tall lived an average of 4.95 years longer than men above this height, and men <170.2 cm (67 inches) lived 7.46 years longer than those of at least 182.9 cm (6 feet tall). An analysis by weight difference revealed a 7.72-year greater longevity for men weighing 63.6 kg (142 pounds) or less compared with those of 90.9 kg (204 pounds) or more. Lower height has been positively correlated with better health in both human and animal studies (Samaras, 2012). Samaras (2012) found that 36 health parameters related to shorter height, including lower cancer risk, less chance of blood clots, atrial fibrillation, and heart health. In 2019, Samaras et al. reported that the fact that women live longer than men is primarily due to their shorter height. Their study documented that men were 7.8% taller, which corresponded to an 8.5% lower life expectancy. Therefore, it can be concluded that, statistically speaking, height is almost directly inversely related to life expectancy.

References

Abdulla, M. R. (2018). Culture, religion, and freedom of religion or belief. *The Review of Faith & International Affairs, 16*(4), 102-115. DOI: 10.1080/15570274.2018.1535033

Abram, D. (1997). The spell of the sensuous: Perception and language in a more-than-human world. New York, NY: Vintage.

Abrams, A. U. (1982). A new light on Benjamin West's Pennsylvania Instruction. *Winterthur Portfolio 17*(4), 243-57.

Abrams, A. U. (1985). The valiant hero: Benjamin West and grand-style history painting. Washington, D.C.: Smithsonian Institution Press.

Abu-Akel, A. & Shamay-Tsoory, S. (2011, Sept.). Neuroanatomical and neurochemical bases of theory of mind. *Neuropsychologia, 49*(11), 2971–84. DOI:10.1016/j.neuropsychologia.2011.07.012. PMID 21803062. S2CID 36226051.

Adler, A., Jelliffe, & S. Ely. (1917). Study of organ inferiority and its psychical compensation: A contribution to clinical medicine. New York, NY: Nervous and Mental Disease Publishing Company.

Adler A. (1956). The individual psychology of Alfred Adler: A systematic presentation in selections from his writings. (Ansbacher H. L. and Ansbacher R. R., Eds.). New York, NY: Basic Books.

Aggrawal, A. (2015). Paraphilias: Exhibitionism. In: A. Jamieson and A. Moenssens (Eds.), *Wiley Encyclopedia of Forensic Science* (Five Volume Set). Wiley, U.S. [Published in an online edition]. http://onlinelibrary.wiley.com/doi/10.1002/9780470061589.fsa1072/pdf [Encyclopedia chapter]

Ainsworth, M., Belhar, M., Waters, E., & Wall, S. (1978). Patterns of attachment: A psychological study of the strange situation. Hillsdale, NJ: Erlbaum.

Allen, J. G., & Coyne, L. (1995). Dissociation and the vulnerability to psychotic experiences. *Journal of Nervous and Mental Disease, 183*, 615–622.

Allen, S. (2020). M to (WT)F: Twenty-six of the funniest moments from my transgender journey. [Audiobook] ASIN B08FTLJCRV

Allen, L. S., & Gorski, R. A. (1990). Sex difference in the bed nucleus of the stria terminalis of the human brain. *Journal of*

Comparative Neurology, 1990(302), 697-706.
https://doi.org/10.1002/cne.903020402

Allison, K. C., Lundgren, J. D., O'Reardon, J. P., Geliebter, A., Gluck, M. E., Vinai, P., Mitchell, J. E., Schenck, C. H., Howell, M. J., Crow, S. J., Engel, S., Latzer, Y., Tzischinsky, O., Mahowald, M. W., & Stunkard, A. J. (2010, April). Proposed diagnostic criteria for night eating syndrome. *International Journal of Eating Disorders, 43*(3), 241-7.

Allison, K. C., Lundgren, J. D., Moore, R. H., O'Reardon, J. P., & Stunkard, A. J. (2010). Cognitive behavior therapy for night eating syndrome: a pilot study. *American Journal of Psychotherapy, 64*(1), 91-106. DOI: 10.1176/appi.psychotherapy.2010.64.1.91. PMID: 20405767.

Allport, G. W. (1954). The nature of prejudice. Reading: Addison-Wesley.

Allport, G. W. (1958). The nature of prejudice. Garden City, NY: Doubleday Anchor Books, Doubleday & Company, Inc.

Allport, G. W. (1960). The individual and his religion. Virginia: MacMillian.

Alós-Ferrer, C., & Shi, F. (2015). Choice-induced preference change and the free-choice paradigm: A clarification. *Judgment and Decision Making, 10*(1), 34-49. DOI:10.1017/S1930297500003168

Alphonso, C. (2000). Bullies push their victims to suicide. *The Globe and Mail, 11*(27). https://www.theglobeandmail.com/news/national/bullies-push-their-victims-to-suicide/article4169325/

Altabe, M., & O'Garo, K-G. N. (2004). Hispanic body images. In T. F. Cash and T. Pruzinsky (Eds.), *Body Image: A Handbook of Theory, Research, and Clinical Practice* (pp. 250-256). New York, NY: The Guilford Press.

Altman, S. E., & Shankman, S. A. (2009). What is the association between obsessive-compulsive disorder and eating disorders? *Clinical Psychological Review, 29*, 638–646. DOI: 10.1016/j.cpr.2009.08.001

Amankwa, J., Obinnim, E., G., Selase, R., & Emefa, A. F. (2016). Skin bleaching and its negative effect on the physical appearance of the black skin: A case study of youthful ladies and women in the Ho municipality in Ghana. *Research on Humanities and Social Sciences, 6*(12), 67-73.

American Psychiatric Association. (2000). Diagnostic and statistical manual of mental disorders (4th ed., text rev.). Washington, DC: Author.

American Psychiatric Association. (2013). Diagnostic and statistical manual of mental disorders (5th ed.). Washington, DC: Author.

American Psychological Association. (2022). Inferiority complex. Retrieved from https://dictionary.apa.org/inferiority-complex

American Psychological Association. (2023a). Selfobject. Retrieved from https://dictionary.apa.org/self-object

American Psychological Association. (2023b). Body-ego. Retrieved from https://dictionary.apa.org/body-ego

American Psychological Association. (2023c). Topics. Retrieved from https://www.apa.org/topics

American Society of Plastic Surgeons. (2023). 2020 statistics. Retrieved from https://www.plasticsurgery.org/news/plastic-surgery-statistics

Amstadter, A. B., & Vernon, L. L. (2008). Emotional reactions during and after trauma: A comparison of trauma types. *Journal of Aggression, Maltreatment & Trauma, 16*, 391–408.

Andersen, B. L., & Cyranowski, J. M. (1994). Women's sexual self-schema. *Journal of Personality and Social Psychology, 67*, 1079-1100. https://doi.org/10.1037/0022-3514.67.6.1079

Andersen, B. L., Cyranowski, J. M., & Espindle, D. (1999). Men's sexual self-schema. *Journal of Personality and Social Psychology, 76*, 645-661.

Andreason, P. J., Zametkin, A. J., Guo, A. C., Baldwin, P., & Coen, R. M. (1994). Gender-related differences in regional cerebral glucose metabolism in normal volunteers. *Psychiatry Research, 1994*(51), 175–83.

Andreotti, A. M., Goiato, M. C., Pellizzer, E. P., Pesqueira, A. A. Guiotti, A. M., Gennari-Filho, H., & dos Santos, D. M. (2014). Phantom eye syndrome: A review of the literature. *ScientificWorldJournal, 686493*. DOI:10.1155/2014/686493. PMC 4273592. PMID 25548790.

Andrew, R., Tiggemann, M., & Clark, L. (2015, Sept.). The protective role of body appreciation against media-induced body dissatisfaction. *Body Image, 15*, 98-104. DOI: 10.1016/j.bodyim.2015.07.005. Epub 2015 Aug 24. PMID: 26311661.

Anketell, C., Dorahy, M. J., Shannon, M., Elder, R., Hamilton, G., Corry, M., MacSherry, A., Curran, D., & O'Rawe, B. (2010). An exploratory analysis of voice hearing in chronic PTSD: Potential associated mechanisms. *Journal of Trauma & Dissociation, 11*(1):93-107. DOI: 10.1080/15299730903143600. PMID: 20063251.

444

Anne L. E., Nayak, M. B., Korcha, R. A., & Greenfield, T. K. (2011). Child physical and sexual abuse: A comprehensive look at alcohol consumption patterns, consequences and dependence from the National Alcohol Survey. *Alcoholism: Clinical and Experimental Research, 35*(2), 317–325.

Argyle, M., & Dean, J. (1965, Sept.). Eye-contact, distance and affiliation. *Sociometry, 28*(3), 289-304. https://www.jstor.org/stable/2786027

Aristotle. (1999). Nicomachean ethics. (Terence Irwin, transl.). Indianapolis, IN: Hackett Publ., Inc.

Armstrong, M. (1991). Career-oriented women with tattoos. *Journal of Nursing Scholarship, 23*, 215-220. DOI: 10.1111/j.1547-5069.1991.tb00674.x

Aron, L. (1998). The clinical body and the reflexive mind. In L. Aron & F. S. Anderson (Eds.), *Relational perspectives on the body* (pp. 3–39). Hillsdale, NJ: Analytic Press.

Arzy, S., Overney, L. S., Landis, T., & Blanke, O. (2006). Neural mechanisms of embodiment. *Archives of Neurology, 63*(7), 1022–5. DOI:10.1001/archneur.63.7.1022. PMID 16831974

Ashelford, J. (1996). The art of dress: clothes and society, 1500-1914. London, UK: National Trust.

Askevold, F. (1975). Measuring body image. *Psychotherapy and Psychosomatics, 26*(2), 71-77.

Asselstine, M. E. (2000). Body experiences of women survivors of child sexual abuse: Implications for therapeutic intervention. *Dissertation Abstract International, Section B: The Sciences and Engineering, 60*(9-b), 43–57.

Astin, J. A. (2004). Mind–body therapies for the management of pain. *The Clinical Journal of Pain, 20*(1), 27-32. Retrieved from http://journals.lww.com/clinicalpain/Fulltext/2004/01000/Mind_Body_Therapies_for_the_Management_of_Pain.6.aspx

Athanasaki, D., Lakoumentas, J., Feketea, G., & Vassilopoulou, E. (2023). The prevalence of orthorexia nervosa among Greek professional dancers. *Nutrients, 15*(2), 379. https://doi.org/10.3390/nu15020379

Atkinson, M. (2002). Pretty in ink: Conformity, resistance, and negotiation in women's tattooing. *Sex Roles, 47*, 219-235. DOI: 10.1023/A:1021330609522

Atkinson, M. (2004). Tattooing and civilizing processes: Body modification as self-control. *Canadian Review of Sociology, 41*, 125-146. DOI: 10.1111/j.1755-618X.2004.tb02173.x

445

Austin, J. L. (1962). How to do things with words. Oxford, UK: Oxford University Press. [Lectures delivered by Austin at Harvard in 1955].

Avicenna (n/d). A compendium on the soul. (Translated by Edward Abbott van Dyck). [Project Gutenberg EBook #58186]. Retrieved from https://www.gutenberg.org/files/58186/58186-0.txt

Ayele, G. M., Atalay, R. T., Mamo, R. T., Hussien, S., Nigussie, B., Fissha, A., & Michael, M. B. (2023, March). Is losing weight worth losing your kidney: Keto diet resulting in renal failure. *Cureus, 15*(3), e36546. DOI: 10.7759/cureus.36546. PMID: 37095796; PMCID: PMC10121483.

Badoud, D., & Tsakiris, M. (2017). From the body's viscera to the body's image: Is there a link between interoception and body image concerns? *Neuroscience and Biobehavioral Reviews, 77*, 237-246 https://doi.org/10.1016/j.neubiorev.2017.03.017

Bae, H. R., Kim, H. D., Park, M., Lee, B., Kim, M., Lee, E., Kyeong, C. K., Kim, S., Im, D., & Chung, H. (2016). β-Hydroxybutyrate suppresses inflammasome formation by ameliorating endoplasmic reticulum stress via AMPK activation. *Oncotarget, 2016*(7), 66444-66454. Retrieved from https://www.oncotarget.com/article/12119/text/

Baier, B., & Karnath, H-O. (2008). Tight link between our sense of limb ownership and self-awareness of actions. *Stroke, 39*, 486-88.

Balint, M. (1968). The basic fault: Therapeutic aspects of regression. London, UK: Tavistock Publications.

Banissy, M., Jonas, C., & Cohen, K. R. (2014). Synesthesia: An introduction. *Frontiers in psychology, 5*, 1414. 10.3389/fpsyg.2014.01414.

Baker-Pitts. (2015). "Look at me… What am I supposed to be?" Women, culture, and cosmetic splitting. In J. Petrucelli (Ed), *Body-States: Interpersonal Relational Perspectives on the Treatment of Eating Disorders* (pp. 104–119). London: Routledge.

Bamji, A. (2013). The First World War and the development of facial surgery. Retrieved from https://www.thepmfajournal.com/features/post/the-first-world-war-and-the-development-of-facial-surgery

Bandura, A. (1982). Self-efficacy mechanism in human agency. *American Psychologist, 37*(2), 122-147.

Bandura, A. (1986). Social foundations of thought and action: A social cognitive theory. Englewood Cliffs, NJ: Prentice Hall.

Bandura, A. (1989). Social cognitive theory. In R. Vasta (Ed.), Annals of child development, Vol. 6, six theories of child development (pp. 1-60). Greenwich, CT: JAI Press.

Bandura, A. (1991). Social cognitive theory of moral thought and action. In W. M. Kurtines & J. L. Gewirtz (Eds.). Handbook of moral behavior and development: Theory, research, and applications (pp. 45–103). Hillsdale, NJ: Lawrence Erlbaum Associates.

Bandura, A. (1993). Perceived self-efficacy in cognitive development and functioning. *Educational Psychologist, 28*(2), 117-149.

Bandura, A. (1994). Self-efficacy. In V.S. Ramachaudran (Ed), Encyclopedia of human behavior. New York, NY: Academic Press, 77-81.

Bandura, A. (1995). Self-efficacy in changing societies. Cambridge, England: Cambridge University Press.

Bandura, A. (1997). Self-efficacy: The exercise of control. New York: Freeman.

Bandura, A. (2001). Social cognitive theory: An agentic perspective. *Annual review of psychology, 52*, 1-26.

Bao, A. M., Hestiantoro, A., Van Someren, E. J., Swaab, D. F., & Zhou, J. N. (2005). Colocalization of corticotrophin releasing hormone and estrogen receptor-alpha in the paraventricular nucleus of the hypothalamus in mood disorders. *Brain, 2005*(128), 1301-13.

Bariso, J. (2022). An FBI agent's 9 ways to read people. Retrieved from https://www.inc.com/justin-bariso/an-fbi-agents-9-ways-to-read-people.html

Barrett, L. F., & Simmons, W. K. (2015, July). Interoceptive predictions in the brain. *Nature Reviews. Neuroscience, 16*(7), 419-29. DOI: 10.1038/nrn3950. Epub 2015 May 28. PMID: 26016744; PMCID: PMC4731102.

Barsalou, L. W., Niedenthal, M. P., Barbey, A. K., & Ruppert, J. A. (2003). Social Embodiment. *The Psychology of Learning and Motivation, 43*, 43–86.

Barthes, R. (1977). Image-music-text. [Essays selected and translated by Stephen Heath.] New York, NY: Noonday.

Bartke, A. (2012). Healthy aging: Is smaller better? *Gerontology, 58*(4), 337-343.

Bartolomeo, P., De Vito, S., & Malkinson, T. S. (2017). Space-related confabulations after right hemisphere damage. *Cortex, 87*, 166-73.

Batista, M., Žigić, A. L., Žaja, O., Jakovina, T., & Begovac, I. (2018, Sept.). Predictors of eating disorder risk in anorexia nervosa

447

adolescents. *Acta Clinica Croatia, 57*(3), 399-410. DOI: 10.20471/acc.2018.57.03.01. PMID: 31168171; PMCID: PMC6536277.

Baudrillard, J. (1976). L'echange symbolique et la mort. Paris, Gallimard.

Baudrillard, J. (1981). Simulacres et simulation. Paris, Galilée.

Baudrillard, J. (1991). La guerre du Golfe n'a pas eu lieu. Paris, Galilée.

Baudrillard, J. (1996). O svádění. Olomouc, CZ: Votobia.

Baumeister, R. F. (2002). Ego depletion and self-control failure: An energy model of the self's executive function. *Self and Identity, 1* (2), 129–136. DOI:10.1080/152988602317319302. S2CID 12823588.

Baumeister, R.F., Bratslavsky, E., Muraven, M., & Tice, D. M. (1998, May). Ego depletion: is the active self a limited resource? *Journal of Personal and Social Psychology, 74*(5),1252-65. DOI: 10.1037//0022-3514.74.5.1252. PMID: 9599441.

Baumeister, R. F., Campbell, J. D., Krueger, J. I., & Vohs, K. D. (2003). Does high self-esteem cause better performance, interpersonal success, happiness, or healthier lifestyles? *Psychological Science in the Public Interest, 4*, 1-44.

BBC. (2018). What's the difference between hijab, niqab, and burqa? Retrieved from https://www.bbc.co.uk/newsround/24118241

BDDFoundation.com. (2023). Information for mental health professionals. Retrieved from https://bddfoundation.org/support/supporting-someone-with-bdd/information-for-mental-health-professionals/

Beans, B. E. (1997). Eagle's plume: The struggle to preserve the life and haunts of America's bald eagle. Omaha, NE: University of Nebraska Press (p. 58.). ISBN 9780803261426.

Becker, S., Navratilova, E., Nees, F., & Van Damme, S. (2018, July). Emotional and motivational pain processing: Current state of knowledge and perspectives in translational research. *Pain Research and Management, 18*, 2018:5457870. DOI: 10.1155/2018/5457870. PMID: 30123398; PMCID: PMC6079355.

Bell, S. (1999). Tattooed: A participant observer's exploration of meaning. *Journal of American Culture, 22*, 53-58. DOI: 10.1111/j.1542-734X.1999.2202_53.x

Belting, H. (2011). An anthropology of images: Picture, medium, body. Princeton, NJ: Princeton University Press.

Belting, H. (2017). Face and mask: A double history. Princeton, NJ: Princeton University Press.

448

Bernal, P. P. (1992). The Huntington Library, art collections, botanical gardens. San Marino, CA: The Huntington Library.

Berne, E. (1964/2004). Games people play: The basic handbook of transactional analysis. New York, NY: Random House.

Berrettini, W. (2004, Nov.). The genetics of eating disorders. *Psychiatry (Edgmont), 1*(3), 18-25. PMID: 21191522; PMCID: PMC3010958.

Berrios, G. E. & Sierra-Siegert, M. (1997). Depersonalization: A conceptual history. *History of psychiatry, 8*(30), 213-29. DOI: 10.1177/0957154X9700803002.

Bessel A., Pelcovitz, D., Roth, S., Mandel, F. S., McFarlane, A., & Herman, J. L. (2022). Dissociation, affect dysregulation and somatization: The complex nature of adaptation to trauma. Harvard, MA: Harvard University Press.

Bessel, Van Der Kolk. (2021). The body keeps the score: Brain, mind, and body in the healing of trauma. [Audiobook.] Audible.com

Biderman, A., & Herman, J. (2003). Was Silas Weir Mitchell really a psychiatrist? *Isr J Psychiatry Relat Sci, 40*(1), 29-35. PMID: 12817667

Bienvenu, O., Samuels, J., Riddle, M., Hoehn-Saric, R., Liang, K., Cullen, B., et al. (2000). The relationship of obsessive-compulsive disorder to possible spectrum disorders: Results from a family study. *Biological Psychiatry, 48*(4), 287-293.

Binet, A. (1977). Alterations of personality: On the double consciousness. (Ed. Daniel N. Robinson. Washington, D.C.). Univ. Publications of America. (Original work published 1890).

Bishop, K. M., & Wahlsten, D. (1997). Sex differences in the human corpus callosum: Myth or reality? *Neuroscience Biobehavioral Review, 21*(5): 58-601.

Blackburn, S. (2016). Oxford dictionary of philosophy (2nd ed.). Oxford, UK: Oxford University Press. Retrieved from https://www.oxfordreference.com/view/10.1093/oi/authority.2 0110803100234623

Blaney, P. H., Krueger, R. F., & Millon, T. (Eds.). (2015). Oxford textbook of psychopathology (3rd ed.). Oxford, UK: Oxford University Press.

Blasi, A. (1980). Bridging moral cognition and moral action: A critical review of the literature. *Psychological Bulletin, 88*(1), 1.

Blasi, A. (1983). Moral cognition and moral action: A theoretical perspective. *Developmental Review, 3*(2), 178–210.

Blasi, A. (1995). Moral understanding and the moral personality: The process of moral integration. In W. M. Kurtines, & J. L.

Gewirtz (Eds.), *Moral Development* (pp. 229–253). Boston, MA: Allyn & Bacon.

Blaszczak-Boxe, A. (2014, July). Taller, fatter, older: How humans have changed in the last 100 years. *Live Science, 7*(14). Retrieved from https://www.livescience.com/46894-how-humans-changed-in-100-years.html

Blaus, B. (2014). Medical gallery of Blausen Medical 2014. *WikiJournal of Medicine, 1*(2). DOI:10.15347/wjm/2014.010. ISSN 2002-4436. Retrieved from https://commons.wikimedia.org/wiki/File:Blausen_0614_LimbicSystem.png

Bloom, A. (1987). The closing of the American mind: How higher education has failed democracy and impoverished the souls of today's students. New York, NY: Simon & Schuster.

Bodybuilding.com. (2019). Female bodybuilders denied? Discriminated against? Retrieved from https://www.bodybuilding.com/fun/other44.htm

Bodybuilding.com. (2020). Is cosmetic surgery ethical in bodybuilding? Retrieved from https://www.bodybuilding.com/fun/topicoftheweek154.htm

Bolar, K. (2022). Mentally ill teen betrayed by health professionals. *Epoch Times, 11*(30). Retrieved from https://www.theepochtimes.com/mentally-ill-teen-betrayed-by-health-professionals-who-recommended-testosterone-and-top-surgery_4895309.html

Bollas, C. (1987). The Shadow of the object: Psychoanalysis of the unknown known. London, UK: Free Association Books.

Bonomi, A. E., Cannon, E. A., Anderson, M. L., Rivara, F. P., & Thompson, R. S. (2008). Association between self-reported health and physical and/or sexual abuse experienced before age 18. *Child Abuse & Neglect, 32*(7), 693–701.

Bonomo, J. (2016). The photograph as an object of mourning: Roland Barthes and the use of photographs in Hughes's birthday letters. Retrieved from https://www.linkedin.com/pulse/photograph-object-mourning-roland-barthes-use-hughess-jon-bonomo/

Book, H. E. (1971, Sept.). Sexual implications of the nose. *Comprehensive Psychiatry, 12*(5), 450-455.

Booth, N. D. (1990). The relationship between height and self-esteem and the mediating effect of self-consciousness. *Journal of Social Psychology, 1990*(130), 609–617.

Boothe, B. (2017). Oedipus complex. In V. Zeigler-Hill, and T. K. Shackelford (Eds.), *Encyclopedia of Personality and*

Individual Differences (pp. 1401-5). University of Zurich, Psychoanalytisch-psychotherapeutische Praxis Bellevue, Zurich, Switzerland: Springer International Publishing, AG. DOI: 10.1007/978-3-319-28099-8_1405-1

Boucher, F. (1987). 20,000 years of fashion: The history of costume and personal adornment. (Expanded Edition). New York, NY: Harry N. Abrams, Inc. (Original work published 1965).

Bourdieu, P. (1986). Distinction: A social critique of the judgement of taste. (1st ed.) (Translated by Richard Nice). London: Routledge Classics. (Original published in 1979).

Bratman, S. (1997, Sept.-Oct.). Health food junkie. *Yoga Journal* [online], pp. 42-50. https://www.beyondveg.com/bratmans/hfj/hf-junkie-1a.shtml

Brausch, A. M., & Gutierrez, P. M. (2009). The role of body image and disordered eating as risk factors for depression and suicidal ideation in adolescents. *Suicide and Life-Threatening Behavior, 39*, 58–71.

Brehm, J. W. (1956, May). Postdecision changes in the desirability of alternatives. *Journal of Abnormal and Social Psychology, 52*(3), 384–389. DOI: 10.1037/h0041006. PMID: 13318848.

Breuer, J., & Freud, S. (1895). Studien über hysterie. Franz Deuticke, Leipzig, Wien.

Bridges, T. S. (2009). Gender capital and male bodybuilders. *Body & Society, 15*(1), 83–107. DOI: 10.1177/1357034X08100148

Briere, J. (2004). Psychological assessment of adult posttraumatic states: Phenomenology, diagnosis and measurement (2nd ed., pp. 175–202). Thousand Oaks, CA: Sage.

Briere, J., & Jordan, C. E. (2004). Violence against women: Outcomes complexity and implications for assessment and treatment. *Journal of Interpersonal Violence, 19*, 1252–1276.

Britannica. (2021). Mona Lisa: The Mona Lisa and its influence. Retrieved from https://www.britannica.com/topic/Mona-Lisa-painting/The-Mona-Lisa-and-its-influence

British Library. (2023). Albert Mehrabian. Retrieved from https://www.bl.uk/people/albert-mehrabian

Britton, A. M. (2012). The beauty industry's influence on women in society. *Honors Theses and Capstones, 86*. [University of New Hampshire Scholar's Repository]. https://scholars.unh.edu/honors/86

Bronfenbrenner, U., & Morris, P. (1998). The ecology of developmental process. *The Handbook of Child Psychology, 1*, 993–1029.

Bronfenbrenner, U. (1979). The ecology of human development. Cambridge: Harvard University Press.

Bronfenbrenner, U. (1986). Ecology of the family as a context for human development: Research perspectives. *Developmental Psychology, 22*(6), 723-742.

Brooke, K. (2021, March). Meet Santiago Lyon: Conflict photographer turned content authenticity expert. Adobe Blog. Retrieved from https://blog.adobe.com/en/publish/2021/03/30/santiago-lyon-conflict-photographer-turned-cai-expert#gs.ghdb1t

Brooks, K., Mond, J., Stevenson, R., & Stephen, I. (2016, Aug.). Body image distortion and exposure to extreme body types: Contingent adaptation and cross adaptation for self and other. *Frontiers in Neuroscience, 1*(10), 1-9. [Article 334] DOI: 10.3389/fnins.2016.00334.

Brown, T. A., Cash, T. F., & Mikulka, P. J. (1990, Fall). Attitudinal body image assessment: factor analysis of the Body-Self Relations Questionnaire. *Journal of Personality Assessment, 55*(1-2), 135-44. DOI: 10.1080/00223891.1990.9674053. PMID: 2231236.

Brytek-Matera, A. (2012). Orthorexia nervosa—an eating disorder, obsessive-compulsive disorder or disturbed eating habit? *Archives of Psychiatry and Psychotherapy, 1*(1), 55–60.

Budiman, A., & Ruiz, N. G. (2021). Key facts about Asian Americans. *Pew Research Center.* Retrieved from https://www.pewresearch.org/fact-tank/2021/04/29/key-facts-about-asian-americans/

Bugiulescu, M. (2021). The concept of soul in Plato and in Patristic thought. [International Multidisciplinary Scientific Conference on the Dialogue between Sciences & Arts, Religion & Education]. *Ideas Forum International Academic and Scientific Association, 2021*(5), 80-84. Retrieved from https://doi.org/10.26520/mcdsare.2021.5.80-84

Bulik, C. (2012). The woman in the mirror. New York, NY: Walker & Company.

Bulwer, J. (1644). Chirologia or the natural language of the hand. Retrieved from https://publicdomainreview.org/collection/chirologia-or-the-natural-language-of-the-hand-1644

Burke, E. (1990). A philosophical enquiry into the origin of our ideas of the sublime and beautiful. New York, NY: Oxford University Press. (Originally published in 1757).

Burton, J. W. (2001). Culture and the human body: An anthropological perspective. Long Grove, IL: Waveland Press, Inc.

Butler-Bowdon, T. (2013). 50 philosophy classics. [audiobook, narrated by Sean Pratt]. Audible.com

Butler, G., & Gaines, C. (1977). Pumping iron. [Movie] (Directed by George Butler and Robert Fiore; Produced by George Butler and Jerome Gary). New Hampshire: White Mountain Films.

Butler, J. (1999). Gender trouble: Feminism and the subversion of identity. London, UK: Routledge. (Originally Published in 1990).

Burnett, C. (1987). Justice: Myth and symbol. *11 Legal Studies File 79, 80.*

Cafri, G., Olivardia, R., & Thompson, J. K. (2008). Symptom characteristics and psychiatric comorbidity among males with muscle dysmorphia. *Comprehensive Psychiatry, 49*(4), 374–379. http://dx.doi.org/10.1016/j.comppsych.2008.01.003

Caldwell, C. (1996). The feminization of America. *Washington Examiner, 12*(22). Retrieved from https://www.washingtonexaminer.com/weekly-standard/the-feminization-of-america

Campbell, W. K., & Baumeister, R. F. (2006). Narcissistic personality disorder. In J. E. Fisher & W. T. O'Donohue (Eds.), *Practitioner's Guide to Evidence-Based Psychotherapy* (pp. 423-431). New York: Springer.

Campbell, W. K., Goodie, A. S., & Foster, J. D. (2004). Narcissism, overconfidence, and risk attitude. *Journal of Behavioral Decision Making, 17*(4), 297–311.

Capetillo-Ventura, N. C., Jalil-Pérez, S. I., & Motilla-Negrete, K. (2017). Gender dysphoria: An overview. *Medicina Universitaria, 17*(66), 53–8. DOI: 10.1016/j.rmu.2014.06.001

Carroll, L., Gilroy, P., & Ryan, J. (2002, Spring). Counseling transgendered, transsexual, and gender-variant clients. *Journal of Counseling and Development, 80*(2). ABI/INFORM Global, pg. 131.

Cartwright, M. (2013, Sept.). The ball game history of Mesoamerica. Retrieved from https://www.worldhistory.org/article/604/the-ball-game-of-mesoamerica/

Cascone, S. (2016). Was the 'Mona Lisa' Leonardo's male lover? Retrieved from https://news.artnet.com/art-world/mona-lisa-leonardos-lover-salai-479783

Casey, L. (2021). The Irish legend of the Pooka. Retrieved from https://www.irishcentral.com/roots/history/irish-legend-pooka#:~:text=The%20Pooka%2C%20or%20in%20Irish%20Puca%2C%20%28goblin%29%20is,its%20name%20from%20Poc%2C%20meaning%20he-goat%20in%20Irish

Cash, T. F. (1990). Body, self, and society: The development of body images. In T. F. Cash & T. Pruzinsky (Eds.), *Body images: Development, Deviance, and Change*. (pp. 51-79). New York, NY: The Guilford Press.

Cash, T. F. (2000). Multidimensional body-self relations questionnaire: MBSRQ user's manual. Norfolk: Old Dominion University.

Cash, T. F. (2004). Beyond traits: Assessing body image states. In T. F. Cash, & T. Pruzinsky (Eds.), *Body Image: A Handbook of Theory, Research, and Clinical Practice* (pp. 163-168). New York, NY: The Guilford Press.

Cash, T. F. (2004). Body image: Past, present, and future. *Body image: An International Journal of Research, 1*, 1–5.

Cash, T. F. (2011). Cognitive-behavioral perspectives on body image. In T. F. Cash & L. Smolak (Eds.), *Body image: A handbook of science, practice, and prevention* (pp. 39–47). New York: Guilford Press.

Cash, T. F. (2012). BESAQ. Retrieved from http://www.body images.com/assessments/besaq.html

Cash, F., & Fleming, E. C. (2004). Body image and social relations. In Thomas Cash & Thomas Pruzinsky (Eds.). *Body Image: A Handbook of Theory, Research, and Clinical Practice* (pp. 277-286). New York, NY: The Guilford Press.

Cash, T. F., Jakatdar, T. A., & Williams, E. F. (2004). The Body Image Quality of Life Inventory: Further validation with college men and women. *Body Image, 1*, 279–287. 10.1016/S1740-1445(03)00023-8

Cash, T. F., & Labarge, A. S. (1996). Development of the Appearance Schemas Inventory: A new cognitive body image assessment. *Cognitive Therapy and Research, 20*, 37–50. 10.1007/BF02229242

Cash, T. F., Maikkula, C. L., & Yamamiya, Y. (2004). Baring the body in the bedroom: Body image, sexual self-schemas, and sexual functioning among college women and men. *Electronic Journal of Human Sexuality, June 29*. Retrieved from. http://www.ejhs.org/volume7/bodyimage.html

Cash, T. F., Melnyk, S., & Hrabosky, J. I. (2004). The assessment of body investment: An extensive revision of the Appearance Schemas Inventory. *International Journal of Eating Disorders, 35*, 305–316.

Cash, T. F., Morrow, J. A., Hrabosky, J. I., & Perry, A. A. (2004). How has body image changed? A cross-sectional study of college women and men from 1983 to 2001. *Journal of Consulting and Clinical Psychology, 72*,1081–1089. 10.1037/0022-006X.72.6.1081

Cash, T. F., Phillips, K. A., Santos, M. T., & Hrabosky, J. I. (2004). Measuring negative body image: Validation of the body image disturbance questionnaire in a non-clinical population. *Body Image, 1*, 363–372. 10.1016/j.bodyim.2004.10.001

Cash, T. F., & Pruzinsky, T. (1990). Body images: Development, deviance, and change. New York, NY: The Guilford Press.

Cash, T. F., & Pruzinsky, T. (2004). Body image: A handbook of theory, research, and clinical practice. New York, NY: The Guilford Press. (Original work published 2002).

Cash, T. F., Santos, M. T., & Williams, E. F. (2005, Feb.) Coping with body image threats and challenges: validation of the Body Image Coping Strategies Inventory. *Journal of Psychosomatic Research, 58*(2), 190-9. DOI: 10.1016/j.jpsychores.2004.07.008. PMID: 15820848.

Cassens, R. G., & Cooper, C. C. (1971). Red and white muscle. (C. O. Chichester, E. M. Mrak, & G. F. Stewart, Eds.). *Advances in Food Research, 19*, 1-74. ISSN 0065-2628. ISBN 9780120164196. https://doi.org/10.1016/S0065-2628(08)60030-0.

Chance, B. (1936). William Porterfield, M.D.: An almost forgotten opticopsychologist. *Archives of Ophthalmology, 16*, 197-207. DOI:10.1001/ARCHOPHT.1936.00840200035003 Corpus ID: 73298062.

Chang, V. W., & Christakis, N. A. (2003, May). Self-perception of weight appropriateness in the United States. *American Journal of Preventive Medicine, 24*(4), 332-9. DOI: 10.1016/s0749-3797(03)00020-5. PMID: 12726871

Chapman, L. J., Chapman, J. P., & Raulin, M. L. (1978). Body image aberration in schizophrenia. *Journal of Abnormal Psychology, 87*, 399–407.

Charcot, J-M. (1889). Clinical lectures on the diseases of the nervous system (3 vols). Trans. Thomas Savill. London, UK: New Sydenham Society.

Cheatham, M. J. (1953). Sheldon's somatotypes and the projective techniques. [Ph.D. dissertation]. Western Reserve University.

Cherry, K. (2022). A historical timeline of modern psychology. Retrieved from https://www.verywellmind.com/timeline-of-modern-psychology-2795599

Chigr, F., Rachidi, F., Segura, S., Mahaut, S., Tardivel, C., Jean, A., Najimi, M., & Moyse, E. (2009). Neurogenesis inhibition in the dorsal vagal complex by chronic immobilization stress in the adult rat. *Neuroscience, 158*(2), 524-36. PMID: 19015004 DOI: 10.1016/j.neuroscience.2008.10.040

Chirisa, S. (2017). Dealing with dissociative disorders. *The Herald,* 7(14).

Chrisman, S. (2013). Victorian secrets: What a corset taught me about the past, the present, and myself. New York, NY: Skyhorse Publishing, 149-150.

Christov-Moore, L., Simpson, E. A., Coudé, G., Grigaityte, K., Iacoboni, M., & Ferrarib, P. F. (2014, Sept.). Empathy: Gender effects in brain and behavior. *Neuroscience and Biobehavioral Reviews, 46*(4): 604–627. DOI: 10.1016/j.neubiorev.2014.09.001 PMCID: PMC5110041 NIHMSID: NIHMS828103 PMID: 25236781

Chu, I., & Vu, M. C. (2022). The nature of the self, self-regulation and moral action: Implications from the Confucian relation self and Buddhist non-self. *Journal of Business Ethics, 180,* 245-262. Retrieved from https://link.springer.com/article/10.1007/s10551-021-04826-z

Ciarrochi, J., Heaven, P. C. L., & Fiona, D. (2007). The impact of hope, self-esteem, and attributional style on adolescents' school grades and emotional well-being: A longitudinal study. *Journal of Research in Personality, 41*, 1161–1178.

Clayton, A. H., McGarvey, E. L., & Clavet, G. J. (1997). The Changes in Sexual Functioning Questionnaire (CSFQ): Development, reliability, and validity. *Psychopharmacological Bulletin, 33*(4), 731-45. PMID: 9493486.

Clark, V. R., Hopkins, W. G., Hawley, J. A., & Burke, L. M. (2000) Placebo effect of carbohydrate feeding during a 4-km cycling time trial. *Medicine and Science in Sport and Exercise 32*, 1642-1647. PMID: 10994918 DOI: 10.1097/00005768-200009000-00019

Clayton, A. H., McGarvey, E. L., Clavet, G. J., & Piazza, L. (1997). Comparison of sexual functioning in clinical and nonclinical populations using the Changes in Sexual Functioning Questionnaire (CSFQ). *Psychopharmacological Bulletin, 33*(4), 747-53. PMID: 9493487.

Clements-Nolle, K., Marx, R., & Katz, M. (2006). Attempted suicide among transgender persons. *Journal of Homosexuality, 51*(3), 53–69. https://doi.org/10.1300/j082v51n03_04

Cogan, J. (2022). Phenomenological reduction. *Internet Encyclopaedia of Philosophy.* Retrieved from https://iep.utm.edu/phen-red/

456

Collins, J. K. (1981). Self-recognition of the body and its parts during late adolescence. *Journal of Youth and Adolescence, 10*, 243–254.

Collins, J. K., Harper, J. F., & Cassel, A. J. (1976). Self-body recognition in late adolescence. *Australian Psychologist, 1976, 11*, 153–157.

Collins, J. K., & LaGanza, S. (1982). Self-recognition of the face: A study of adolescent narcissism. *Journal of Youth and Adolescence, 11*, 317–328.

Collins, J. K., & Propert, D. S. (1983). A developmental study of body recognition in adolescent girls. *Adolescence, 28*, 767–774.

Collura, T. F. (2020). Rorschach – Reliability and validity. Retrieved from https://brainmaster.com/kb-entry/id489/

Condor-Fisher, S. (2018). Immigration and diversity. Los Angeles, CA: Independent Publishing.

Condor-Fisher, S. (2021). Bullying and harassment. Los Angeles, CA: Fisher Publishing, Inc.

Connell, R. W. (1987). Gender and Power. Stanford, CA: Stanford University Press.

Connell, R. W. (1990). An iron man: The body and some contradictions of hegemonic masculinity. In M. Messner and D. Sabo (Eds.), *Sport, Men and the Gender Order.* Champaign, IL: Human Kinetic Books.

Connell, R. W. (1995). Masculinities. Berkeley, CA: University of California Press.

Cooper, M-B. (2023). The birthplace of basketball. Retrieved from https://springfield.edu/where-basketball-was-invented-the-birthplace-of-basketball

Cooper, P. J., Taylor, M. J., Cooper, Z., & Fairburn, C. G. (1987). The development and validation of the Body Shape Questionnaire. *International Journal of Eating Disorders, 6*(4), 485–494. https://doi.org/10.1002/1098-108X(198707)6:4<485::AID-EAT2260060405>3.0.CO;2-O

Costill, D. L., Daniels, J., Evans, W., Fink, W., Krahenbuhl, G., & Saltin, B. (1976, Feb.). Skeletal muscle enzymes and fiber composition in male and female track athletes. *Journal of Applied Physiology, 40*(2), 149-54. DOI: 10.1152/jappl.1976.40.2.149. PMID: 129449.

Craighead, W. E., & Nemeroff, C. B. (Eds.) (2022) The concise Corsini encyclopedia of psychology and behavioral science (3rd ed.). Wiley. Credo Reference: https://proxy.lirn.net/WilliamHowardTaftUniv?qurl=https%3A%2F%2Fsearch.credoreference.com%2Fcontent%2Fentry%

2Fwileypsych%2Fsomatosensory_function%2F0%3Finstitutio nId%3D103

Compte, E. J., Sepulveda, A. R., & Torrente, F. (2015). A two-stage epidemiological study of eating disorders and muscle dysmorphia in male university students in Buenos Aires. *International Journal of Eating Disorders, 48*(8), 1092–1101. http://dx.doi.org/10.1002/eat.22448

Condor-Fisher, S. (2021). Bullying and harassment. Los Angeles, CA: Independent Publishing.

Costa, S. N., Alves, A. S., & Melo-Neto, J. S. (2022, June). Effects of dance therapy in women with breast cancer: A systematic review protocol. *Public Library of Science, 17*(6), e0257948. DOI: 10.1371/journal.pone.0257948

Costa, P. T., McCrae, R. R., & Holland, J. L. (1984). Personality and vocational interests in an adult sample. *Journal of Applied Psychology, 69*, 390–400.

Costeris, C., Petridou, M., & Ioannou, Y. (2021). Psychological Impact of Skin Disorders on patients' self-esteem and Perceived Social Support. *Journal of Dermatological and Skin Science, 3*(1), 14-22.

Craig, A. D. (2002). How do you feel? Interoception: the sense of the physiological condition of the body. *Nature Reviews. Neuroscience, 3*(8), 655–666. DOI: 10.1038/nrn894. PMID 12154366. S2CID 17829407

Crofutt, G. (1873). American progress. Retrieved from https://www.loc.gov/pictures/item/97507547/

Crossley, N. (2004). The circuit trainer's habitus. *Body & Society, 10*(1), 37–69.

Crossley, N. (2005). Mapping reflexive body techniques. *Body & Society 11*(1), 1–35.

Csikszentmihalyi, M. (1990). Flow: The psychology of optimal experience. New York, NY: Harper and Row.

Csikszentmihalyi, M. (2002). Flow: The psychology of happiness: The classic work on how to achieve happiness. London, UK: Rider.

Csikszentmihalyi, M. (2014). Flow and the foundations of positive psychology: The collected works of Mihaly Csikszentmihalyi. Claremont, CA: Springer.

Csoboth, C. T., Birkas, E., & Gyorgy, P. (2005). Living in fear of experiencing physical and sexual abuse in association with severe depressive symptomatology among young women. *Journal of Women's Health, 14*, 441–448.

Cunningham, M. L., Castle, D., & Mitchison, D. (2017, Nov.). Muscle dysmorphia: An overview of clinical features and treatment options. *Journal of Cognitive Psychotherapy, 31*(4), 255-272. https://www.researchgate.net/publication/321145066

Cyranowski, J. M., Frank, E., Young, E., & Shear, M. K. (2000, Jan.). Adolescent onset of the gender difference in lifetime rates of major depression: A theoretical model. *Archives of General Psychiatry, 57*(1), 21-7. DOI: 10.1001/archpsyc.57.1.21. PMID: 10632229.

Dacey, J., & Kenny, M. (1994). Adolescent development. Madison, WI: Brown & Benchmark.

Dafermos, M. (2014). Psyche. Retrieved from: https://www.researchgate.net/publication/261985599 DOI: 10.1007/978-1-4614-5583-7_241

Damasio, A. (2010). Self comes to mind: Constructing the conscious brain. New York, NY: Pantheon Books, 2010.

Darwin, C. (1872). The expression of the emotion in man and animals. London: John Murray. (Transcribed for John van Wyhe 2002, corrections 2003, 8.2006. Proofread and corrected by Sue Asscher, 2.2008, corrections by John van Wyhe 10.2022. RN6). Retrieved from http://darwin-online.org.uk/content/frameset?pageseq=1&itemID=F1142&viewtype=text

Daubenmier, J. J. (2005). The relationship of yoga, body awareness, and body responsiveness to self-objectification and disordered eating. *Psychology of Women Quarterly, 29*(2), 207–219. https://doi.org/10.1111/j.1471-6402.2005.00183.x

Davey, C., & Bishop, J. (2006). Muscle dysmorphia among college men: An emerging gender-related counseling concern. *Journal of College Counseling, 9*, 171–180. http://dx.doi.org/10.1002/j.2161-1882.2006.tb00104.x

Davies, C. (2007). Reflexive ethnography: A guide to researching selves and others. (2nd Ed.). London: Routledge.

Davies, H., Schmidt, U., & Tchanturia, K. (2013, Nov.). Emotional facial expression in women recovered from anorexia nervosa. *BMC Psychiatry, 2013 Nov 7*(13), 291. DOI: 10.1186/1471-244X-13-291. PMID: 24200423; PMCID: PMC4226259.

Davies, K. (2021). Marie Antoinette fashions. *BA Fashion Marketing*. Retrieved from https://womens-fashion.lovetoknow.com/fashion-tips-women/marie-antoinette-fashions

Davis, C., & Katzman, M. (1997). Charting new territory: Body esteem, weight satisfaction, depression and self-esteem among

Chinese males and females in Hong Kong. *Sex Roles, 36,* 449-459. https://doi.org/10.1007/BF02766683

Davison, T. E., & McCabe, M. P. (2006, Feb.). Adolescent body image and psychosocial functioning. *The Journal of Social Psychology, 146*(1), 15-30.

Dawes, G.W. (2017, Winter). Ancient and medieval empiricism. In Edward N. Zalta (Ed.). *The Stanford Encyclopedia of Philosophy*. Retrieved from https://plato.stanford.edu/archives/win2017/entries/empiricism -ancient-medieval/

DeBlaere, C., & Brewster, M. E. (2017). A confirmation of the drive for muscularity scale with sexual minority men. *Psychology of Sexual Orientation and Gender Diversity, 4*(2), 227–232. 2329-0382/17/$12.00 http://dx.doi.org/10.1037/sgd0000224

Deckersbach, T., Savage, C., Phillips, K., Wilhelm, S., Buhlmann, U., Rauch, S., et al. (2000). Characteristics of memory dysfunction in body dysmorphic disorder. *Journal of the International Neuropsychological Society, 6*(6), 673-681.

Delahoy, R., Davey, C. G., Jamieson, A. J. Finlayson-Short, L., Savage, H. S., Steward, T., & Harrison, B. J. (2022). Modulation of the brain's core-self network by self-appraisal processes. *Neuroimage, 251,* 118980.

Demasio, A. (2010). Self comes to mind: Constructing the conscious brain. New York, NY: Random House.

DeMello, M. (2004). Not just for bikers anymore: Popular representations of American tattooing. *Journal of Popular Culture, 29*, 37-52. DOI: 10.1111/j.0022-3840.1995.00037.x

Deogracias, J. J., Johnson, L. J., Meyer-Bahlburg, H. F. L., Kessler, S. J., Schober, J. M., & Zucker, K. J. (2007). The gender identity/gender dysphoria questionnaire for adolescents and adults. *The Journal of Sex Research, 44*(4), 370-379. DOI: 10.1080/00224490701586730

De Quincey, T. (1968). A brief appraisal of the Greek literature in its foremost pretensions. In D. Masson (Ed.), *The Collected Writings of Thomas De Quincey.* (Vol. 10, pp. 300–301). AMS Press, New York, NY: AMS Press. (Originally published in 1838).

Derrida, J. (1978). Writing and difference. Chicago, IL: Chicago University Press.

Descartes, R. (1990). Meditations on first philosophy. [Meditationes de prima philosophia]. (Transl. by George Heffernan). Notre Dame: University of Notre Dame Press. (A literal translation

of the six Meditations proper, with facing-page Latin;
originally published in 1641).

Descartes, R. (1998). Meditations and other metaphysical writings.
(Transl. by Desmond M. Clarke). London, England: Penguin.

Díaz, P., Bellucci, A., Yuan, C-W., & Aedo, I. (2018). Augmented
experiences in cultural spaces through social participation.
Journal on Computing and Cultural Heritage, 11(4), 1–18.
https://doi.org/10.1145/3230675

Dibbell-Hope, S. (2000, Dec.). The use of dance/movement therapy in
psychological adaptation to breast cancer. *The Arts in
Psychotherapy, 27*(1), 51-68. DOI: 10.1016/S0197-
4556(99)00032-5

Diemer, E. W., Grant, J. D., Munn-Chernoff, M. A., Patterson, D. A.,
& Duncan, A. E. (2015). Gender identity, sexual orientation,
and eating-related pathology in a national sample of college
students. *Journal of Adolescent Health,57*(2), 144-149.
https://doi.org/10.1016/j.jadohealth.2015.03.003

Dietrich, S., & Hernandez, E. (2022). Languages we speak in the
United States. Retrieved from
https://www.census.gov/library/stories/2022/12/languages-we-
speak-in-united-states.html

Dijkerman, & de Haan, E. H. F. (2007). Somatosensory processes
subserving perception and action. *Behavioral and brain
sciences, 30*, 189-239. DOI: 10.1017/S0140525X07001392

Dillon, J. & Gerson, L. P. (2004). Neoplatonic philosophy.
Indianapolis, IN: Hackett Publishing Company, Inc.

Donker B., & Burmanje P. (2012). Short men. [Kleine mannetjes].
Amsterdam, The Netherlands: Atlas Contact, Uitgeverij.

Doris, E. , Westwood, H. , Mandy, W. & Tchanturia, K. (2014). A
qualitative study of friendship in patients with anorexia
nervosa and possible autism spectrum disorder. *Psychology, 5*,
1338-1349. DOI: 10.4236/psych.2014.511144.

Dowd, J. J., & Dowd, L. A. (2003, Jan.). The center holds: From
subcultures to social worlds. *Teaching Sociology, 31*(1), pp.
20-37. American Sociological Association.
https://www.jstor.org/stable/3211422

Drapela, V. J. (1995). A review of personality theories. Springfield, Il:
Charles C. Thomas Publishing.

Drug Enforcement Administration. (2020). Drug fact sheet: Steroids.
Retrieved from https://www.dea.gov/files/steroids

Duarte, R. A., & Argoff, C. E. (2009). Pain management secrets (3rd
Ed.). Elsevier, Inc. https://doi.org/10.1016/B978-0-323-04019-
8.X0001-7

Dubner, R., & Ke, R. (1999, Aug.). Endogenous mechanisms of sensory modulation. *Pain, 82*(),S45-S53. DOI: 10.1016/S0304-3959(99)00137-2

Duggan, J. J. (1976). A guide to studies on the Chanson de Roland. Retrieved from https://books.google.com/books?id=W9jM8ky77_sC&pg=PA53#v=onepage&q&f=false

Durkheim, É. (1979). Suicide: A study in sociology. [Trans. Spaulding, J. A.]. New York, NY: The Free Press. (Original work published 1897).

Durkheim, É. (1995). The elementary forms of religious life. (Trans. Karen E. Fields]. New York, NY: The Free Press.

Dutta, S., Chawla, S., & Kumar, S. (2018, Feb.). Psoriasis: A review of existing therapies and recent advances in treatment. *Journal of Rational Pharmacotherapy, 4*(1), 1-12.

Eakin, E. (2003, April). I feel therefore I am. *New York Times.* Retrieved from https://www.nytimes.com/2003/04/19/books/i-feel-therefore-i-am.html

Eastern Star. (2023). Order of the Eastern Star: History. Retrieved from https://easternstar.org/about-oes/our-history/

Eatingdisorders.org. (2023). Ben's story. Retrieved from https://www.eatingdisorders.org.au/story/young-professional-male-and-living-with-an-eating-disorder/

Eco, U. (Ed.). (2005). History of beauty. (Transl. by Alastair McEwen). New York, NY: Rizzoli Publishing. (Originally published in 2004).

Eddy, K. T., Thomas, J. J., Hastings, E., Edkins, K., Lamont, E., Nevins, C. M., Patterson, R. M., Murray, H. B., Bryant-Waugh, R., & Becker, A. E. (2015). Prevalence of DSM-5 avoidant/restrictive food intake disorder in a pediatric gastroenterology healthcare network. *International Journal of Eating Disorders, 48*(5), 464-70.

Ede-Osifo, U., & Wilson, L. (2023). Leg-lengthening surgery is gaining popularity among men seeking to be taller, doctors say. [Online article: NBC News, April, 23, 2023] Retrieved from https://www.nbcnews.com/health/mens-health/leg-lengthening-surgery-gains-popularity-men-seeking-taller-rcna79819

Edgerton, M. (2006). Foreword. In Sarwer et al. *Psychological Aspects of Reconstructive and Cosmetic Plastic Surgery* (p. vii). Baltimore: MD, Lippincott Williams & Wilkins.

Edwards, S.B., & Henkel, C.K. (1978). Superior colliculus connections with the extraocular motor nuclei in the cat. *Journal of Comparative Neurology, 179*(2), 451-67. Retrieved from https://pubmed.ncbi.nlm.nih.gov/641226/

Egret. (2023). The symbol of a star. Retrieved from https://egretjewellery.co.uk/blogs/jewellery-reflections/the-symbol-of-a-star-and-their-meanings

Eibl-Eibesfeldt, I. (1989). Human Ethology: The biology of behavior. New York, NY: Aldine de Gruyter. ISBN 0-202-020304

Eichenbaum, I. (2012). Roundtable: The changing landscape of female desire: The growing chasm between "hotness" and sexual obsolescence in a digitized, surgicized, and pornographized world. *Psychoanalytic Perspectives, 9,* 163-202.

Eisenberger, N., & Lieberman, M. D. (2005). Why it hurts to be left out: The neurocognitive overlap between physical and social pain. In D. Williams Kipling, & Joseph P. Forgas (Eds.). *The social outcast: Ostracism, social exclusion, rejection, and bullying*. New York, NY: Psychology Press.

Ekman, P. (2023). FACS. Retrieved from https://www.paulekman.com/facial-action-coding-system/

Ekman, P., Sorenson, E. R., & Friesen, W. V. (1969). Pan-cultural elements in facial displays of emotion. *Science, 164*(3875), 86–88. https://doi.org/10.1126/science.164.3875.86

Eliade, M. (1965). The two and the one. New York, NY: Harper and Row.

Elson, M., & Kohut, M. (Eds.). (1987). The Kohut seminars on self psychology and psychotherapy with adolescents and young adults. New York, NY: W. W. Norton & Co.

Emerson, R. W. (1841). Essays: Self-Reliance. Retrieved from https://www.google.com/url?sa=t&rct=j&q=&esrc=s&source=web&cd=&ved=2ahUKEwjpsJSSuu36AhWaHkQIHdoqCSEQFnoECA4QAQ&url=https%3A%2F%2Fmath.dartmouth.edu%2F~doyle%2Fdocs%2Fself%2Fself.pdf&usg=AOvVaw0b-JwZ-JPKLr9bvjLSf4od

Engelke, M. (2018). How to think like an anthropologist. Princeton, NJ: Princeton University Press.

Entrenas-Yepez, V. G. (2000). The effects of emotional, physical and sexual abuse on Latina body image. Dissertation Abstracts International: Section B: The Sciences and Engineering, 4219.

Erickson, J. (2022). Revisioning the animal psyche. *Journal of Jungian Scholarly Studies, Vol. 17*(7), 7–22. https://doi.org/10.29173/jjs175s

463

Erikson, E. H. (1956). The problem of ego identity. *American Journal of Psychoanalytic Association, 4*, 56–118.

Erikson, E. H. (1963). Childhood and society (2nd Ed.). London, UK: Vintage Press.

Erikson, E. H. (1994). Identity: Youth and crisis. New York, NY: W. W. Norton & Co. (Original published 1968).

Esposito, G., Van Horn, J. D., Weinberger, D. R., & Berman, K. F. (1996). Gender differences in cerebral blood flow as a function of cognitive state with PET. *Journal of Nuclear Medicine, 1996*(37),559–64.

Etchegoyen, R.H. (1985). Identification and its vicissitudes. *International Journal of Psychoanalysis, 66*(Pt. 1), 3-18. PMID: 4066167.

Etzel, J. C. (2006). A diagnostic exemplar of experiential avoidance: Examining shame and selfharm in battered women with PTSD. *Dissertation Abstracts International: Section B: The Sciences and Engineering, 66*(8-B), 4480.

Etymonline. (2021). Normal. Retrived from https://www.etymonline.com/word/normal

Etymonline. (2023). Idea. Retrieved from https://www.etymonline.com/word/idea

Etymonline. (2023a). Tattoo. Retrieved from https://www.etymonline.com/word/tattoo

Eubanks, J. R., Kenkel, M. Y., & Gardner, R.M. (2006). Body-size perception, body-esteem and parenting history in college women reporting a history of child abuse. *Perceptual and Motor Skills, 102*, 485–497.

Evans, C. (2023). BSQ. Retrieved from https://www.psyctc.org/psyctc/root/tools/bsq/bsq-english-download/

Evans, D. (2003) Placebo: The belief effect. London, UK: Harper Collins.

Ezhumalai, S., Muralidhar, D., Dhanasekarapandian, R., & Nikketha, B. S. (2018, Feb.). Group interventions. *Indian Journal of Psychiatry, 60*(Suppl 4), S514-S521. DOI: 10.4103/psychiatry.IndianJPsychiatry_42_18. PMID: 29540924; PMCID: PMC5844165.

Faculty of Physical Education and Sport, Charles University. (2023). Kinanthropology. [PhD Course Description]. Retrieved from https://ftvs.cuni.cz/FTVSEN-122.html

Faith, M. S., & Schare, M. L. (1993, Aug.). The role of body image in sexually avoidant behavior. *Archives of Sexual Behavior, 22*(4), 345-56. DOI: 10.1007/BF01542123. PMID: 8368917.

464

Fawkner, H. J., & McMurray, N. E. (2002). Body image in men: Self-reported thoughts, feelings, and behaviors in response to media images. *International Journal of Mens Health, 1*, 137-162. DOI: 10.3149/jmh.0102.137

Federn, P. (1952). Ego psychology and the psychoses. New York, NY: Basic Books.

Feingold, A. (1994). Gender differences in personality: A meta-analysis. *Psychological Bulletin, 116*, 429–456.

Feinstein, A. R. (1970). Pre-therapeutic classification of co-morbidity in chronic disease. *Journal of Chronic Diseases, 23*(7), 455–468.

Feldman, H. O., Dalgleish, T., & Mobbs, D. (2013). Alexithymia decreases altruism in real social decisions. Cortex, 49 (3): 899–904. DOI:10.1016/j.cortex.2012.10.015. PMID 23245426. S2CID 32358430

Feldman, M. (1997). Projective identification: The analyst's involvement. *International Journal of Psychoanalysis, 78*(Pt. 2), 227–242. PMID: 9152752.

Ferguson, H. (2000). Modernity and subjectivity : Body, soul, spirit. Charlottesville, VA: University of Virginia Press.

Fergusson, D. M., Boden, J. M., & Horwood, L. J. (2008). Exposure to childhood sexual and physical abuse and adjustment in early adulthood. *Child Abuse & Neglect, 32*(6), 607–619.

Ferioli, M., Zauli, G., Martelli, A. M., Vitale, M., McCubrey, J. A., Ultimo, S., Capitani, S., & Neri, L. M. (2018). Impact of physical exercise in cancer survivors during and after antineoplastic treatments. *Oncotarget, 9*, 14005-14034. Retrieved from https://www.oncotarget.com/article/24456/text/

Fernando, J. (2022, Oct.) Compound Annual Growth Rate (CAGR) formula and calculation: How reinvesting your profits at the end of the year can impact your investments. (Reviewed by Julius Mansa; fact checked by Pete Rathburn). *Investopedia.* Retrieved from https://www.investopedia.com/terms/c/cagr.asp

Festinger, L. (1957). A theory of cognitive dissonance. Evanston, IL: Row, Peterson.

Feusner, J. D., Hembacher, E., Moller, H., & Moody, T. D. (2011). Abnormalities of object visual processing in body dysmorphic disorder. *Psychological Medicine*, 1-13.

Feusner, J. D., Moody, T., Townsend, J., McKinley, M., Hembacher, E., Moller, H., et al. (2010). Abnormalities of visual processing and frontostriatal systems in body dysmorphic disorder. *Archives of General Psychiatry, 67*(2), 197-205.

Feusner, J. D., Townsend, J., Bystritsky, A., & Bookheimer, S. (2007). Visual information processing of faces in body dysmorphic disorder. *Archives of General Psychiatry, 64*(12), 1417-1425.

Fidan, T., Ertekin, V., Işikay, S., & Kirpinar, I. (2010). Prevalence of orthorexia among medical students in Erzurum, Turkey. *Comprehensive Psychiatry, 51*(1): 49–54.

Filipas, H. H., & Ullman, S. E. (2006). Child sexual abuse, coping responses, self-blame, posttraumatic stress disorder and adult sexual revictimization. *Journal of Interpersonal Violence, 21*, 652–672.

Fina, D. (2022). The origins of Eros: Myth of the androgynous by Aristophanes in Symposium. Retrieved from https://www.damianofina.it/en/the-origins-of-eros-myth-of-the-androgynous-by-arisotphanes-in-symposium/

Finnegan, R., Shaw, M. & Becker, S. (2017). Restricted Boltzmann Machine models of hippocampal coding and neurogenesis. In Arjen van Ooyen, and Markus Butz-Ostendorf (Eds.), *The Rewiring Brain* (Chpt. 21, pp. 443-461). ISBN 9780128037843 https://doi.org/10.1016/B978-0-12-803784-3.00021-4.

Fisher, G. T., Stark, R. B., & Fisher, J. B. (1984). Aesthetic plastic surgery: The body image. Boston, MA: Little, Brown and Company.

Fisher, G. T. (2001). Carpal tunnel syndrome: In the place of internal neurolysis in current therapy. Los Alamitos, CA: Premier Press.

Fisher, G. T. (2017). Conversations. [Audiotaped conversations and interviews with Dr. Gregory T. Fisher, F.A.C.S., conducted by Author.]

Fisher, S. (1990). Evolution of psychological concepts about the body. In T. F. Cash & T. Pruzinsky, *Body images: Development, Deviance, and Change*. (pp. 1-20). New York, NY: The Guilford Press.

Fisher, S. (2014). Development and structure of the body image. (2nd Ed. 2 vols.) New York, NY: Psychology Press. (First published by Lawrence Earlbaum Associates Inc., 1986).

Fisher, S., & Cleveland, S. E. (1968). Body image and personality (Rev. Ed.). New York, NY: Dover Press.

Flor, H., & FLOR, H. (2002). Phantom limb pain. In V. S. Ramachandran, *Encyclopedia of the human brain*. Elsevier Science & Technology. Credo Reference. Retrieved from

466

https://proxy.lirn.net/WilliamHowardTaftUniv?qurl=https%3
A%2F%2Fsearch.credoreference.com%2Fcontent%2Fentry%
2Festhumanbrain%2Fphantom_limb_pain%2F0%3Finstitutio
nId%3D10361

Foster, G. D., & Matz, P. E. (2004). Weight loss and changes in body image. In T. F. Cash and T. Pruzinsky (Eds.), *Body Image: A Handbook of Theory, Research, and Clinical Practice* (pp. 405-413). New York, NY: The Guilford Press.

Foucault, M. (1970). Les mots et les choses. Paris, Gallimard. English translation: The order of things. London, Tavistock. (Original work published in 1966).

Foucault, M. (1980). Power/Knowledge. Brighton, England: Harvester.

Foucault, M. (1995). Discipline and punish: The birth of the prison (2nd ed.). New York, NY: Vintage Books.

Fox-Davies (2012). A complete guide to heraldry. London, UK: Graham Johnston. (Original published 1909). Retrieved from https://www.gutenberg.org/files/41617/41617-h/41617-h.htm

Franko, D. L., & Keel, P. K. (2006). Suicidality in eating disorders: Occurrence, correlates, and clinical implications. *Clinical Psychology Review, 26*, 769–782.

Frazer, J. G. (1920). The golden bough: A study in magic and religion (3rd ed.). New York and London: MacMillan and Co.

Frederikse, M.E., Lu, A., Aylward, E., Barta, P., & Pearlson, G. (1999, Dec.). Sex differences in the inferior parietal lobule. *Cerebral Cortex, 9*(8), 896-901. DOI: 10.1093/cercor/9.8.896. PMID: 10601007.

Fredrickson, B. L., & Roberts, T. A. (1997). Objectification theory. *Psychology of Women Quarterly, 21*(2), 173-206.

Freedenthal, S. (2017). Language matters: Committed suicide vs. completed suicide vs. died by suicide: Speaking of suicide. Retrieved from https://www.speakingofsuicide.com/2017/09/21/suicide-language/

Freedman, R. (1990). Cognitive-behavioral perspectives on body image change. In T. F. Cash & T. Pruzinsky (Eds.), *Body images* (pp. 272–295). New York, NY: Guilford Press.

Freud, A. (1937). The Ego and the mechanisms of defense. London, UK: Hogarth Press and Institute of Psycho-Analysis.

Freud, S. (1920). Beyond the pleasure principle. In J. Strachey (Ed. & Trans.), *Standard Edition of the Complete Psychological Works of Sigmund Freud,* XIIX (pp. 7-64). London, UK: Hogarth Press.

Freud, S. (1921). Group psychology and the analysis of the ego. In J. Strachey (Ed. & Trans.), *Standard Edition of the Complete Psychological Works of Sigmund Freud*, XIIX (pp. 69-143). London, UK: Hogarth Press.

Freud, S. (1923). The ego and the id. In J. Strachey (Ed. & Trans.), *Standard Edition of the Complete Psychological Works of Sigmund Freud*, XIX (pp. 12-66). London, UK: Hogarth Press.

Freud, S. (1927). Fetishism. In *Miscellaneous Papers, 1888-1938* (Vol. 5 of Collected Papers). London: Hogarth and Institute of Psycho-Analysis (1924-1950), 198-204.

Freud, S. (1953). The interpretation of dreams. In J. Strachey (Ed. & Trans.) *The standard edition of the complete psychological works of Sigmund Freud* (Vols. 4 & 5, pp. 1-627). London, UK: Hogarth. (Original work published in 1900).

Freud, S. (1957). The unconscious. In J. Strachey (Ed. & Trans.) *The standard edition of the complete psychological works of Sigmund Freud* (Vol. 14, pp. 159-215). London, UK: Hogarth. (Original work published in 1915).

Freud, S. (1977). Introductory lectures on psychoanalysis. (J. Strachey, Transl.). New York, London: W. W. Norton & Co. (Originally published in 1920).

Friedan, B. (2006). The feminine mystique. (10th Anniversary Edition). New York, NY: W. W. Norton & Company. (Originally published in 1963).

Fromm, E. (2006). The art of being. Blackstone Audio, Inc. [audiobook]

Fryd, V. G. (1995, Spring). Rereading the Indian in Benjamin West's 'Death of General Wolfe.' *American Art, 9*(1), 72-85. http://links.jstor.org/sici?sici=1073-9300(199521)9:1<72:RTIIBW>2.0.CO;2-J)

Fukutake, T., Kawamura, M., Sakakibara, R., & Hirayama, K. (1993, Feb.). Alloesthesia without impairment of consciousness after right putaminal small hemorrhage. *Rinsho Shinkeigaku, 33*(2), 130-3. PMID: 8319382

Gabbard, G. O. (1996). Lessons to be learned from the study of sexual boundary violations. *American Journal of Psychotherapy, 50*, 311–322.

Gabbard, G. O. (2004). Long-term psychodynamic psychotherapy. Washington, DC: American Psychiatric Publishing.

Galioto R., & Crowther, J.H. (2013). The effects of exposure to slender and muscular images on male body dissatisfaction. *Body Image, 2013*(10), 566-573. DOI: http://dx.doi.org/10.1016/j.bodyim.2013.07.009

Galmiche, M., Déchelotte, P., Lambert, G., & Tavolacci, M. P. (2019, May). Prevalence of eating disorders over the 2000-2018 period: A systematic literature review. *American Journal of Clinical Nutrition, 109*(5), 1402-1413. DOI: 10.1093/ajcn/nqy342. PMID: 31051507.

Galvez-Sánchez, C. M., Duschek, S., & Reyes Del Paso, G. A. (2019, Feb.). Psychological impact of fibromyalgia: Current perspectives. *Psychology Research and Behavior Management, 2019 Feb 13*(12), 117-127. DOI: 10.2147/PRBM.S178240. PMID: 30858740; PMCID: PMC6386210.

Gandola, M., Invernizzi, P., Sedda, A., Ferrè, E. R., Sterzi, R., Sberna, M., Paulesu, E., & Bottini, G. (2011, June). An anatomical account of somatoparaphrenia. *Cortex, 48*(9), 1165-78. DOI: 10.1016/j.cortex.2011.06.012. Epub 2011 Jun 22.

Ganeri, J. (2015). The natural self. Retrieved from https://philosophyofbrains.com/2015/03/31/the-natural-self.aspx#:~:text=A%20natural%20self%20is%20metaphysica lly%20dependent%20on%20the,self%20reducible%20to%20p hysical%20states%20of%20the%20body

Ganesha, S. (2023). Astrology: Jupiter. Retrieved from https://www.ganeshaspeaks.com/astrology/planets/jupiter/

Garcia, T., & Pintrich, P. (1994). Regulating motivation and cognition in the classroom: The role of self-schemas and self-regulatory strategies. In D. Schunk & B. J. Zimmerman (Eds.), *Self-Regulation of Learning and Performance: Issues and Educational Applications.* (pp.127-153). Hillsdale, NJ: Lawrence Erlbaum.

Gard, G., Nyboe, L., & Gyllensten, A. L. (2019): Clinical reasoning and clinical use of basic body awareness therapy in physiotherapy – a qualitative study. *Journal of Bodywork and Movement Therapies 23*(4), 1-7. DOI: 10.1080/21679169.2018.1549592 https://doi.org/10.1080/21679169.2018.1549592

Gardner, A. (1862). Bodies of Confederate artillerymen near Dunker church. [Photograph. Sharpsburg, MD]. Retrieved from the Library of Congress: https://www.loc.gov/item/2012647801

Gardner, R. M. (1996). Methodological issues in assessment of the perceptual component of body image disturbance. *British Journal of Psychology, 87*, 327-337.

Gardner, R. M., & Boice, R. (2004). A computer program for measuring body size distortion and body dissatisfaction.

Behavior Research Methods, Instruments, and Computers, 36, 89-95.

Gardner, R. M., Jappe, L. M., & Gardner, L. (2009, Jan.). Development and validation of a new figural drawing scale for body image assessment: The BIAS-BD. *Journal of Clinical Psychology, 65*(1), 113–122. Wiley Periodicals, Inc. [www.interscience.wiley.com]. DOI: 10.1002/jclp.20526.

Garner, D. M. (2004). Body image and anorexia nervosa. In T. F. Cash and T. Pruzinsky (Eds.), *Body Image: A Handbook of Theory, Research, and Clinical Practice* (pp. 295-303). New York, NY: The Guilford Press.

Garner, D. M., & Garfinkel, P. E. (1979) The Eating Attitudes Test. An index of symptoms of anorexia nervosa. *Psychological Medicine, 9,* 273-279. http://dx.doi.org/10.1017/S0033291700030762

Garner, D. M., Olmsted, M. P., & Polivy, J. (1983). Development and validation of a multidimensional Eating Disorder Inventory for anorexia nervosa and bulimia. *International Journal of Eating Disorders, 2,* 17–36.

Gaymard, B., François, C., Ploner, C. J., Condy, C., & Rivaud-Péchoux, S. (2003). A direct prefrontotectal tract against distractibility in the human brain. *Annals of Neurology, 53*(4), 542-5. Retrieved from https://pubmed.ncbi.nlm.nih.gov/12666125/

Gelfand, M. J., Nishii, L. H., and Raver, J. L. (2006). On the nature and importance of cultural tightness-looseness. *Journal of Applied Psychology, 91*(6), 1225-44.

Gelfand, M. J., Raver, L. J., Nishii, L., Leslie, L. M., Lun, J., Lim, C. B., & Duan, L. (2011). Differences between tight and loose cultures: A 33-Nation Study. *Science, 332*(6033), 1100-104.

Genis-Mendoza, A. D. , Ruiz-Ramos, D. , López-Narvaez, M. L. , Tovilla-Zárate, C. A. , Rosa García, A. , Cortes Meda, G. , … Nicolini, H. (2019, July). Genetic association analysis of 5-HTR2A gene variants in eating disorders in a Mexican population. *Brain and Behavior, 9*(7), e01286. DOI: 10.1002/brb3.1286. Epub 2019 Jun 14. PMID: 31199591; PMCID: PMC6625474.

Gershon, L. (2021). Why does the Bible forbid tattoos. *JSTOR Daily, 2021*(2). Retrieved from https://daily.jstor.org/why-does-the-bible-forbid-tattoos/

Gervais, S., et. al. (2013, Dec.). My eyes are up here: The nature of the objectifying gaze toward women. *Sex Roles, 69*(11), 557-570.

Gethin, R. (1998). The foundations of Buddhism. Oxford, UK: Oxford University Press.

Getty. (2008). Lessons from Bernard Rudofsky. Getty Museum. Retrieved from https://www.getty.edu/art/exhibitions/rudofsky/

Gieler, U., Gieler, T., Peters, E. M. J., & Linder, D. (2020, Nov.). Skin and psychosomatics – Psychodermatology today. *Journal der Deutschen Dermatologischen Gesellschaft, 18*(11): 1280–1298. (*Journal of the German Society of Dermatology*). DOI: 10.1111/ddg.14328 PMCID: PMC7756276 PMID: 33251751

Gitnux. (2023). Tattoo industry statistics. Retrieved from https://blog.gitnux.com/tattoo-industry-statistics/

Glucksman, M. L., & Hirsch, J. (1969, Jan.). The response of obese patients to weight reduction. III. The perception of body size *Psychosomatic Medicine, 31*(1), 1-7.

Glynn, M. A., & Abzug, R. (2002, Feb.). Institutionalizing identity: Symbolic isomorphism and organizational names. *The Academy of Management Journal, 45*(1), 267-280.

Goetz, C. G. (1997). Jean-Martin Charcot and Silas Weir Mitchell. *Neurology, 48*(4), 1128-32. PMID: 9109917; DOI: 10.1212/wnl.48.4.1128

Goldberg, A. (1980). Self psychology and the distinctiveness of psychotherapy. *International Journal of Psychotherapy, 8*, 57-70.

Golden, R. L., & Oransky, M. (2019). An intersectional approach to therapy with transgender adolescents and their families. *Archives of Sexual Behavior, 48*(7), 2011–2025. https://doi.org/10.1007/s10508-018-1354-9

Goldfield, G. S., Moore, C., Henderson, K., Buchholz, A., Obeid, N., Flament, M. F. (2010, April). Body dissatisfaction, dietary restraint, depression, and weight status in adolescents. *Journal of School Health, 80*(4), 186-92. DOI: 10.1111/j.1746-1561.2009.00485.x. PMID: 20433644

Goldstein, J. M., Seidman, L. J., Horton, N. J., Makris, N., Kennedy, D. N., Caviness Jr., V. S., Faraone, S. V., Tsuang, M. T. (2001, June). Normal sexual dimorphism of the adult human brain assessed by in vivo magnetic resonance imaging. *Cerebelum Cortex, 11*(6), 490-7. PMID: 11375910 DOI: 10.1093/cercor/11.6.490

Goldwyn, R. M. (2006). Psychological aspects of plastic surgery: A surgeon's observations and reflections. In Sarwer et al. (Eds.), *Psychological Aspects of Reconstructive and Cosmetic Plastic*

Surgery: Clinical, Empirical, and Ethical Perspectives (pp. 13-23). Baltimore: MD, Lippincott Williams & Wilkins.

Gomez-Marin, A., Paton, J. J, Kampff, A. R., Costa, R. M., & Mainen, Z. F. (2014, Oct.). Big behavioral data: Psychology, ethology and the foundations of neuroscience. *Nature Neuroscience, 17*(11), 1455–1462. DOI: 10.1038/nn.3812. ISSN 1097-6256. PMID 25349912 S2CID 10300952

Gomez-Marin, A., Stephens, G. J., & Louis, M. (2011). Active sampling and decision making in Drosophila chemotaxis. *Natural Communication, 2*(441).

Gorbet, D.J., & Sergio, L.E. (2007). Preliminary sex differences in human cortical BOLD fMRI activity during the preparation of increasingly complex visually guided movements. *European Journal of Neuroscience, 25*(4), 1228-39. DOI: 10.1111/j.1460-9568.2007.05358.x. PMID: 17331218.

Goulding, C., Follett, J., Saren, M., & MacLaren, P. (2004) Process of meaning in "getting a tattoo." *Advances in Consumer Research, 31*, 279-284.

Grabe S., Ward L. M., & Hyde, J. S. (2008). The role of the media in body image concerns among women: A meta-analysis of experimental and correlational studies. *Psychological Bulletin, 134*, 460-476. DOI: org/http://dx.doi.org/10.1037/0033-2909.134.3.460 Retrieved from: https://www.researchgate.net/publication/320671751_Beauty_Body_Image_and_the_Media

Graumann, C. (1996). Psyche and her descendants. In C. Graumann & K. Gergen (Eds.), *Historical Dimensions of Psychological Discourse* (pp. 83–102). New York, NY: Cambridge University Press.

Great Seal. (2023a). Great seal. Retrieved from http://www.greatseal.com/committees/firstcomm/index.html

Great Seal. (2023b). First selfie. Retrieved from http://www.greatseal.com/committees/firstcomm/firstselfie.html

Great Seal. (2023c). Eye of Providence. Retrieved from http://www.greatseal.com/symbols/eye.html

Green, C. (1987). Cubism and its enemies: Modern movements and reaction in French art, 1916-1928. New Haven, CT: Yale University Press.

Greenberg, J. L. (2021). What is body dysmorphic disorder? Retrieved from https://bdd.iocdf.org/professionals/what-is-bdd/

Greenwald, A. G., & Pratkanis, A. R. (1984). The self. In R. S. Wyer & T. K. Srull (Eds.), *Handbook of Social Cognition.* (Vol. 3, pp. 129-178). Hillsdale, NJ: Erlbaum.

Griffiths, S., Hay, P., Mitchison, D., Mond, J. M., McLean, S., Rodgers, B., . . . Paxton, S. J. (2016). Sex differences in the relationships between body dissatisfaction, quality of life and psychological distress. *Australian and New Zealand Journal of Public Health, 40*(6), 518–522. http://dx.doi.org/10.1111/1753-6405.12538

Griffiths, S., Henshaw, R., McKay, F. H., & Dunn, M. (2017). Post-cycle therapy for performance and image enhancing drug users: A qualitative investigation. *Performance Enhancement & Health, 5*(3), 103–107. http://dx.doi.org/10.1016/j.peh.2016.11.002

Griffiths, S., Mond, J. M., Murray, S. B., & Touyz, S. (2015). Positive beliefs about anorexia nervosa and muscle dysmorphia are associated with eating disorder symptomatology. *Australian & New Zealand Journal of Psychiatry, 49*, 812–820. http://dx.doi.org/10.1177/0004867415572412

Griffiths, S., & Murray, S. B. (2017). Muscle dysmorphia: Strategies for treating a muscularity-oriented eating disorder. In L. K. Anderson, S. B. Murray, W. H. Kaye (Eds.), *The Clinical Handbook of Complex and Atypical Eating Disorders* (pp. 235–252). London, UK: Oxford University Press.

Griffiths, S., Murray, S. B., Mitchison, D., & Mond, J. M. (2016). Anabolic steroids: Lots of muscle in the short-term, potentially devastating health consequences in the long-term. *Drug and Alcohol Review, 35*, 375–376. http://dx.doi.org/10.1111/dar.12433

Griffiths, S., Murray, S. B., & Touyz, S. (2015). Extending the masculinity hypothesis: An investigation of gender role conformity, body dissatisfaction, and disordered eating in young heterosexual men. *Psychology of Men & Masculinity, 16*, 108–114.

Griffiths, S., & Yager, Z. (2019, April). Gender, embodiment, and eating disorders. *Journal of Adolescent Health*, *64*(4), 425-426. DOI: 10.1016/j.jadohealth.2019.01.016. PMID: 30904090.

Groesz, L. M., Levine, M.P., & Murnen, S. K. (2002). The effect of experimental presentation of thin media images on body satisfaction: A meta-analytic review. *International Journal of Eating Disorders, 31*, 1-16. DOI: org/10.1002/eat.10005 Retrieved from:

https://www.researchgate.net/publication/320671751_Beauty_Body_Image_and_the_Media

Grosse, V. (2021, Jan.). Transgender youths and eating disorders. [Web article]. Retrieved from http://www.societyforpsychotherapy.org/transgender-youths-and-eating-disorders

Gschwandtner, C. (2021). Faith, religion, and spirituality: A phenomenological and hermeneutic contribution to parsing the distinctions. *Religions 12*(476), 1-23. https://doi.org/10.3390/rel12070476

Guillaume, J. (2015). 9 stories of women's complicated relationship with their bodies. Retrieved from https://www.buzzfeed.com/jennaguillaume/stories-of-womens-body image-struggle

Gupta, M. A., & Gupta, A. K. (2013, Jan-Feb). Evaluation of cutaneous body image dissatisfaction in the dermatology patient. *Clinical Dermatology, 31*(1), 72-9. DOI: 10.1016/j.clindermatol.2011.11.010. PMID: 23245977.

Gur, R. C., Mozley, L. H., & Mozley, P. D. (1995). Sex differences in regional cerebral glucose metabolism during a resting state. *Science, 1995*(267), 528–31.

Guss, C. E., Williams, D. N., Reisner, S. L., Austin, S. B., & Katz-Wise, S. L. (2017). Disordered weight management behaviors, nonprescription steroid use, and weight perception in transgender youth. *Journal of Adolescent Health, 60*(1), 17-22. ISSN 1054-139X. https://doi.org/10.1016/j.jadohealth.2016.08.027. https://www.sciencedirect.com/science/article/pii/S1054139X16303214

GVR. (2023). Cosmetic surgery and procedure market report: 2022-2030. Retrieved from https://www.grandviewresearch.com/industry-analysis/cosmetic-surgery-procedure-market

Hagelquist, J. (2015). The mentalization guidebook. Karnac Books. Retrieved from https://www.centerformentalization.com/mentalization/

Haggard, P., & Wolpert, D. (2005). Disorders of body schema. High-order motor disorders: from neuroanatomy and neurobiology to clinical neurology. Oxford, UK: Oxford University Press.

Haiken, E. (1999). Venus envy: A history of cosmetic surgery. Baltimore, MD: Johns Hopkins University Press.

Haizlip, K. M., Harrison, B. C., & Leinwand, L. A. (2015). Sex-based differences in skeletal muscle kinetics and fiber-type composition. *Physiology, 2015*(30), 30–39. DOI:10.1152/physiol.00024.20141548-9213/15

Halliwell, E., & Dittmar, H. (2004). Does size matter? The impact of model's body size on women's body-focused anxiety and advertising effectiveness. *Journal of Social and Clinical Psychology, 23*(1), 104-22.

Halsted, E. (2015). "Stretched to the limit:" The elastic body image in the reflexive mind. In J. Petrucelli (Ed.), *Body-states: Interpersonal/Relational Perspectives on the Treatment of Eating Disorders* (pp. 79–91). London: Routledge.

Hamshaw, G. (2011). Green recovery: One dancer's harrowing story. Retrieved from https://www.thefullhelping.com/green-recovery-one-dancers-harrowing-story/

Harici, F. (2006). Masonic origins of the United States. Retrieved from https://masonlar.org/masonlar_forum/index.php?topic=320.0

Harmon-Jones, E., & Mills, J. (2019). An introduction to cognitive dissonance theory and an overview of current perspectives on the theory. In E. Harmon-Jones (Ed.), *Cognitive Dissonance: Reexamining a Pivotal Theory in Psychology* (pp. 3–24). American Psychological Association. https://doi.org/10.1037/0000135-001

Harper, D. (2022). Etymonline: Consciousness. Retrieved from https://www.etymonline.com/word/consciousness

Hasan, S. (2013). Mass communication: Principles and concepts. (2nd Ed.). New Delhi: CBS Publishers & Distributors.

Haupt, H. A., & Rovere, G. D. (1984). Anabolic steroids: A review of the literature. *American Journal of Sports Medicine, 12*, 469–484.

Hay, P., Girosi, F., & Mond, J. (2015). Prevalence and sociodemographic correlates of DSM-5 eating disorders in the Australian population. *Journal of Eating Disorders, 3*(1), 1-7.

Head, H., & Holmes, G. (1911). Sensory disturbances from cerebral lesions. *Brain, 34*(2–3), 102. DOI:10.1093/brain/34.2-3.102

Hedstrom, O. (2010). Depersonalization: Self and sensation. Retrieved from https://www.academia.edu/8117366/Depersonalization_Self_and_Sensation

Heidegger, M. (2010). Being and time. Albany, NY: New York University Press. (Originally published by Verlag, 1953).

Heidegger, M. (2001). Poetry, language, thought. (Albert Hofstadter, transl.). New York, NY: Harper. (Originally published in 1971).

Heidelberg. (2011). Mona Lisa: Heidelberg discovery confirms identity. Retrieved from https://web.archive.org/web/20131105050239/http://www.ub.uni-heidelberg.de/Englisch/news/monalisa.html

Heilbrun, C. G. (1973). Toward a recognition of androgyny. New York, NY: Knopf.

Heine, S. J., & Lehman, D. R. (1999). Culture, self-discrepancies, and self-satisfaction. *Personality and Social Psychology Bulletin, 25*(8), 915-25.

Hess, C. L. (2021). Seven countries with the most cosmetic surgeries. Retrieved from https://www.hessplasticsurgery.com/blog/the-seven-countries-with-the-most-cosmetic-surgeries/

Hetzel, M. D., & McCanne, T. R. (2005). The roles of peritraumatic dissociation, child physical abuse and child sexual abuse in the development of posttraumatic stress disorder and adult victimization. *Child Abuse and Neglect, 29*, 915–930.

Hildebrandt, T., Shope, S., Varangis, E., Klein, D., Pfaff, D. W., & Yehuda, R. (2014, March). Exercise reinforcement, stress, and β-endorphins: An initial examination of exercise in anabolic-androgenic steroid dependence. *Drug and Alcohol Dependence, 6*(139), 86-92. DOI: 10.1016/j.drugalcdep.2014.03.008. Epub 2014 Mar 19. PMID: 24690349; PMCID: PMC4039319.

Hinchy, J. (2019). Governing gender and sexuality in colonial India: The Hijra, c.1850–1900. Cambridge, UK: Cambridge University Press. ISBN 9781108492553.

History.com. (2023). Uncle Sam. (Amanda Onion, Missy Sullivan, Matt Mullen, Christian Zapata, Eds.). Retrieved from https://www.history.com/this-day-in-history/united-states-nicknamed-uncle-sam

Ho, S. G., & Goh, C. L. (2015, May). Laser tattoo removal: A clinical update. *Journal of Cutaneous and Aesthetic Surgery 8*(1), 9-15. DOI: 10.4103/0974-2077.155066 License CC BY-NC-SA 3.0. Source: PubMed.

Hohmann, L., Bradt, J., Stegemann, T., & Koelsch, S. (2017). Effects of music therapy and music-based interventions in the treatment of substance use disorders: A systematic review. *Public Library of Science, 12*(11), e0187363. https://doi.org/10.1371/journal.pone.0187363 PMID: 29141012

Hoffman, E. (1988). The right to be human: A biography of Abraham Maslow. Los Angeles, CA: Jeremy P. Tarcher, Inc.

Holden, C. (2005, Jan.). Sex and the suffering brain. *Science, 10*(308), 1574. DOI: 10.1126/science.308.5728.1574. PMID: 15947170.

Holweck, F. (1912). The five sacred wounds. In *The Catholic Encyclopedia*. New York, NY: Robert Appleton Company. Retrieved March 13, 2023 from New Advent: http://www.newadvent.org/cathen/15714a.htm

Honour, H., & Fleming, J. (1982). A world history of art. London, UK: Macmillan Reference Books.

Horney, K. (1942). Self-analysis. New York, NY: Norton.

Horney, K. (1950). Neurosis and human growth. New York, NY: Norton.

Hosseini, S. A., & Padhy, R. K. (2022). Body image distortion. In: StatPearls [Internet]. Treasure Island, FL: StatPearls Publishing. Retrieved from https://www.ncbi.nlm.nih.gov/books/NBK546582/

Hudson, J. I., Hiripi, E., Pope H. G. Jr., and Kessler, R. C. (2007). The prevalence and correlates of eating disorders in the National Comorbidity Survey Replication. *Biological Psychiatry 61*, 348–358. DOI: 10.1016/j.biopsych.2006.03.040

Humphreys, S. (2010, Sept.). The unethical use of BMI in contemporary general practice. *British Journal of General Medicine, 60*(578): 696–697. DOI: 10.3399/bjgp10X515548. PMCID: PMC2930234. PMID: 20849708.

Hussain, L. S., Reddy, V., & Maani, C. V. (2023). Physiology, noradrenergic synapse. [Updated 2023 May 1]. In: *StatPearls* [Internet]. Treasure Island, FL: StatPearls Publishing. Retrieved from: https://www.ncbi.nlm.nih.gov/books/NBK540977/

Husserl, E. (1989). Ideas pertaining to a pure phenomenology and to a phenomenological philosophy: Second book studies in the phenomenology of constitution. Berlin/Heidelberg, Germany: Springer Science & Business Media. (Manuscript edited in 1928, originally published posthumously by Husserl-Archives, in 1952).

Husserl, E. (1999). The idea of phenomenology. Trans. Lee Hardy. Dordrecht: Kluwer. (Originally published 1907).

Husserl, E. (2001). Logical investigations. Ed. Dermot Moran. (2nd ed. 2 vols.) London, UK: Routledge. (Originally published in 1900).

Hutchinson, D. M., Rapee, R. M., & Taylor, A. (2010). Body dissatisfaction and eating disturbance in early adolescence: A structural modeling investigation examining negative affect and peer factors. *The Journal of Early Adolescence, 30*, 489–517.

Ivey, G. (1993). The psychology of satanic worship. *South African Journal of Psychology, 23*(4), 180-185. DOI:10.1177/008124639302300404

Jackson, B., & Eagle, L. (1988). The book of black beauty. London, UK: Macmillan Publishers Ltd.

Jackson, S. A. (1995). Factors influencing the occurrence of flow state in elite athletes. *Journal of applied sport psychology, 7*(2), 138-166.

Jafferany, M. (2007). Psychodermatology: A guide to understanding common psychocutaneous disorders. Primary Care Companion. *Journal of Clinical Psychiatry, 9*(3), 203-13. DOI: 10.4088/pcc.v09n0306. PMID: 17632653; PMCID: PMC1911167.

Jakatdar, T. A., Cash, T. F., Engle, E. K. (2006, Dec.). Body image thought processes: The development and initial validation of the Assessment of Body image Cognitive Distortions. *Body Image, 3*(4), 325-33. DOI: 10.1016/j.bodyim.2006.09.001. Epub 2006 Nov 2. PMID: 18089236.

James, H. (2006). The portrait of a lady. Boston, MA: Houghton, Mifflin & Co. (Originally published 1881).

James, W. (1896, June). The will to believe. [Address to the Philosophical Clubs of Yale and Brown Universities. Published in *The New World*.]. Retrieved from http://krypton.mnsu.edu/~jp6372me/THE%20WILL%20TO%20BELIEVE%20.pdf

James, S., Herman, J., Rankin, S., Keisling, M., Mottet, L., & Anafi, M. A. (2016). The Report of the 2015 US transgender survey. Retrieved from http://www.ustranssurvey.org/reports

Jefferson, Y. (2004). Facial beauty: Establishing a universal standard. *International Journal of Orthodontics, 15*, 9–22.

Jirásek, I. (2009). Nakedness and movement culture. *Physical Culture and Sport. Studies and Research, 1*(12). DOI: 10.2478/v10141-009-0036-7 Retrieved from: https://www.researchgate.net/publication/239057562

Johnson, M. (1987). The body in the mind. Chicago, IL: The University of Chicago Press.

Johnson, T. W., Brett, M. A., Roberts, L. F., & Wassersug, R. J. (2007, July). Eunuchs in contemporary society: characterizing men who are voluntarily castrated (part I). *Journal of Sexual Medicine, 4*(4), 930-45. PMID: 17627740 DOI: 10.1111/j.17436109.2007.00521.x

478

Jonckheere, F. (1954, April-June). L'Eunuque dans l'Égypte pharaonique. *Revue d'Histoire des Sciences, 7*(2), 139-155.

Jones, E. E. (1985). Major developments in social psychology during the past five decades. In G. Lindzey & E. Aronson (Eds.), *The handbook of social psychology* (3rd ed., pp. 47–108). New York, NY: Random House.

Jones, L. (2016). Things are going great in my absence. Divine Openings. Retrieved from https://www.divineopenings.com/best-spiritual-awakening-enlightenment-books

Jones, B. A., Haycraft, E., Bouman, W. P., Brewin, N., Claes, L., & Arcelus, J. (2018). Risk factors for eating disorder psychopathology within the treatment seeking transgender population: The role of cross-sex hormone treatment. *European Eating Disorders Review, 26*(2), 120-128. https://doi.org/10.1002/erv.2576

Jones, B. A., Haycraft, E., Murjan, S., & Arcelus, J. (2015). Body dissatisfaction and disordered eating in trans people: A systematic review of the literature. *International Review of Psychiatry, 28*(1), 81-94. https://doi.org/10.3109/09540261.2015.1089217

Joseph, B. (1989). Psychic equilibrium and psychic change: Selected papers of Betty Joseph. (Edited by M. Feldman, & E. B. Spillius). London, UK: Routledge.

Josephs, R., Markus, H., & Tafarodi, R. (1992). Gender and self-esteem. *Journal of Personality and Social Psychology, 63*(3), 391-402. https://doi.org/10.1037/0022-3514.63.3.391

Joshi, S., Ostfeld, R. J., & McMacken, M. (2019, Sept.). The ketogenic diet for obesity and diabetes-enthusiasm outpaces evidence. *JAMA Internal Medicine, 179*(9), 1163-1164. DOI: 10.1001/jamainternmed.2019.2633. PMID: 31305866.

Judge, T. A., & Cable, D. M. (2004). The effect of physical height on workplace success and Income: Preliminary test of a theoretical model. *Journal of Applied Psychology, 89*(3), 428–441. https://doi.org/10.1037/0021-9010.89.3.428

Jung, C. G. (1960). The nature of the psyche (R. F. C. Hull, Trans.). In H. Read, et al. (Series Eds.), *The collected works of C. G. Jung* (Vol. 8, 2nd ed., pp. 159–324). Princeton, NJ: Princeton University Press. (Originally published in 1946).

Jung, C. G. (1990). The archetypes and the collective unconscious. In Sir Herbert Read & Gerhard Adler (Eds.), *Collected Works* (Vol. 9, Pt. 1, 10th Printing). Princeton, NJ: Princeton University Press. (Originally published in 1959).

479

Jung, C. G. (1992). Analytical psychology: Notes of the seminar given in 1925. (William McGuire, Ed.). London, UK: Routledge. (Originally published in 1926).

Jung, J., & Seung-Hee, L. (2006). Cross-cultural comparisons of appearance self-schema, body image, self-esteem, and dieting behavior between Korean and U.S. women. *Journal of Family and Consumer Sciences, 34*(4), 350-356. DOI: 10.1177/1077727X06286419 Retrieved from https://www.researchgate.net/publication/227945936

Juraska, J. M. (1991). Sex differences in 'cognitive' regions of the rat brain. *Psychoneuroendocrinology, 16*, 105-9.

Justia. (2023). Trade dress. Retrieved from https://www.justia.com/intellectual-property/trademarks/trade-dress/

Kajantie, E., & Phillips, D. I. (2005, Sept.). The effects of sex and hormonal status on the physiological response to acute psychosocial stress. *Psychoneuroendocrinology, 31*(2), 151-78. DOI: 10.1016/j.psyneuen.2005.07.002. Epub 2005 Sep 1. PMID: 16139959.

Kammers, M. P., Kootker, J. A., Hogendoorn, H., & Dijkerman, C. H. (2010). How many motoric body representations can we grasp? *Experimental Brain Research, 202*, 203–212. DOI: 10.1007/s00221-009-2124-7

Kant, I. (1914). Critique of judgment. (Trans. J. H. Bernard.) London, UK: MacMillan & Co. Retrieved from https://www.gutenberg.org/files/48433/48433-h/48433-h.htm#s17 (Originally published 1790).

Kant, I. (1929). Critique of pure reason. (Trans. Norman Kemp Smith.) London, UK: Macmillan. (Originally published 1781).

Kara, T., & Topkarcı, Z. (2018, May-June). Interactions between – posttraumatic stress disorder and alopecia areata in child with trauma exposure: Two case reports. *International Journal of Trichology, 10*(3), 131-134. DOI: 10.4103/ijt.ijt_2_18. PMID: 30034194; PMCID: PMC6028996.

Karaferi, S., Papaliagka, M. N., Tolia, M., Poultsidi, A., Felemegas, P. D., & Bonotis, K. (2022). Dance movement psychotherapy in breast cancer: Throwing the ball to Mount Olympus. *Psychology, 4*, 281–291. https://doi.org/10.3390/psych4020025

Kark, R. (2022). Androgyny. *The Springer Encyclopedia of Personality and Individual Differences*. The Department of Psychology, Bar-Ilan University, Ramat Gan, Israel. Retrieved from https://www.academia.edu/31239664/Androgyny

Kawamura, K. Y. (2004). Asian American body images. In T. F. Cash and T. Pruzinsky (Eds.), *Body Image: A Handbook of Theory, Research, and Clinical Practice* (pp. 243-249). New York, NY: The Guilford Press.

Kawamura, M., Hirayama, K., Shinohara, Y., Watanabe, Y., & Sugishita, M. (1987, Feb.). Alloaesthesia. *Brain, 110*(1): 225-36. PMID: 3801852 DOI: 10.1093/brain/110.1.225

Kaye, W. H., Bulik, C. M., Thornton, L., Barbarich, N., Masters, K., & Group, P. F. C. (2004). Comorbidity of anxiety disorders with anorexia and bulimia nervosa. *American Journal of Psychiatry, 161*, 2215–2221. DOI: 10.1176/appi.ajp.161.12.2215

Keizer, A., Smeets, M. A. M., Dijkerman, H. C, Hout, M., Klugkist, I., Elburg, A., & Postma, A. (2011, Nov.). Tactile body image disturbance in anorexia nervosa. *Psychiatry Research, 190*(1), 115-120. ISSN 0165-1781. https://doi.org/10.1016/j.psychres.2011.04.031

Keizer, A., Smeets, M. A. M., Dijkerman, H. C, Hout, M., Klugkist, I., Elburg, A., & Postma, A. (2012, Dec.). Aberrant somatosensory perception in Anorexia Nervosa. *Psychiatry Research, 200*(2–3), 530-537. ISSN 0165-1781. https://doi.org/10.1016/j.psychres.2012.05.001

Kelvin, W. T. (1879). The sorting demon of Maxwell. [Abstract of a Friday evening lecture before the Royal Institution of Great Britain, Feb. 28, Proc. R.I. vol. ix. P. 113]. In *Popular Lectures and Addresses by William Thomson Kelvin* (pp.144-48), London, UK: MacMillan and Co.

Kendroud, S., Fitzgerald, L. A., & Murray IV, et al. (2022). Physiology, nociceptive pathways. [Updated 2022 Sep 26]. In: StatPearls [Internet]. Treasure Island, FL: StatPearls Publishing. Retrieved from: https://www.ncbi.nlm.nih.gov/books/NBK470255/

Kendzierski, D. (1988). Self-schemata and exercise. *Basic and Applied Social Psychology, 9*(1), 45-59. https://doi.org/10.1207/s15324834basp0901_4

Kenton, W. (2021, Oct. 7). Going concern: Definition and examples. *Investopedia*. Retrieved from https://www.investopedia.com/terms/g/goingconcern.asp

Kernberg, O. F. (1984). Severe personality disorders. New Haven, CT: Yale University Press.

Kernberg, O. F., & Caligor, E. (2005). A psychoanalytic theory of personality disorders. In M. F. Lenzenweger & J. F. Clarkin

(Eds.), *Major theories of personality disorder* (2nd ed., pp. 115-156). New York: Guilford.

Kerry, E. (2023). Confession of a body image bully: Featuring Erin Kerry. Retrieved from https://comparedtowho.me/confession-of-a-body image-bully/

Khalsa, S. S., & Lapidus, R. C. (2016). Can interoception improve the pragmatic search for biomarkers in psychiatry?. *Frontiers in Psychiatry, 7*, 121. DOI: 10.3389/fpsyt.2016.00121. ISSN 1664-0640. PMC 4958623. PMID 27504098.

Kimmel, M. S. (1989). The contemporary 'crisis' of masculinity in historical perspective. In Harry Brod (Ed.). *The Making of Masculinities* (pp. 121–53). Boston, MA: Allen and Unwin.

Kimmel, M. S. (2006). Manhood in America (2nd Ed.). New York, NY: Oxford University Press.

Kimmel, M. S. (2007). Gender and society (3rd Ed.) New York, NY: Oxford University Press.

King, A. J. (2004). The superior colliculus. *Current Biology, 14*(9), R335-8. Retrieved from https://pubmed.ncbi.nlm.nih.gov/15120083/

Kinz, K. (2023). The finger: Symbolism. Retrieved from https://kinzkanaan.com/pages/finger-symbolism

Kioulachoglou, A. (2022). The origins of the doctrine of the "immortality of the soul." Retrieved from https://www.jba.gr/The-origins-of-the-doctrine-of-the-immortality-of-the-soul.htm

Kirkham, N. Z., Slemmer, J. A., & Johnson, S. P. (2002) Visual statistical learning in infancy: Evidence for a domain general learning mechanism. *Cognition, 83*, B35-B42.

Kleck, R., & Strenta, A. (1980, Nov.). Perceptions of the impact of negatively valued characteristics on social interaction. *Journal of Personality and Social Psychology, 39*(5), 861-873. DOI: 10.1037/0022-3514.39.5.861

Klein, A. M. (1993). Little big men. Albany, NY: State University of New York.

Klein, C. (2018, Oct.). World War I veterans' ravaged faces restored by innovative plastic surgery. Retrieved from https://www.history.com/news/world-war-i-plastic-surgery-innovations-gillies

Klein, M. (1960). Early stages of the Oedipus conflict and of super-ego formation. In *The Psychoanalysis of Children* (pp. 179-209). New York, NY: Grove Press. (Original work published 1932). Retrieved from:

https://www.researchgate.net/publication/313167434_Introject
ion

Knapen, J. E. P., Blaker, N. M., & Van Vugt, M. (2018, July). The Napoleon complex: When shorter men take more. *Psychological Science, 29*(7), 1134-1144 https://doi.org/10.1177/0956797618772822

Knight, D. J., Langmeyer, D., & Lundgren, D. C. (1973, Sept.). Eye-contact, distance, and affiliation: The role of observer bias. *Sociometry, 36*(3), 390-401. https://www.jstor.org/stable/2786340

Knopp, L. (2006). Canadian teen convicted of bullying friend into suicide. Retrieved from https://komonews.com/archive/canadian-teen-convicted-of-bullying-friend-into-suicide

Kohut, H. (1971). The Analysis of the self. New York, NY: International University Press.

Kohut, H. (1987). The Kohut seminars on self psychology and psychotherapy with adolescents and young adults. (Miriam Elson, Ed.). New York, NY: W. W. Norton & Company.

Kohut, H., & Wolf, E. S. (1978). The disorders of the self and their treatment: On outline. *International Journal of Psycho-Analysis, 59*, 413-425.

Koide, R., Iizuka, S., Fujihara, K., & Morita, N. (2003). Body image symptoms and insight in schizophrenia. *Psychiatry and Clinical Neurosciences, 56*, 9–15. DOI:10.1046/j.1440-1819.2002.00925.x

Kolbinger, W., Trepel, M., Beyer, C., Pilgrim, C., & Reisert, I. (1991). The influence of genetic sex on sexual differentiation of diencephalic dopaminergic neurons in vitro and in vivo. *Brain Research, 544*(2), 349-52.

Konradsen, H. (2012, Jan.). Body image and cancer. In: Hanne Konradsen, *Topics in Cancer Survivorship* (pp. 12-26). Gentofte University Hospital, Denmark: InTech Publishing. Retrieved from https://www.researchgate.net/publication/221923133_Body_Image_and_Cancer

Kosut, M. (2000). Tattoo narratives: The intersection of the body, self-identity and society. *Visual Sociology, 15*, 79-100. DOI: 10.1080/14725860008583817

Kosut, M. (2006). An ironic fad: The commodification and consumption of tattoos. *The Journal of Popular Culture, 39*, 1035-1048. DOI:10.1111/j.1540-5931.2006.00333.x

Kristeva, J. (2002). The subject in signifying practice. In Kelly Oliver (Ed.), *Portable Kristeva* (pp. 23-129). New York, NY: Columbia University Press.

Krueger, D. W. (2001). Body self: Development, psychopathologies, and psychoanalytic significance. *Psychoanalytic Studies in the Child, 56,* 238-259.

Krueger, D. W. (2002). Integrating body self and psychological self. New York, NY: Brunner-Routledge.

Krueger, D. W. (2004). Psychodynamic approaches to changing body image. In T. F. Cash and T. Pruzinsky (Eds.) (2002, 2004). *Body Image: A Handbook of Theory, Research, and Clinical Practice* (pp. 461-468). New York, NY: The Guilford Press.

Kruijver, F. P., Zhou, J. N., Pool, C. W., Hofman, M. A., Gooren, L. J. & Swaab, D. F. (2000). Male-to-female transsexuals have female neuron numbers in a limbic nucleus. *The Journal of Clinical Endocrinology and Metabolism, 85*(2000), pp. 2034-2041. PMID: 10843193 DOI: 10.1210/jcem.85.5.6564

Krystal, H. (1979). Alexithymia and psychotherapy. *American Journal of Psychotherapy, 33*, 17–31.

Kudielka, B. M., Kirschbaum, C. (2004, April). Sex differences in HPA axis responses to stress: a review. *Biological Psychology, 69*(1), 113-32. DOI: 10.1016/j.biopsycho.2004.11.009. Epub 2004 Dec 25. PMID: 15740829.

Kuhnke, E. (2007). Body language for dummies. Chichester, England: John Wiley & Sons. [e-book]

Kun, G., Chang, H. L., & Hettie, R. (2011). I know you are beautiful even without looking at you: Discrimination of facial beauty in peripheral vision. *Perception, 40*(2), 191–195.

Kunst, J. (2023). Michael Phelps: On addiction and recovery. Retrieved from https://www.amethystrecovery.org/michael-phelps-on-addiction-and-recovery/

Lacan, J. (1953). Some reflections on the ego. *Introduction Journal of Psychological Analysis, 34,* 13.

Lacan, J. (1977). Écrits: A selection. Trans. Alan Sheridan. London: Tavistock Publications.

Lacan, J. (1993). The seminar. Book III. The psychoses, 1955-56. Trans. Russell Grigg. London: Routledge.

Lai, T. M., Li, W., & Feusner, J. (2021). The neurobiology of body dysmorphic disorder. Retrieved from https://bdd.iocdf.org/professionals/neurobiology-of-bdd/

Langworth, R. M. (2011). Drunk and ugly: The rumor mill. Retrieved from https://winstonchurchill.org/publications/churchill-bulletin/bulletin-031-jan-2011/drunk-and-ugly-the-rumor-mill/

Lanius, R. A., Vermetten, E., Loewenstein, R. J., Brand, B., Schmahl, C., Bremner, J. D., & Spiegel, D. (2010, June). Emotion modulation in PTSD: Clinical and neurobiological evidence for a dissociative subtype. *American Journal of Psychiatry, 167*(6), 640-7. DOI: 10.1176/appi.ajp.2009.09081168. Epub 2010 Apr 1. PMID: 20360318; PMCID: PMC3226703.

Laplanche, J., & Pontalis, J-B. (1983). The language of psycho-analysis. London: Hogarth.

Lapras, C., Bognar, L., Turjman, F., Villanyi, E., Mottolese, C., Fischer, C., Jouvet, A., & Guyotat, J. (1994). Tectal plate gliomas. Part I: Microsurgery of the tectal plate gliomas. *Acta Neurochirugica, 126*(2-4), 76-83. Retrieved from https://pubmed.ncbi.nlm.nih.gov/8042559/

La Rose, L. (2011, May). Boys not immune to body image issues, pressures, say researchers. Toronto, Canada: The Canadian Press.

Lasch, C. (1979). The culture of narcissism: American life in an age of diminishing expectations. New York, NY: W. W. Norton & Co.

Lasson, C., Rousseau, A., Vicente, S., Goutaudier, K., Romo, L., Roncero, M. & Barrada, J. R. (2023, April). Orthorexic eating behaviors are not all pathological: A French validation of the Teruel Orthorexia Scale (TOS). *Journal of Eating Disorders, 11*(65), 1-13. DOI: 10.1186/s40337-023-00764-5

Laver, J. (2020/1969). World of art: Costume and fashion. (6th ed.). London, UK: Thames & Hudson.

Laviajera, S. (2019). Confessions of a late 20-something: Body image and self-esteem. Retrieved from https://sarahlaviajera.com/2018/11/30/confessions-of-a-late-20-something-body image-and-self-esteem/

Lebowitz, E. A. (2010). Negative body image bias in college women as a function of self-awareness and self-reported body dissatisfaction. Dissertation Abstracts International: Section B: The Sciences and Engineering, 2690.

Lecrubier, Y. (2001). The influence of comorbidity on the prevalence of suicidal behaviour. *European Psychiatry, 16*(7), 395-399. ISSN 0924-9338. https://doi.org/10.1016/S0924-9338(01)00596-X

Lee, K., Kim, D., & Cho, Y. (2018). Exploratory factor analysis of the Beck Anxiety Inventory and the Beck Depression Inventory-II in a psychiatric outpatient population. *Journal of Korean Medical Science, 33*(16), e128. DOI:

10.3346/jkms.2018.33.e128. PMID: 29651821; PMCID: PMC5897159.

Leibniz, G. W. (1765). Nouveaux essais. (Livre II. Des Idées, Chptr. 1, § 6). Retrieved from https://archive.org/details/nouveauxessaissu0000leib

Lenroot, R. K., & Giedd, J. N. (2009, Nov.) Sex differences in the adolescent brain. *Brain and Cognition,72*(1), 46. DOI: 10.1016/j.bandc.2009.10.008 PMCID: PMC2818549 NIHMSID: NIHMS160271 PMID: 19913969

Leonard, C. M., Towler, S., Welcome, S., Halderman, L. K., Otto, R., Eckert, M. A., & Chiarello, C. (2008). Size matters: Cerebral volume influences sex differences in neuroanatomy. *Cerebral Cortex,18*(12), 2920-31. PMID: 18440950 PMCID: PMC2583156 DOI: 10.1093/cercor/bhn052

Leone, J. E., Mullin, E. M., Maurer-Starks, S. S., & Rovito, M. J. (2014, Sept.). The adolescent body image satisfaction scale for males: Exploratory factor analysis and implications for strength and conditioning professionals. *Journal of Strength and Conditioning Research, 28*(9), 2657–2668.

Levenson, E. A. (1982). Follow the fox—An inquiry into the vicissitudes of psychoanalytic supervision. *Contemporary psychoanalysis, 18*, 1–15.

Levenson, E. A. (1987). The purloined self. *Journal of the American Academy of Psychoanalysis, 15*, 481–490.

Levenson, E. A. (1988). The Pursuit of the particular—On the psychoanalytic inquiry. *Contemporary Psychoanalysis, 24*, 1–16.

Levine, M., & Smolak, L. (2008). Body image development in adolescence. In T. F. Cash & T. Pruzinsky (Eds.), *Body image* (pp. 74–82). New York: Guilford Press.

Lévi-Strauss, C. (1963). Structural anthropology. New York, NY: Basic Books.

Lévi-Strauss, C. (1972). Structuralism and ecology. Barnard College New York, NY: Gildersleeve Lecture (delivered March 28, 1972.).

Lewin, K. (1951). Field Theory in social science: Selected theoretical papers. New York, NY: Harper & Row.

Lewis, M., & Brooks-Gunn, J. (1984). The development of early visual self-recognition. *Developmental Review, 4*(3), 215-39.

Li, E. P., Min, H. J., Belk, R. W., Kimura, J., Bahl, S. (2008). Skin lightening and beauty in four Asian cultures. *Advances in Consumer Research, 2008*(35), 444-449.

Liebman, S. J., Porcerelli, J., & Abell, S. C. (2005). Reliability and validity of Rorschach aggression variables with a sample of adjudicated adolescents. *Journal Of Personality Assessment, 85*(1), 33-39. DOI:10.1207/s15327752jpa8501_03

Limbert, C. (2004). The Eating Disorder Inventory: A test of the factor structure and the internal consistency in a nonclinical sample. *Health Care for Women International, 25*, 165–178. https://doi.org/10.1080/07399330490267486

Linderová, N., Gregor, T, & Sciranka, J. (2019). Attitudes analysis about tattoo of students from Faculty of Physical Education and Sports of Comenius University in Bratislava. *Psychologie a její kontexty, 10*(1), 65–74. DOI: 10.15452/PsyX.2019.10.0005

Linkenauger, S. A., Wong, H. Y., Geuss, M., Stefanucci, J. K., McCulloch, K. C., Bülthoff, H. H., Mohler, B. J., & Proffitt, D. R. (2015). The perceptual homunculus: The perception of the relative proportions of the human body. *Journal of Experimental Psychology: General, 144*(1), 103–113. https://doi.org/10.1037/xge0000028

Liu, A. P. Y., Harreld, J. H., Jacola, L. M., Gero, M., Acharya, S., Ghazwani, Y., Wu, S., Li, X., Klimo, P., Gajjar, A., Chiang, J., & Qaddoumi, I. (2018). Tectal glioma as a distinct diagnostic entity: a comprehensive clinical, imaging, histologic and molecular analysis. *Acta Neuropathologica Communications, 6*(1), 101. Retrieved from https://www.ncbi.nlm.nih.gov/pmc/articles/PMC6154813/

Liu, Y. (2018). A semiotic interpretation of online selfie culture. *Chinese Semiotic Studies, 14*(4), 419–34. https://doi.org/10.1515/css-2018-0024

Lizana-Calderón, P. F., Alvarado, J. M., Cruzat-Mandich, C., Díaz-Castrillón, F. & Quevedo, S. (2023). Psychometric Properties of the Multidimensional Body–Self Relations Questionnaire—Appearance Scales (MBSRQ-AS) in Chilean Youth. *International Journal of Environmental Research of Public Health, 20*(1), 628. https://doi.org/10.3390/ijerph20010628

Lobbestael, J., Arntz, A., & Bernstein, D. P. (2010). Disentangling the relationship between different types of childhood maltreatment and personality disorders. *Journal of Personality Disorders, 24*, 285–295.

Lokko, H. N., & Stern, T. A. (2015, May). Regression, diagnosis, evaluation, and management. *Prim Care Companion, 17*(3). DOI: 10.4088/PCC.14f01761 PMCID: PMC4578899 PMID: 26644947. Retrieved from

https://www.ncbi.nlm.nih.gov/pmc/articles/PMC4578899/#bib
1

Longinus. (2006). On the sublime. (Transl. H. L. Havell). Retrieved
from https://www.gutenberg.org/files/17957/17957-h/17957-
h.htm (Original ca. 1st cent. A.D.).

Loucks, J., Mutschler, C., & Meltzoff, A. N. (2017). Children's
representation and imitation of events: How goal organization
influences 3-year-old children's memory for action sequences.
Cognitive Science, 41, 1904–1933. ISSN: 0364-0213 print /
1551-6709 online DOI: 10.1111/cogs.12446

Love, B. (1992). The encyclopedia of unusual sex practices. New York,
NY: Barricade Press, Inc.

Lown, E. A., & Vega, W. A. (2001). Prevalence and predictor of
physical partner abuse among Mexican American women.
American Journal of Public Health, 91(3), 441–445.

Lucado, D. (2013). Britney Spears: The bigger, the better. Retrieved
from https://www.justjared.com/2013/08/02/britney-spears-
the-bigger-the-better/ [Photographs placed in public domain
by FameFlynet, AKM-GSI].

Lugli, U. (2014). The concept of myth. *Journal of Studies in Social
Sciences, 6*(1), 38-57.

Lundberg, U. (2005, Nov.). Stress hormones in health and illness: the
roles of work and gender. *Psychoneuroendocrinology,
30*(10):1017-21. DOI: 10.1016/j.psyneuen.2005.03.014.
PMID: 15963652.

Lynn, R. and Martin, T. (1997). Gender differences in extraversion,
neuroticism, and psychoticism in 37 countries. *Journal of
Social Psychology, 137*, 369–373.

Lyotard, J.-F. (1984/1979). La condition postmoderne. Paris: Minuit.
[English translation: The Postmodern Condition, trans. by G.
Bennington and B. Massumi. Minneapolis, MI: University of
Minnesota Press.]

MacDonald, G., & Leary, M. (2005). Why does social exclusion hurt?
The relationship between social and physical pain.
Psychological Bulletin, 131(2), 202-223.

MacLean, D. P. (1990). The triune brain in evolution: Role in
paleocerebral functions. New York, NY: Plenum.

MacKinnon, L., & James, K. (1992). Raising the stakes in child-at-risk
cases: Eliciting and maintaining parent motivation. *Australian
& New Zealand Journal of Family Therapy, 13*, 59–70.

Macroni, C. (2018). The Oxford handbook of Greek and Roman art and
architecture. Oxford, UK: Oxford University Press.

Madan, S., Basu, S., Ng, S., & Lim, E. A. C. (2018). Impact of culture on the pursuit of beauty: Evidence from five countries. *Journal of International Marketing, 26*(4), 54-68. DOI: 10.1177/106903(X)8805493

Mahapatra, D. (2014). The Supreme Court recognizes transgenders as third gender. Retrieved from https://timesofindia.indiatimes.com/india/Supreme-Court-recognizes-transgenders-as-third-gender/articleshow/33767900.cms

Main, M., & Solomon, J. (1990). Procedures for identifying infants as disorganized/disorientated during the Ainsworth strange Situation. In M. Geenberg, D. Cicchetti, and E. Cummings (Eds.), *Attachment in the Preschool Years: Theory, Research, and Intervention* (pp. 121-160). Chicago, IL: University of Chicago Press.

Maine, M., & Kelly, J. (2005). The body myth. New Jersey: Wiley.

Malancharuvil, J.M. (2004, Dec.). Projection, introjection, and projective identification: a reformulation. *American Journal of Psychoanalysis, 64*(4), 375-82. DOI: 10.1007/s11231-004-4325-y. PMID: 15577283.

Malden, J. (2020). Hannah Arendt: On standing up to the banality of evil. Retrieved from https://philosophybreak.com/articles/hannah-arendt-on-standing-up-to-the-banality-of-evil/#:~:text=T%20he%20%E2%80%9Cbanality%20of%20evil%E2%80%9D%20is%20the%20idea,people.%20Evil%20becomes%20commonplace%3B%20it%20becomes%20the%20everyday

Malinowski, B. (2005). Introduction: The subject, method and scope of this inquiry. *Argonauts of the Western Pacific, 1-19*. London: Routledge. (Originally published in 1922).

Malpas, J., Pellicane, M.J., & Glaeser, E. (2021). Family-Based Interventions with Transgender and Gender Expansive Youth: Systematic Review and Best Practice Recommendations. *Transgender Health, 7*(1), 7-29 .

Maltsberger, J. T. (1993). Confusion of the body, the self and others in suicide states. In A. Leenaars (Ed.), Suicidology: *Essays in honor of Edwin S. Shneidman* (pp. 148–171). Northrale, NJ: Jonson Aronson.

Mancini, F., Bauleo, A., Cole, J., Lui, F., Porro, C. A., & Haggard, P. (2014). Whole-body mapping of spatial acuity for pain and touch. *Annals of Neurology, 75*(6), 917-924. https://doi.org/10.1002/ana.2417

Mangweth, B., Pope, H. G., Kemmler, G., Ebenbichler, C. et al. (2001). Body image and psychopathology in male bodybuilders. *Psychotherapy and Psychosomatics, 70*(1).

Maniscalco, E., La Marca, L., Faldetta, N., Fabbiano, F., & Verderame, F. (2022, April). Maladaptive personality features, alexithymia, and traumatic events as risk factors for patients with cancer diagnosis. *Journal of Mental Health Counseling; 44*(2), 153-172. DOI:10.l7744/mehc.44.2.04

Maravelias, C., Dona, A., Stefanidou, M., & Spiliopoulou, C. (2005). Adverse effects of anabolic steroids in athletes. A constantthreat. *Toxicology Letters, 158*(3), 167-75.

Marbach, J. J. & Raphael, K. G. (2000). Phantom tooth pain: A new look at an old dilemma. *Pain Medicine, 1*(1), 68–77. DOI: 10.1046/j.1526-4637.2000.00012.x. PMID 15101965.

Marcus, H. (1977). Self-schemata and processing information about the self. *Journal of Personal Social Psychology, 35*(63-78).

Markus, H., Crane, M., Bernstein, S., & Siladi, M. (1982). Self-schemas and gender. *Journal of Personality and Social Psychology, 42*, 38-50.

Markus, H., Cross, S., & Wurf, E. (1990). The role of the self-system in competence. In R.J. Stenberg & J. Kolligian (Eds.), *Competence Considered*. (pp. 205-225). New Haven, CT: Yale University Press.

Markus, H., Hamill, R., & Sentis, K. (1987). Thinking fat: Self-schemas for body weight and the processing of weight relevant information. *Journal of Applied Social Psychology, 17*, 50-71.

Markus, H., & Sentis, K. (1982). The self in social information processing. In J. Suls (Ed.), *Social Psychological Perspectives on the Self* (pp. 41-70). Hillsdale, NJ: Erlbaum.

Markus, H., & Wurf, E. (1987). The dynamic self-concept: A social psychological perspective. In M.R. Rosenweig & L.W. Porter (Eds.), *Annual Review of Psychology, 38*, 299-337.

Markus, H., & Zajonc, R. B. (1985). The cognitive perspective in social psychology. In G. Lindzey & E. Aronson (Eds.), *Handbook of Social Psychology* (3rd Ed., pp. 137-229). New York, NY: Random House.

Marsh, H. W., & Richards, G.E. (1988). Tennessee Self-concept Scale: Reliability, internal structure, and construct validity. *Journal of Personality and Social Psychology, 55*, 612-624.

Marcus, S. (1997). Media and self-reference: The forgotten initial state. In W. Noth (Ed.), *Semiotics of the media*, 15–45. Berlin: Mouton de Gruyter.

490

Martin, K. A., & Lichtenberger, C. M. (2004). Fitness enhancement and changes in body image. In T. F. Cash and T. Pruzinsky (Eds.), *Body Image: A Handbook of Theory, Research, and Clinical Practice* (pp. 414-421). New York, NY: The Guilford Press.

Martinez, E. T., & Spinetti, M. (1997). Behaviour therapy in Argentina. *The Behaviourist Therapist, 20,* 171-174.

Maslow, A. (1965). Humanistic science and transcendent experiences. *Journal of Humanistic Psychology, 5*(2), 219-227.

Maslow, A. (1970). Motivation and personality. San Francisco, CA: Harper & Row. (Originally published in 1954.)

Maslow, A. (1971). The farther reaches of human nature. New York, NY: Viking.

Maslow, A. (2011). Toward a psychology of being. Blackburg, VA: Wilder Publications.

Masood, W., Annamaraju, P., Khan Suheb, M. Z., & Uppaluri, K. R. (2023, June). Ketogenic diet. Treasure Island, FL: StatPearls Publishing. PMID: 29763005.

Matamala-Gomez, M., Diaz Gonzalez, A. M., Slater, M., & Sanchez-Vives, M. V. (2019). Decreasing pain ratings in chronic arm pain through changing a virtual body: Different strategies for different pain types. *Journal of Pain, 20,* 685–697. DOI: 10.1016/j.jpain.2018.12.001

Matamala-Gomez, M., Nierula, B., Donegan, T., Slater, M., & Sanchez-Vives, M. V. (2020). Manipulating the perceived shape and color of a virtual limb can modulate pain responses. *Journal of Clinical Medicine, 9,* 291. DOI: 10.3390/jcm9020291

Mathews, S. & Herzog, H. (1997). Personality and attitudes toward the treatment of animals. *Society & Animals, 5,* 169-175.

Matthews, A. (1908). Uncle Sam. *American Antiquarian Society, 4,* 21-65. Retrieved from https://www.google.com/url?sa=t&rct=j&q=&esrc=s&source=web&cd=&ved=2ahUKEwj4yo_Rpub9AhXUOkQIHWi8BX8QFnoECCcQAQ&url=https%3A%2F%2Fwww.americana ntiquarian.org%2Fproceedings%2F44806541.pdf&usg=AOvVaw1J9dQDoRsHkPZclaFcMmWx

Matusik, A., Grajek, M., Szlacheta, P., & Korzonek-Szlacheta, I. (2022, Aug.). Comparison of the prevalence of eating disorders among dietetics students and students of other fields of study at selected universities (Silesia, Poland). *Nutrients, 14*(15), 3210. DOI: 10.3390/nu14153210. PMID: 35956386; PMCID: PMC9370438.

Maxwell, J. (1867). Letter to Peter Guthrie Tait (11 Dec). In P. M. Harman (Ed.), *The Scientific Letters and Papers of James Clerk Maxwell* (1995), Vol. 2, 331-2.

Mayo Clinic Staff (2023). Glioma. Retrieved from https://www.mayoclinic.org/diseases-conditions/glioma/symptoms-causes/syc-20350251

McCaw, B., Golding, J. M., Farley, M., & Minkoff, J. R. (2007). Domestic violence and abuse, health status and social functioning. *Women and Health, 45*, 1–23.

McCrae, R. R. & Costa, P. T. (2008). Empirical and theoretical status of the five-factor model of personality traits. In G. J. Boyle, G. Matthews, & D. H. Saklofske (Eds.), *The Sage handbook of personality theory and assessment*. (Vol. 1) *Personality theories and models.* London: Sage.

McCuen-Wurst, C., Ruggieri, M., & Allison, K. C. (2018, Jan.). Disordered eating and obesity: Associations between binge-eating disorder, night-eating syndrome, and weight-related comorbidities. *Annals of the New York Academy of Sciences, 1411*(1), 96-105. DOI: 10.1111/nyas.13467.

McDougal, J. (1989). Theaters of the body. New York, NY: W.W. Norton.

McGuire, R. J., Carlisle, J. M. & Young, B. G. (1965). Sexual deviations as conditioned behaviour: A hypothesis. *Behaviour Research and Therapy, 3*, 185–19. PMID: 14253217 DOI: 10.1016/0005-7967(64)90014-2

McInnis, R. (2022). Harold Delf Gillies (1882-1960). *Embryo Project Encyclopedia* (2022-05-31). ISSN: 1940-5030 http://embryo.asu.edu/handle/10776/13336

McLeod, S. (2019). Sensorimotor stage of cognitive development. Retrieved from https://www.simplypsychology.org/sensorimotor.html

McQuail, D. (2007). Mass Communication Theory (5th Ed.). LosAngeles, CA: Sage.

McWilliams, N. (2020). Primary defensive processes. In *Psychoanalytic Diagnosis: Understanding Personality Structure in the Clinical Process* (2 ed.), p. 111. New York, NY: The Guilford Press. p. 111. ISBN 978-1462543694. (Originally published in 2011).

Mee, S., Bunney, B. G., Reist, C., Potkin, S., & Bunney, W. E. (2007, Jan.). Psychological pain: A review of evidence. *Journal of Psychiatric Research 40*(8), 680-90. DOI: 10.1016/j.jpsychires.2006.03.003

Meerwijk, E. L., & Sevelius, J. M. (2017, Feb.). Transgender population size in the United States: A meta-regression of population-based probability samples. *American Journal of Public Health, 107*(2), e1-e8. DOI: 10.2105/AJPH.2016.303578. PMID: 28075632; PMCID: PMC5227946.

Mehmood, A. (2023, Feb.). Body dysmorphic disorder and depression. *Middle East Current Psychiatry, 30*(1), 1-11. DOI: 10.1186/s43045-023-00283-8

Meltzoff, A. N., & Moore, M. K. (1999) Imitation of facial and manual gestures by human neonates and resolving the debate about early imitation. In A. Slater and D. Muir (Eds.), *The Blackwell Reader in Developmental Psychology*. (Pt. 3, Chpt. 12). Oxford, England: Blackwell Press.

Melzack, R. (1990) Phantom limbs and the concept of a neuromatrix. *Trends Neurosci 13*, 88–92.

Melzack, R., Israel, R., Lacroix, R., & Schultz, G. (1997). Phantom limbs in people with congenital limb deficiency or amputation in early childhood. *Brain, 120*, 1603–1620.

Merleau-Ponty, M. (1962) Phenomenology of perception. London and New York: Routledge.

MerriamWebster. (2021). Mediation. Retrieved from https://www.merriam-webster.com/dictionary/mediation

MerriamWebster. (2022a). Fat. Retrieved from https://www.merriam-webster.com/dictionary/fat

MerriamWebster. (2022b). 395 synonyms and antonyms of fat. Retrieved from https://www.merriam-webster.com/thesaurus/fat

MerriamWebster. (2022c). Myth. Retrieved from https://www.merriam-webster.com/dictionary/myth

MerriamWebster. (2023). Nativism. Retrieved from https://www.merriam-webster.com/dictionary/nativism

MerriamWebster. (2023a). Acculturation. Retrieved from https://www.merriam-webster.com/dictionary/acculturation

Messinger, P. R., Xin, G., Smirnov, K., Stroulia, E., & Lyons, K. (2019). Reflections of the extended self: Visual self-representation in avatar-mediated environments. *Journal of Business Research, 100*, 531–46. https://doi.org/10.1016/j.jbusres.2018.12.020

Mikkelson, D. (2010, January 12). Raised finger: Origin. https://www.snopes.com/fact-check/church-key-2/

Milbank, C. R. (1997). Couture, the great designers. New York, NY: Stewart Tabori & Chang.

493

Milkie, M. A. (1999). Social comparisons, reflected appraisals, and mass media: The impact of pervasive beauty images on black and white girls' self-concepts. *Social Psychology Quarterly, 62*(2), 190-210.

Miller, C. C. (1907). The correction of featural imperfection. Chicago, IL: Oak Printing Co.

Millière, R., Carhart-Harris, R.L., Roseman, L., Trautwein, F.-M., & Berkovich-Ohana, A. (2018). Psychedelics, meditation, and self-consciousness. *Frontiers of Psychology 9*, 1475.

Mills, J. S., Shannon, A., & Hogue, J. (2017, Oct.). Beauty, body image, and the media. In Martha Peaslee Levine, Ed., *Perception of Beauty* (Ch. 8). Pennsylvania State College of Medicine. Retrieved from https://www.researchgate.net/publication/320671751_Beauty_Body_Image_and_the_Media DOI: 10.5772/intechopen.68944

Miner, E. (1972). The wild man through the looking glass. In Edward Dudley and Maximillian Novak (Eds.), *The Wild Man Within: An Image in Western Thought from the Renaissance to Romanticism* (p. 106). Philadelphia, PA: University of Pittsburgh Press. ISBN 9780822975991

Miranda, P. (2014). Body and soul relations: Marion Woodman and C. G. Jung. *Jung Bulletin: Uitgave van C.G. Jung Vereniging Nederland – IVAP, 1*(31), 16-19.

Mitchell, N. (2022). Body image pressures as a cisgendered gay man. Retrieved from https://butterfly.org.au/body image-pressures-as-a-cisgendered-gay-man/

Mitchell, R. W. (1997). A comparison of the self-awareness and kinesthetic-visual matching theories of self-recognition: Autistic children and others. *Annals of the New York Academy of Sciences, 818*, 38–62.

Mitzman, A. (1970). The iron cage: An historical interpretation of Max Weber. New York, NY: Alfred A. Knopf, Inc.

Molden, D. C. (2014). What is "social priming?" Understanding priming effects in social psychology: What is social priming and how does it occur? *Social Cognition, 32* [Special Issue], 1–11.

Monton, B., & Mohler, C. (2021, Summer). Constructive Empiricism. In Edward N. Zalta (Ed.). *The Stanford Encyclopedia of Philosophy*. Retrieved from https://plato.stanford.edu/archives/sum2021/entries/constructive-empiricism/

Monzani, B., Krebs, G., Anson, M., Veale, D., & Mataix-Cols, D. (2013). Holistic versus detailed visual processing in body dysmorphic disorder: Testing the inversion, composite and global precedence effects. *Psychiatry research, 210*(3), 994-999.

Morgan, J. F. (2008). The invisible man: A self-help guide for men with eating disorders, compulsive exercise and bigorexia. East Sussex, UK: Routledge.

Morin, J. W., & Levenson, J. S. (2008). Exhibitionism: Assessment and treatment. In D. R. Laws & W. O'Donohue (Eds.), *Sexual Deviance* (2nd Ed.). New York, NY: Guilford Press.

Morley, S. (2021). A short history of the sublime. *The MIT Press Reader, 3*(22). Retrieved from https://thereader.mitpress.mit.edu/a-short-history-of-the-sublime/

Morris, D. (1970). The naked ape (8th printing). London, England: Jonathan Cape Ltd. (First published 1967).

Mort, F. (1988). Boys own? Masculinity, style and popular culture. In R. Chapman & J. Rutherford (Eds.), *Male Order: Unwrapping Masculinity*. London: Lawrence and Wishart.

Mosley, P. (2009). Bigorexia: Bodybuilding and muscle dysmorphia. *European Eating Disorders Review, 17*(3), 191–198. http://dx.doi.org/10.1002/erv.897

Moss, D. (1989). Brain, body and the world: Body image and the psychology of the body. In R. S. Valle & H. S. Halling (Eds.), *existential phenomenological perspectives in psychology* (pp. 63–82). New York, NY: Plenum Press.

Mubarak, H. (2009). "Burqa". In John L. Esposito (Ed.). *The Oxford encyclopedia of the Islamic world*. Oxford: Oxford University Press.

Müllerová, J., Hansen, M., Contractor, A. A., Elhai, J. D., & Armour, C. (2016). Dissociative features in posttraumatic stress disorder: A latent profile analysis. *Psychological Trauma: Theory, Research, Practice, and Policy, 8*(5), 601–608. https://doi.org/10.1037/tra0000148.

Murata, A., Gallese, V., Luppino, G., Kaseda, M. & Sakata, H. (2000). Selectivity for the shape, size, and orientation of objects for grasping in neurons of monkey parietal area AIP. *Journal of Neurophysiology, 83*, 2580– 601.

Murray, S. B. (2017). Gender identity and eating disorders: The need to delineate novel pathways for eating disorder symptomatology. *Journal of Adolescent Health, 60*(2017), 1-2. DOI: https://doi.org/10.1016/j.jadohealth.2016.10.004.

Murray, S. B., Boon, E., & Touyz, S. W. (2012, Dec.). Diverging eating psychopathology in transgendered eating disorder patients: A report of two cases. *The Journal of Treatment & Prevention, 21*(1), 70-74. https://doi.org/10.1080/10640266.2013.741989

Murray, S. B., Griffiths, S., Mitchison, D., & Mond, J. M. (2017). The transition from thinness-oriented to muscularity-oriented disordered eating in adolescent males: A clinical observation. *The Journal of Adolescent Health, 60*(3), 353–355. http://dx.doi.org/10.1016/j.jadohealth.2016.10.014

Murray, C. D., Macdonald, S., & Fox, J. (2008). Body satisfaction, eating disorders and suicide ideation in an internet sample of self-harmers reporting and not reporting childhood sexual abuse. *Psychology, Health & Medicine, 13*, 29–42.

Murray, S. B., Rieger, E., Touyz, S. W., & García, G., L. Y. (2010). Muscle dysmorphia and the DSM-V conundrum: Where does it belong? A review paper. *The International Journal of Eating Disorders, 43*(6), 483–491. http://dx.doi.org/10.1002/eat.20828

Mussap, A. J., & Salton, N. (2006). A 'rubber-hand' illusion reveals a relationship between perceptual body image and unhealthy body change. *Journal of Health Psychology, 11*, 627–639.

Myowa-Yamakoshi, M. & Takeshita, H. (2006). Do human fetuses anticipate self-oriented actions? A study by four-dimensional (4D) ultrasonography. *Infancy, 10*, 289-301.

Nadler, S. (2020). Baruch Spinoza. In Edward N. Zalta (Ed.), *The Stanford encyclopedia of philosophy*. Retrieved from https://plato.stanford.edu/archives/sum2020/entries/spinoza/

Nagata, J. M., Ganson, K. T., & Austin, S. B. (2020). Emerging trends in eating disorders among sexual and gender minorities. *Current Opinion in Psychiatry, 33*(6), 562-567. https://doi.org/10.1097/yco.0000000000000645

NAM. (2022). The birth of plastic surgery. Retrieved from https://www.nam.ac.uk/explore/birth-plastic-surgery

National Cancer Institute. (2023). Adjuvant therapy. Retrieved from https://www.cancer.gov/publications/dictionaries/cancer-terms/def/adjuvant-therapy

National Park Service. (2023). Secret symbol of the Lincoln Memorial. Retrieved from https://www.nps.gov/articles/secret-symbol-of-the-lincoln-memorial.htm#:~:text=What%20do%20fasces%20represent%3F%20In%20ancient%20times%2C%20fasces,that%20a%20man%20held%20imperium%2C%20or%20executive%20authority.

496

Nave, O., Trautwein, F.-M., Ataria, Y., Dor-Ziderman, Y., Schweitzer, Y., Fulder, S., & Berkovich-Ohana, A. (2021) Self-boundary dissolution in meditation: A phenomenological Investigation. *Brain Science 11*(819), 1-32. https://doi.org/10.3390/brainsci11060819

Neda. (2022). Orthorexia. Retrieved from https://www.nationaleatingdisorders.org/learn/by-eating-disorder/other/orthorexia

NEDC. (2023). Body image fact sheet. Retrieved from https://www.confidentbody.net/uploads/1/7/0/2/17022536/nedc_body_image_fact_sheet.pdf

Nelson, R. J. & Liu, Y. (2009). Somatosensory cortex: Functional architecture. In Larry R. Squire (Ed.), *Encyclopedia of Neuroscience* (pp. 79-84). Academic Press. ISBN 9780080450469. https://doi.org/10.1016/B978-008045046-9.01910-0

Nergiz-Unal, R., Bilgiç, P., & Yabancı, N. (2014, Dec.). High tendency to the substantial concern on body shape and eating disorders risk of the students majoring Nutrition or Sport Sciences. *Nutrition Research and Practice, 8*(6), 713-8. DOI: 10.4162/nrp.2014.8.6.713. Epub 2014 Nov 5. PMID: 25489412; PMCID: PMC4252532

Newman, J. C., & Verdin, E. (2017). B-hydroxybutyrate: A signaling metabolite. *Annual Review of Nutrition, 37*, 51-76.

Nicholls, M. E. R., Orr, C. A., Okubo, M., & Loftus, A. (2006). Satisfaction guaranteed: The effect of spatial biases on responses to Likert scales. *Psychological Science, 17*, 1027-1028. https://doi.org/10.1111/j.1467-9280.2006.01822.x

Nickerson, C. (2022). Personality types. Retrieved from https://www.simplypsychology.org/sheldon-constitutional-theory-somatotyping.html

Nietzsche, F. (2016). The birth of tragedy: Or Hellenism and Pessimism. (Translated by William August Haussmann). Retrieved from https://www.gutenberg.org/files/51356/51356-h/51356-h.htm (Originally published in 1872).

NIH. (2023). Encepalopathy. Retrieved from https://www.ninds.nih.gov/health-information/disorders/encephalopathy

Nuñez, C. (2009). The self portrait, a powerful tool for self-therapy. *European Journal of Psychotherapy & Counselling 11*(1), 51–61. https://doi.org/10.1080/13642530902723157

Obong, U. N. (2019). Television and Nigerian cultural values: the symbiosis and social impacts. *Equatorial Journal of Communication Technology, 2*(1), 9–19.

OED. (2023). Beauty. Retrieved from https://www.oxfordlearnersdictionaries.com/us/definition/american_english/beauty

Ogden, P., Minton, K., & Pain, C. (2006). Trauma and the body. New York & London: W.W. Norton & Company.

Ogden, P. (2015). I can see clearly now the rain has gone: The role of the body in forecasting the future. In Jean Petrucelli (Ed.), *Body-States: Interpersonal Relational Perspectives on the Treatment of Eating Disorders* (pp. 92-103). London, UK: Routledge.

Ogden, T. H. (1979). On projective identification. *International Journal of Psychoanalysis, 60*(Pt.3), 357–373. PMID: 533737

Ogden, T. H. (1992a). The dialectically constituted/decentred subject of psychoanalysis. I. The Freudian subject. *International Journal of Psychoanalysis, 73*, 517–526.

Ogden, T. H. (1992b). The dialectically constituted/decentred subject of psychoanalysis. II. The contributions of Klein and Winnicott. *International Journal of Psychoanalysis, 73*, 613–626.

Olivardia, R. (2001). Mirror, mirror on the wall, who's the largest of them all? The features and phenomenology of muscle dysmorphia. *Harvard Review of Psychiatry, 9*(5), 254–259.

Olivardia, R., Pope, H. G., Jr., & Hudson, J. (2000). Muscle dysmorphia in male weightlifters: A case-control study. *The American Journal of Psychiatry, 157*(8), 1291–1296. http://dx.doi.org/10.1176/appi.ajp.157.8.1291

Oravec, J. A. (1998). Every picture tells a story: Digital video and photography issues in business ethics classrooms. *Teaching Business Ethics, 3*(3), 269–82. https://doi.org/10.1023/A:1009869905418

Oravec, J. A. (2012a). Digital image manipulation and avatar configuration: Implications for inclusive classrooms. *Journal of Research in Special Educational Needs, 12*(4), 245–51. https://doi.org/10.1111/j.1471-3802.2012.01232.x

Oravec, J. A. (2012b). bullying and mobbing in academe: Challenges for distance education and social media applications. *Journal of Academic Administration in Higher Education, 8*(1): 49–58. https://doi.org/10.1111/j.1471-3802.2012.01232.x

Oravec, J. A. (2019). Changing the face of higher education: Digital image manipulation and avatars in identity management.

Ubiquitous Learning, 13(2), 1-18.
http://doi.org/10.18848/1835-9795/CGP

Orbach, I. (1994). Dissociation, physical pain and suicide: A hypothesis. *Suicide and Life Threatening Behavior, 24*, 68–78.

Orbach, S. (1993). Hunger strike. London, UK: Penguin.

Orbach, S. (2006). How Can We Have a Body? Desires and Corporeality. *Studies in Gender and Sexuality, 7*(1), 89-111.

Orbach, S. (2009). Bodies. New York, NY: Picador.

Orbach, I., & Mikulincer, M. (1998). The body investment scale: Construction and validation of a body experience scale. *Psychological Assessment, 104*, 415–425.

Ortlieb, S. A., Fischer, U. C., & Carbon C-C. (2016, April). Enquiry into the origin of our ideas of the sublime and beautiful: Is there a male gaze in empirical aesthetics? *Art & Perception 4*(3), 205-224. DOI: 10.1163/22134913-00002051

O'Shaughnessy, B. (1980) The will: A dual aspect theory. Vol. 1. Cambridge, UK: Cambridge University Press.

Osmond, H., Mullaly, R., & Bisbee, C. (1984). The pain of depression compared with physical pain. *Practitioner, 228*, 849–53.

Oswald, A., Chapman, J., & Wilson, C. (2017). Do interoceptive awareness and interoceptive responsiveness mediate the relationship between body appreciation and intuitive eating in young women? *Appetite, 109*, 66-72.
https://doi.org/10.1016/j.appet.2016.11.019

Otte, C., Hart, S., Neylan, T. C., Marmar, C. R., Yaffe, K., & Mohr, D. C. (2005, Jan.). A meta-analysis of cortisol response to challenge in human aging: importance of gender. *Psychoneuroendocrinology, 30*(1), 80-91. DOI: 10.1016/j.psyneuen.2004.06.002. PMID: 15358445.

Oyserman, D., Coon, H. M., & Kemmelmeier, M. (2002), Rethinking individualism and collectivism: Evaluation of theoretical assumptions and meta-analyses. *Psychological Bulletin, 128*(1), 3-72.

Padfield, D., Chadwick, T., & Omand, H. (2017). The body as image: Image as body. *The Lancet, 389*, 1177–78.

Paillard, J. (1999) Body schema and body image: A double dissociation in deafferented patients. In G. N. Gantchev, S. Mori & J. Massion (Eds.), *Motor control, today and tomorrow* (pp. 197-214). Academic Publishing House.

Paillard, J., Michel, F. & Stelmach, G. (1983) Localization without content: A tactile analogue of 'blind sight.' *Archives of Neurology 40*, 548-51.

Palamar, J. J., Kiang, M. V., & Halkitis, P. N. (2011). Development and psychometric evaluation of scales that assess stigma associated with illicit drug users. *Substance Use & Misuse, 46*(12), 1457–1467. http://dx.doi.org/10.3109/10826084.2011.596606

Paolacci, S., Kiani, A. K., Manara, E., Beccari, T., Ceccarini, M. R., Stuppia, L., Chiurazzi, P., Ragione, D. L., & Bertelli, M. (2020, July). Genetic contributions to the etiology of anorexia nervosa: New perspectives in molecular diagnosis and treatment. *Molecular Genetics and Genomic Medicine, 8*(7):e1244. DOI: 10.1002/mgg3.1244. Epub 2020 May 5. PMID: 32368866; PMCID: PMC7336737.

Parisi, R., Symmons, D. P. M., Griffiths, C. E. M., & Ashcroft, D. M. (2013). The identification and management of Psoriasis and associated comorbidity project team. Global epidemiology of psoriasis: A systematic review of incidence and prevalence. *Journal of Investigative Dermatology, 133*(2), 377-85. DOI: 10.1038/jid.2012.339.

Parker, L. L., & Harriger, J. A. (2020). Eating disorders and disordered eating behaviors in the LGBT population: A review of the literature. *Journal of Eating Disorders, 8*(51), 1-20. https://doi.org/10.1186/s40337-020-00327-y

Parker, R. (2011). On Greek religion. Ithaca, New York: Cornell University Press. ISBN 978-0-8014-7735-5.

Patton, M. Q. (1990). Qualitative evaluation methods. Newbury Park, CA: Sage.

Patton, G. C., Selzer, R., Coffey, C., Carlin, J. B., & Wolfe, R. (1999, March). Onset of adolescent eating disorders: population based cohort study over 3 years. *British Medical Journal, 318*(7186), 765-8. DOI: 10.1136/bmj.318.7186.765. PMID: 10082698; PMCID: PMC27789.

Patwardhan, B., Mutalik, G., & Tillu, G. (2015). Integrative approaches for health: Biomedical research, Ayurveda and Yoga. Cambridge, MA: Academic Press.

Pavlov, I. P. (1927). Conditioned reflexes: An investigation of the physiological activity of the cerebral cortex. Oxford, England: Oxford University Press.

PBS. (2017). What does it mean to be American: The answer depends on your politics, study says. Retrieved from https://www.pbs.org/newshour/politics/mean-american-answer-depends-politics-study-says

Peacocke, C. (2014). The mirror of the world: Subjects, consciousness, and self-consciousness. Oxford, UK: Oxford University Press.

Peacocke, C. (2017). Philosophical reflections on the first person, the body, and agency. In Frédérique de Vignemont and Adrian J. T. Alsmith (Eds.), *The Subject's Matter: Self-Consciousness and the Body*. Cambridge, MA: MIT Press, 289-310.

Pearsall, P., Schwartz, G. E. R., & Russek, L. G. S. (2002). Changes in heart transplant recipients that parallel the personalities of their donors. *Journal of Near-Death Studies, 20*(3), 191-206. Human Sciences Press, Inc.

Pease, A. (1988). Body language: How to read others' thoughts by their gestures (10th Impression). North Sydney, Australia: Camel Publishing. [e-book] (Originally published in 1981).

Pease, A., & Pease B. (2004). The definitive book of body language. Buderim, Australia: Pease International. [e-book]

Peirce, C. S. (1931–1966). Collected Papers of Charles Sanders Peirce, (8 vols). Charles Hartshorne, Paul Weiss, and A. W. Burks (Eds.). Cambridge, MA: Harvard University Press.

Penfield, W., & Rasmussen, T. (1950). The cerebral cortex of man: A clinical study of localization of function. New York, NY: Macmillan.

Pereda, N., Guilera, G., Forns, M., & Gomez-Benito, J. (2009). The international epidemiology of child sexual abuse: A continuation of Finkelhor (1994). *Child Abuse & Neglect, 33*(6), 331–342.

Pereira, A. (2012). Body, possibility, and biographical interpretation. *QSR, VIII*(36), 64-86.

Perona-Garcelán, S., Cuevas-Yust, C., García-Montes, J. M., Pérez-Alvarez, M., Ductor-Recuerda, M. J., Salas-Azcona, R., Gómez-Gómez, M. T., & Rodríguez-Martín, B. (2008). Relationship between self-focused attention and dissociation in patients with and without auditory hallucinations. *The Journal of Nervous and Mental Disease, 196*(3), 190–197.

Perona-Garcelán, S., Perez-Alverez, M., Garcia-Montes, J. M., & Cangas, A. J. (2015). Auditory verbal hallucinations as dialogical experiences. *Journal of Constructivist Psychology, 28*(3), 264-280.

Persico, N., Postlewaite, A., & Silverman, D. (2004). The effect of adolescent experience on labor market outcomes: The case of height. *Journal of Political Economy, 2004*(112), 1019–1053.

Perraudin, F. (2018). How tattoos went from subculture to pop-culture. *The Guardian, 11*(26). Retrieved from https://www.theguardian.com/fashion/2018/oct/26/how-tattoos-went-from-subculture-to-pop-culture

Perret, D. I., May, K. A., & Yoshikava, S. (1994). Facial shape and judgements of female attractiveness. *Nature, 368*, 239–242.

Peterson, J. (1999). Maps of meaning: The architecture of belief. New York, NY: Routledge.

Petrucelli, J. (Ed.). (2015), Body-states: Interpersonal relational perspectives on the treatment of eating disorders. London: Routledge.

Petrucelli, J. (2016). Body-states, body image and dissociation: When Not-Me is "Not Body." *Clin Soc Work J, 44*, 18–26.

Phenomenology. (2002). In A. Flew (Ed.), *A dictionary of philosophy*, MacMillan (3rd ed.). Macmillan Publishers Ltd. Retrieved from: https://proxy.lirn.net/WilliamHowardTaftUniv?qurl=https%3A%2F%2Fsearch.credoreference.com%2Fcontent%2Fentry%2Fmacdphil%2Fphenomenology%2F0%3FinstitutionId%3D10361

Phillips, K., Didie, E., Feusner, J., & Wilhelm, S. (2008). Body dysmorphic disorder: treating an underrecognized disorder. *American Journal of Psychiatry, 165*(9), 1111-1118.

Phillips, K. (2021). Prevalence of BDD. *International OCD Foundation.* Retrieved from https://bdd.iocdf.org/professionals/prevalence/#:~:text=This%20means%20that%20more%20than%205%20million%20people,reluctant%20to%20reveal%20their%20BDD%20symptoms%20to%20others

Piaget, J. (1946). Play, dreams, and imitation in childhood. New York, NY: Norton.

Piccardi, L., Iaria, G., Ricci, M., Bianchini, F., Zompanti, L., & Guariglia, C. (2008, Feb.). Walking in the Corsi test: Which type of memory do you need? *Neuroscience Letters, 20*;432(2), 127-31. DOI: 10.1016/j.neulet.2007.12.044. Epub 2008 Jan 15. PMID: 18226450.

Piacentino, D., Kotzalidis, G., del Casale, A., Aromatario, D. M., Pomara, C., Girardi, P., et al. (2015). Anabolic-androgenic steroid use and psychopathology in athletes. A systematic review. *Current Neuropharmacology, 13*(1), 101-21. http://www.ingentaconnect.com/content/ben/cn/2015/00000013/00000001/art00011

Plato. (n/d)). The Project Gutenberg e-book of Phaedo. Sue Asscher, & David Widger (Eds.). [Transl. by Benjamin Jowett]. Retrieved from https://www.gutenberg.org/files/1658/1658-h/1658-h.htm

Plato. (360 BC). Timaeus. Retrieved from
https://www.gutenberg.org/files/1572/1572-h/1572-h.htm

Plato. (370 BC). Phaedrus. Retrieved from
https://freeclassicebooks.com/Plato/Phaedrus.pdf

Pohanka, S. (2001). The hidden obvious. [Interview conducted by the author with Dr. Sylvia Pohanka, Department of Dermatology, Charles University, Prague.]

Polidoro, P. (2019). Image schemas in visual semiotics: Looking for an origin of plastic language. *Cognitive Semiotics, 2019,* 1-11. Rome, Italy: LUMSA University.

Pollatos, O., Kurz, A-L., Albrecht, J., Schreder, T., Kleemann, A. M., Schöpf, V., Kopietz, R., Wiesmann, M., & Schandry, R. (2008). Reduced perception of bodily signals in anorexia nervosa. *Eating Behaviors, 9*(4), 381-388. ISSN 1471-0153. https://doi.org/10.1016/j.eatbeh.2008.02.001.

Pollock, S. E., Taylor, S., Oyerinde, O., ...Kourosh, S. A. (2020, Sept.). The dark side of skin lightening: An international collaboration and review of a public health issue affecting dermatology. *International Journal of Women's Dermatology, 7*(2), 1-22. DOI: 10.1016/j.ijwd.2020.09.006

Pope, H. G., Jr., & Brower, K. J. (2000). Anabolic-androgenic steroid abuse. In B. J. Sadock & V. A. Sadock (Eds.), *Comprehensive Textbook of Psychiatry* (Vol. VII), (pp. 1419–1431). Philadelphia, PA: Lippincott Williams & Wilkins.

Pope, H. G., Gruber, A. J., Choi, P., Olivardia, R., & Phillips, K. A. (1997). Muscle dysmorphia: An unrecognized form of body dysmorphic disorder? *Psychosomatics, 38,* 548-557. http://dx.doi.org/10.1016/S0033-3182(97)71400-2

Pope, H. G., Jr., Katz, D. L., & Hudson, J. I. (1993). Anorexia nervosa and "reverse anorexia" among 108 male body builders. *Comprehensive Psychiatry, 34,* 406-409.

Pope, H. G., Jr., Olivardia, R., Gruber, A., & Borowiecki, J. (1999). Evolving ideals of male body image as seen through action toys. *International Journal of Eating Disorders, 26,* 65-72.

Pope, H. G., Jr., Phillips, K. A., & Olivardia, R. (2000). The Adonis complex: The secret crisis of male body obsession. New York: The Free Press.

Pope, C., Pope, H. G., Jr., Menard, W., Fay, C., Olivardia, R., & Phillips, K. (2005). Clinical features of muscle dysmorphia among males with body dysmorphic disorder. *Body Image, 2,* 395–400. http://dx.doi.org/10.1016/j.bodyim.2005.09.001

Porcelli, P., & Mihura, J. L. (2010). Assessment of alexithymia with the Rorschach comprehensive system: The Rorschach

Alexithymia Scale (RAS). *Journal Of Personality Assessment, 92*(2), 128-136. DOI:10.1080/00223890903508146

Posavac, H. D., Posavac, S. S., & Weigel, R. G. (2001, Sept.) Reducing the impact of media images on women at risk for body image disturbance: Three targeted interventions. *Journal of Social and Clinical Psychology, 20*(3), 324-340. DOI: 10.1521/jscp.20.3.324.22308

PRC. (2023). Religious landscape study. Retrieved from https://www.pewresearch.org/religion/religious-landscape-study/

Pressly, W. L. (1985). Review of the valiant hero: Benjamin West and grand-style history painting, by Abrams. *Archives of American Art Journal 25*(3), 27-29.

Price, C. J. (2004). Body oriented therapy in sexual abuse recovery: A study of efficacy, dissociation and process. *Dissertation Abstracts International: Section B: The Sciences and Engineering, 65*(5-B), 2646.

Price, E. H. (2006, June). A critical review of congenital phantom limb cases and a developmental theory for the basis of body image. *Conscious Cogn., 15*(2), 310-22. PMID: 16182566; DOI: 10.1016/j.concog.2005.07.003

Prince, M. (1906). The dissociation of a personality. New York, NY: Longman, Green and Co.

Probst, M., Vandereycken, W., Van Coppenolle, H., & Pieters, G. (1998). Body size estimation in anorexia nervosa patients: The significance of overestimation. *Journal of Psychosomatic Research, 44*(3–4), 451-456. https://doi.org/10.1016/S0022-3999(97)00270-5

Psychologytoday. (2022). Depersonalization. Retrieved from https://www.psychologytoday.com/us/conditions/depersonalizationderealization-disorder

Purves, D., Augustine, G. J., Fitzpatrick, D., et al. (Eds.). Neuroscience (2nd Ed.). Sunderland, MA: Sinauer Associates. [Neuroglial Cells]. Available from: https://www.ncbi.nlm.nih.gov/books/NBK10869/

Quigley, R. (2020, March). BHB (beta-hydroxy butyrate) benefits and side effects. Retrieved from https://community.bulksupplements.com/bhb-beta-hydroxybutyrate/

Quinn, N. P., Toone, B., Lang, A. E., Marsden, C. D. & Parkes, J. D. (1983). Dopa dose-dependent sexual deviation. *British Journal of Psychiatry, 142*, 296–298.

Quirk, R., Greenbaum, S., Leech, G., & Svartvik, J. (2003). A comprehensive grammar of the English language. (Edited by David Crystal). Halow, England: Pearson Education. Longman. (Originally published in 1985).

Rabinowicz, T. D., & Courten-Myers, J., McD-C. (1999). Gender differences in the human cerebral cortex: More neurons in males, more processes in females. *Journal of Child Neurology, 14*, 98–107.

Rabinowicz, T., MacDonald-Comber, J., Gartside, P. S., Sheyn, D., Sheyn, T., & Courten-Myers, J., McD-C. (2002, Jan.). Structure of the cerebral cortex in men and women. *Journal of Neuropathology & Experimental Neurology, Volume 61*(1), 46–57. https://doi.org/10.1093/jnen/61.1.46

Rabstejnek, Carl. (2015). A brief review of self psychology. Retrieved from https://www.researchgate.net/publication/284898645_A_Brief_Review_of_Self_Psychology

Radika, L. M., & Hayslip, B. (2004). Projective techniques to assess body image. In T. F. Cash and T. Pruzinsky (Eds.), *Body Image: A Handbook of Theory, Research, and Clinical Practice* (pp. 155-162). New York, NY: The Guilford Press.

Rainville, P. (2002, April). Brain mechanisms of pain affect and pain modulation. *Current Opinion in Neurobiology, 12*(2), 195-204. DOI: 10.1016/s0959-4388(02)00313-6. PMID: 12015237.

Rakel, D. (Ed.). (2007). Integrative medicine (2nd Ed.). Philadelphia, PA: WB Saunders, an imprint of Elsevier.

Ramachandran, V. S. (2008). Phantom penises in transsexuals. *Journal of Consciousness Studies, 15*(1), 5-16.

Ramos, G. (2023). What is sarcoplasmic and myofibrillar muscle hypertrophy? Retrieved from https://seriouslystrongtraining.com/what-is-sarcoplasmic-myofibrillar-muscle-hypertrophy/

Rao, R. M., Amritanshu, R., Vinutha, H. T., Vaishnaruby, S., Deepashree, S., Megha, M., et al. (2017). Role of yoga in cancer patients: Expectations, benefits, and risks: A review. *Indian Journal of Palliative Care, 23*, 225-30.

Rasmussen, D. M., Hansen, H. P., & Elverdam, B. (2010). How cancer survivors experience their changed body encountering others. *European Journal of Oncology Nursing 14*, 154–159.

Ratcliff, J. J., & Lassiter, G. D. (2007). On the induction and consequences of variation in behavior perception. *Current Psychology, 26*(1), 16–36. DOI:10.1007/s12144-007-9003-9

Rhodes, G. (2006). The evolutionary psychology of facial beauty. *Annual Review of Psychology, 57*, 199–226.

Rhodes, G., Yoshikawa, S., Palerm, R., Simmons, L. W., Peters, M. C., Lee, K., . . . Crawford, J. R. (2007). Perceived health contributes to the attractiveness of facial symmetry, averageness, and sexual dimorphism. *Perception, 36*, 1244–1252.

Rhodes, G., Zebrowitz, L. A., Clark, A., Kalick, S. M., Hightower, A., & McKay, R. (2001). Do facial averageness and symmetry signal health. *Evolution and Human Behavior, 22*(1), 31–46.

Rhymezone.com. (2022). Fat. Full-sized. Retrieved from https://www.rhymezone.com/r/rhyme.cgi?Word=fat&typeofrhyme=syn&org1=syl&org2=l&org3=y

Richter, M., Tharmalingam, S., Burroughs, E., King, N., Menard, W., Kennedy, J., et al. (2004). A preliminary genetic investigation of the relationship between body dysmorphic disorder and OCD. *Neuropsychopharmacology, 29*, S200-S200.

Riddle, J. E. (1838). English Latin dictionary. London, England: Longman, Orme, Brown, Green, and Lognmans, Paternoster-Row; and John Murray. Retrieved from www.archive.com

Riedweg, C. (2005). Pythagoras: His life, teaching and influence. Ithaca, NY: Cornell University Press.

Rizzolatti, G., & Craighero, L. (2004) The mirror neuron system. *Annual Review of Neuroscience, 27*, 169-192.

Robinson, H. (2020, Fall). Dualism. In Edward N. Zalta (Ed.), *The Stanford encyclopedia of philosophy*. Retrieved from https://plato.stanford.edu/archives/fall2020/entries/dualism/

Rodman, G. (2006). Mass media in changing world: History, industry and controversy. Boston: McGraw-Hill.

Roeder, A. (2015). Advertising's toxic effect on eating and body image. School of Public Health, Harvard University. Retrieved from https://www.hsph.harvard.edu/news/features/advertisings-toxic-effect-on-eating-and-body image/

Rogers, B. O. (1971). A brief history of cosmetic surgery. *Surgical Chronicles of North America, 51*(2), 265-288.

Rojas-Morales, P., Tapia, E., & Pedraza-Chaverri, J. (2016). B-hydroxybutyrate: A signaling metabolite in starvation response? *Cellular Signaling, 28,* 917-923.

Rosenberg, M. (1965). Society and the adolescent self-image. Princeton, NJ: Princeton University Press.

Rosenberg, M. (1979). Conceiving the self. New York, NY: Basic Books.

Rosenthal, A. M. (1964). Thirty-eight witnesses. New York: McGraw Hill.

Ross, C. A. (2021). Problems with the dissociative subtype of posttraumatic stress disorder in DSM-5. *European Journal of Trauma and Dissociation, 5*(4), 100081. https://doi.org/10.1016/j.ejtd.2018.08.005

Ross, J. G. (1975, Feb.). The concept of androgyny. [Conference paper]. J. Sherwood Williams, Allan M. Schwartzbaum, and Rodney F. Ganey (Eds.), *Sociological Research Symposium V*. Richmond, VA: University of Virginia Press.

Rugbyfootballhistory.com. (2023). Origins of rugby. Retrieved from http://www.rugbyfootballhistory.com/originsofrugby.htm

Russon, M-A. (2014). China photo story: The last survivors of crippling foot binding tradition. Retrieved from https://www.ibtimes.co.uk/china-photo-story-last-survivors-crippling-foot-binding-tradition-1451949

Ryan, T. A., & Morrison, T. G. (2014, Sept.). Psychometric properties of the drive for muscularity attitudes questionnaire among Irish men. *Sage Open, 4*(3), 1-7. DOI: 10.1177/2158244014551526

Sabbatini, R. M. E. (1997). Are there differences between the brains of males and females? Retrieved from https://cerebromente.org.br/n11/mente/eisntein/cerebro-homens.html

Sadibolova, R., Ferre, E. R., Linkenauger, S. A., & Longo, M. R. (2019, Feb.). Distortions of perceived volume and length of body parts. *Cortex, 111*, 74-86. https://doi.org/10.1016/j.cortex.2018.10.016

Sadove, M. S., & Cassels, W. H., (1947). Endotracheal anesthesia. *Archives of Surgery, 55*(4), 493–497. doi:10.1001/archsurg.1947.01230080501009

Sakson-Obada, O., Chudzikiewicz, P., Pankowski, D., & Jarema, M. (2016, Nov.). Body image and body experience disturbances in schizophrenia: An attempt to introduce the concept of body delf as a conceptual framework. *Current Psychology, 37*, 390–400. DOI: 10.1007/s12144-016-9526-z

Saltin, B., Henriksson, J., Nygaard, E., Andersen, P., & Jansson, E. (1977). Fiber types and metabolic potentials of skeletal muscles in sedentary man and endurance runners. *Annals of the New York Academy of Sciences, 301*, 3-29. DOI: 10.1111/j.1749-6632.1977.tb38182.x. PMID: 73362.

Sam, N. (2018). Rorschach test. In PsychologyDictionary.org. Retrieved from https://psychologydictionary.org/rorschach-test/

Sam, N. (2022). What is priming? Retrieved from https://psychologydictionary.org/priming/

Sam, N. (2023). Allopsyche. Retrieved from https://psychologydictionary.org/allopsychic/

Samaras, T. T. (2012). How height is related to our health and longevity: a review. *Nutrition and Health, 21*(4), 247-261.

Samaras, T. T. (2017). Biological parameters explain why shorter or smaller people have lower cardiovascular disease and greater longevity. *JSRR, 15*(1), 1-16; Article no. JSRR.34729.2.

Samaras, T. T., Marson, S. M., & Lillis, J. P. (2019). International data demonstrating the inverse height and life expectancy between the sexes. *Journal of Social Science, 4*, 2581-6.

Samaras, T. T., & Storms, L. H. (1992). Impact of height and weight on life span. *Bulletin of the World Health Organization, 70*(2), 259-267.

Sansone, R. A., Chu, J. W., & Wiederman, M. W. (2010, Nov-Dec.). Body image and borderline personality disorder among psychiatric inpatients. *Comprehensive Psychiatry, 51*(6), 579-84. DOI: 10.1016/j.comppsych.2010.04.001. PMID: 20965303.

Santonastaso, P., Favaro, A., Ferrara, S., Sala, A., & Zanetti, T. (1995). Prevalence of body image disturbance in a female adolescent sample: A longitudinal study. *Eating Disorders: The Journal of Treatment & Prevention, 3*(4), 342–350. https://doi.org/10.1080/10640269508250064

Sapolsky, R. M. (2004). Why zebras don't get ulcers. New York, NY: Holt Paperbacks, LLC.

Sartwell, C. (2022). Beauty. In Edward N. Zalta (Ed.), *The Stanford Encyclopedia of Philosophy* (Summer 2022 Edition). Retrieved from https://plato.stanford.edu/archives/sum2022/entries/beauty

Sarwer, D. B., Pruzinsky, T., Cash, F. T., Goldwyn, R. M, Persing, J. A., & Whitaker, L. A. (2006). Psychological aspects of reconstructive and cosmetic plastic surgery: Clinical, empirical, and ethical perspectives. Baltimore: MD, Lippincott Williams & Wilkins.

Saussure, F. (1959). Course in general linguistics. (Transl. by Wade Baskin). New York, NY: Philosophical Library, Inc. (Originally published in 1916).

Schamberg, K., & Barker, K. (2007, March). The not-so-simple story of Barack Obama's youth. *Chicago Tribune, 3*(25). Retrieved from https://www.chicagotribune.com/chi-070325obama-youth-story-archive-story.html

Schein, M., Biderman, A., Baras, M., Bennet, L., Bisharat, B., Borken, J., & Kitai, E. (2000). The prevalence of a history of child sexual abuse among adults visiting family practitioners in Israel. *Child Abuse & Neglect, 24*, 667–675.

Scheerer, E., et al. (1992). Repräsentation. In J. Ritter & K. Grunder (Eds.) *Historisches wörterbuch der philosophie* (Vol. 8, 790–852). Basel: Schwabe.

Schieman, S., Bierman, A., Upenieks, L., & Ellison, C. G. (2017, March). Love thy self? How belief in a supportive God shapes self-esteem. *Review of Religious Research, 59*(1), 1-26. DOI: 10.1007/s13644-017-0292-7

Schilder, P. (1923). Das koerperschema. Berlin: Spirnger.

Schilder, P. (1935). The image and appereance of the human body. London, UK: Kegan, Paul.

Schilder, P. (1942). Mind, perception, and thought in their construction aspects. New York, NY: Columbia University Press.

Schilder, P. (1950). The image and appearance of the human body. New York, NY: International Universities Press.

Schilder, P. (1964/1935). The image and appearance of the human body: Studies in the constructive energies of the psyche. New York, NY: John Wiley and Sons.

Schilder, P. (1999). The image and appearance of the human body. London, United Kingdom: Kegan Paul, Trench, Trubner & Co.

Schmidt S. (2013). Tattoos: An historical essay. *Travel Medicine and Infectious Disease, 11*, 444-447.

Schneiderman, S. (1980). Returning to Freud: Clinical psychoanalysis in the school of Lacan. New Haven, CT: Yale University Press.

Schöen, S. (2015). "You're the one that I want:" Appetite, agency and the gendered self. In J. Petrucelli (Ed.), *Body-States: Interpersonal Relational Perspectives on the Treatment of Eating Disorders* (pp. 59-78). London, New York, NY: Routledge.

Schopenhauer, A. (1818). The world as will and representation. In Christopher Janaway (Ed.), *Introduction: The world as will and representation.* Cambridge University Press. Retrieved from

https://assets.cambridge.org/97805218/71846/frontmatter/978
0521871846_frontmatter.pdf

Schore, A. (2003). Affect dysregulation and disorders of the self. New York, NY: Norton.

Schroeder, J. L. (1998). The Vestal and the fasces: Hegel, Lacan, property, and the feminine. Los Angeles, CA: University of California Press. ISBN 978-0-520-21145-2.

Schroth, J. (2019). Ethical deontology. *Oxford Bibliographies.* Retrieved from https://www.oxfordbibliographies.com/display/document/obo-9780195396577/obo-9780195396577-0383.xml

Schwekendiek, D. (2009, Jan.). Height and weight differences between North and South Korea. *Journal of Biosocial Science 41*(1), 51-5. DOI:10.1017/S002193200800299X

Segal, B. (2001). Responding to victimized Alaska native women in treatment for substance use. *Substance Use and Misuse, 36*, 845–865.

Segal, Z. V., Williams, J. M. G., & Teasdale, J.D. (2002) Mindfulness-based cognitive therapy for depression: A new approach to preventing relapse. New York, NY: Guilford Press.

Senra, M. S., & Wollenberg, A. (2014). Psychodermatological aspects of atopic dermatitis. *British Journal of Dermatology, 170*, 38–43. DOI: 10.1111/bjd.13084

Senseney, M. (2019, May). The ancient tradition of neck elongation explained. *Urbo.* Retrieved from https://www.urbo.com/content/the-ancient-tradition-of-neck-elongation-explained

Sepulveda, A., Botella, J., & Leon, A. (2002). Body image disturbance in eating disorders: A meta-analysis. *Psychology in Spain, 6*, 83-9.

Serafino G. M. (2016). Body image inflexibility mediates the relationship between body image evaluation and maladaptive body image coping strategies. *Body Image, 16*, 28-31. ISSN 1740-1445. https://doi.org/10.1016/j.bodyim.2015.10.003. https://www.sciencedirect.com/science/article/pii/S174014451500128X

Sevilla-Liu, A. (2022). Understanding self-compassion within narrative identity: The struggles of Japanese students with measuring up. *The Qualitative Report, 27*(10), 2230-2250. Fukuoka, Japan: Kyushu University. https://doi.org/10.46743/2160-3715/2022.5602

Shani-Sela, M. (2000). Body attitudes and body experiences in suicidal adolescents. *Suicide and Life Threatening Behavior, 31*, 237–249.

Sharhabani-Arzy, R., Amir, M., Kotler, M., & Liran, R. (2003). The toll of domestic violence: PTSD among battered women in an Israeli sample. *Journal of Interpersonal Violence, 18*, 1335–1346.

Sharman, R. (1997). The anthropology of aesthetics: A cross-cultural approach. *Journal of Anthropological Society, 28*(2), 177-192. Retrieved from https://www.anthro.ox.ac.uk/sites/default/files/anthro/docume nts/media/jaso28_2_1997_177_192.pdf

Shaywitz, B. A., Shaywitz, S. E., Pugh, K. R., Constable, R. T., Skudlarski, P., Fulbright, R. K., Bronen, R. A., Fletcher, J. M., Shankweiler, D. P., Katz, L., et al. (1995, Feb.). Sex differences in the functional organization of the brain for language. *Nature, 16*(373)(6515), 607-9. DOI: 10.1038/373607a0. PMID: 7854416 DOI: 10.1038/373607a0

Sheerha, A. & Mukta, S. (2016). How does positive visualization affect people's level of happiness and perception of their physical body image? *Indian Journal of Positive Psychology, 7*(4), 472-479.

Shenefelt, P. D. (2003). Biofeedback, cognitive-behavioral methods, and hypnosis in dermatology: Is it all in your mind? *Dermatologic Therapy, 16*(2), 114-22. DOI: 10.1046/j.1529-8019.2003.01620.x. PMID: 12919113.

Shenefelt, P. D. (2018, July). Mindfulness-based cognitive hypnotherapy and skin disorders. *American Journal of Clinical Hypnosis, 61*(1), 34-44. DOI: 10.1080/00029157.2017.1419457. PMID: 29771216.

Sheng, Y. (2006). Dharma drum: The life and heart of Chan practice. London, UK: Shambhala.

Shevlin, M., McElroy, E., & Murphy, J. (2014). Loneliness mediates the relationship between childhood trauma and adult psychopathology: Evidence from the adult psychiatric morbidity survey. *Social Psychiatry and Psychiatric Epidemiology, 50*(4), 591-601.

Shiff, R. (2012, Sept.) Regarding art and art history: Unexplained. *The Art Bulletin, 94*(3).

Shukla, U. (2017). Selling skinny: Marketing, social media, and female body image. [TC 660H, Plan II Honors Program, The University of Texas at Austin]. Retrieved from

https://repositories.lib.utexas.edu/bitstream/handle/2152/7518
7/shuklaunnati_THESIS.pdf?sequence=1

Siegel, D. J., Schore, A. N., & Cozolino, L. (2021). Interpersonal
neurobiology and clinical practice. New York, NY: W.W.
Norton & Co.

Silverstein, J. L. (1996). Exhibitionism as countershame.
Sexual Addiction & Compulsivity 3(1), 33–42.

Simon, H. A. (1956). Rational choice and the structure of the
environment. *Psychological Review, 63*(2), 129–138.
CiteSeerX 10.1.1.545.5116. DOI:10.1037/h0042769. PMID
13310708. S2CID 8503301.

Singh, A. R., & Veale, D. (2019). Understanding and treating body
dysmorphic disorder. *Indian Journal of Psychiatry, 1*(2019),
S131-S135. DOI:
10.4103/psychiatry.IndianJPsychiatry_528_18

Slade, P. D., Dewey, M. E., Newton, T. & Brodie, D. A. (1990).
Development and preliminary validation of the Body
Satisfaction Scale (BSS). *Psychology and Health, 4*, 213-220.

Slade, P. D. & Russell, G. F. M. (1973). Awareness of body
dimensions in anorexia nervosa: Cross-sectional and
longitudinal studies. *Psychological Medicine, 3*, 188-199.

Slater, M., Perez-Marcos, D., Ehrsson, H. H., & Sanchez-Vives, M. V.
(2008). Towards a digital body: The virtual arm illusion.
Frontiers of Human Neuroscience. 2(6). DOI:
10.3389/neuro.09.006.2008

Sloman, S. (April 2013). Gainsborough's 'Blue Boy'. *The Burlington
Magazine, 155*, 231–237.

Smart, N. (1979). The philosophy of religion. New York, NY: Oxford
University Press.

Smith, A. (2006). Cognitive empathy and emotional empathy–affective
empathy in human behavior and evolution. *Psychological
Record, 56*(1), 3–21.

Smith, G. A., Rotolo, M., & Tevington, P. (2022, Oct.). 45% of
Americans say U.S. should be a 'Christian Nation.' Retrieved
from https://www.pewresearch.org/religion/2022/10/27/45-of-
americans-say-u-s-should-be-a-christian-nation/

Smith, S. R., Chang, J., Kochinski, S., Patz, S., & Nowinski, L. A.
(2010). Initial validity of the logical Rorschach in the
assessment of trauma. *Journal Of Personality Assessment,
92*(3), 222-231. DOI:10.1080/00223891003670174

Snowden, R. J. & Freeman, T. C. A. (2004). The visual perception of
motion. *Current Biology, 14*(19), R828-R831. Retrieved from

512

https://www.cell.com/current-biology/pdf/S0960-9822(04)00716-X.pdf

Soldz, S., & Vaillant, G. E. (1999). The big five personality traits and the life course: A 45-year longitudinal study. *Journal of Research in Personality, 33*, 208–232.

Somatosensory function. (2004). In W. E. Craighead, & C. B. Nemeroff (Eds.), *The concise Corsini encyclopedia of psychology and behavioral science* (3rd ed.). Wiley. Credo Reference: https://proxy.lirn.net/WilliamHowardTaftUniv?qurl=https%3A%2F%2Fsearch.credoreference.com%2Fcontent%2Fentry%2Fwileypsych%2Fsomatosensory_function%2F0%3Finstitutionid%3D103.

Somer, E. (2003). Prediction of abstinence from heroin addiction by childhood trauma, dissociation and extent of psychosocial treatment. *Addiction Research and Theory, 11*, 339–348.

Somer, E. (2004). Between pleasure and pain: The sexuality of sexual assault victims. Retrieved from http://www.tdil.org/atricale-3.html.

Sorabji, R. (2005). The philosophy of the commentators, 200-600 AD (in English and Ancient Greek). Vol. 1: Psychology (with Ethics and Religion). Ithaca, New York, NY: Cornell University Press.

Sörös, P., Vo, O., Husstedt, I.-W., Evers, S., & Gerding, H. (2003). Phantom eye syndrome: Its prevalence, phenomenology, and putative mechanisms. *Neurology, 60*(9), 1542–1543. DOI: 10.1212/01. wnl.0000059547.68899.f5. PMID 12743251. S2CID 27474612.

Sparkes, A. C. (1996). The fatal flaw: A Narrative of the fragile body-self. *Qualitative Inquiry, 2*(4), 463–494. https://doi.org/10.1177/107780049600200405

Spillius, E. B. (1992). Clinical experiences of projective identification, in Clinical Lectures on Klein and Bion. (Edited by R. Anderson). London, UK: Tavistock/Routledge.

Spivey, L. A., & Edwards-Leeper, L. (2019). Future directions in affirmative psychological interventions with transgender children and adolescents. *Journal of Clinical Child and Adolescent Psychology, 48*(2), 343–356. https://doi.org/10.1080/15374416.2018.1534207

Splavski, B., Rotim, K, Boop, F. A., Gienapp, A. J., & Kenan, I. A. (2019). Ambroise Paré: His contribution to the future advancement of neurosurgery and the hardships of his times affecting his life and brilliant career. *World Neurosurg, Feb*

(34), 233-239. PMID: 31706970. DOI: 10.1016/j.wneu.2019.10.187

Spocter, M.A., Hopkins, W. D., Barks, S. K., Bianchi, S., Hehmeyer, A. E., Anderson. S. M., Stimpson, C. D., Fobbs, A. J., Hof, P. R., & Sherwood, C. C. (2012, Sept.). Neuropil distribution in the cerebral cortex differs between humans and chimpanzees. *The Journal of Comparative Neurology, 520*(13), 2917-29. DOI: 10.1002/cne.23074. PMID: 22350926; PMCID: PMC3556724.

Squires, N. (2016, April). Mona Lisa based on Da Vinci's gay lover, art detective claims. Retrieved from https://www.telegraph.co.uk/news/2016/04/20/mona-lisa-based-on-da-vincis-gay-lover-art-detective-claims/

Sta, M., & Elaine, E. (2005). Intentions in self harm behavior in an emergency population: Can they be distinguished based upon a history of childhood physical and sexual abuse? *Dissertation Abstracts International Section B 66*(6-B), 3063.

Stanford.edu. (2023). Civil War photographs. [Lesson plan]. Stanford History Education Group. Retrieved from https://sheg.stanford.edu/sites/default/files/download-pdf/Civil%20War%20Photographs%20Teacher%20Materials.pdf

Stanghellini, G., Ballerini, M., Blasi, S., Mancini, M., Presenza, S., Raballo, A., & Cutting, J. (2014). The bodily self: a qualitative study of abnormal bodily phenomena in persons with schizophrenia. *Comprehensive Psychiatry, 55*, 1703–1711.

Stark, R. B. (1975, Oct.). The history of plastic surgery in wartime. *Clinics in Plastic Surgery, 2*(4), 509-510.

Steel, J. L., & Herlitz, C. A. (2005). The association between childhood and adolescent sexual abuse and proxies for sexual risk behavior: A random sample of the general population of Sweden. *Child Abuse and Neglect, 29*, 1141–1153.

Stein, K. F. (1994). Complexity of the self-schema and responses to disconfirming feedback. *Journal of Cognitive Research and Therapy, 18*, 161-178.

Stein, K. F. (1995). Schema model of the self-concept. *Journal of Nursing Scholarship, 27*(3), 187-193. Retrieved from https://deepblue.lib.umich.edu/bitstream/handle/2027.42/69219/Schema20Model20of20the20Self-Concept.pdf?sequence=1

Stern, D. (1985). The interpersonal world of the infant. USA: Basic Books.

Stice, E. (2004). Body image and bulimia nervosa. In T. F. Cash and T. Pruzinsky (Eds.), *Body Image: A Handbook of Theory,*

Research, and Clinical Practice (pp. 305-311). New York, NY: The Guilford Press.

Stice, E., Marti, C. N., & Rohde, P. (2013). Prevalence, incidence, impairment, and course of the proposed DSM-5 eating disorder diagnoses in an 8-year prospective community study of young women. *Journal of Abnormal Psychology, 122*, 445. DOI: 10.1037/a0030679

Stokke, K. & Selboe, E. (2009). Symbolic representation as political practice. Retrieved from https://www.researchgate.net/publication/248707010_Symbolic_Representation_as_Political_Practice DOI: 10.1057/9780230102095_4

Strachey, J., Freud, A., Strachey, A., & Tyson, A. (Eds. & Transl.). (1953-74). The complete psychological works of Sigmund Freud (14 vols). London, UK: Hogarth Press and the Institute of Psycho-Analysis.

Straus, M. (1988). Abuse and victimization across the life span. London, United Kingdom: The Johns Hopkins Press.

Strauss, C-L. (1963). Structural anthropology. New York, NY: Basic Books.

Striegel-Moore, R. H., Rosselli, F., Perrin, N., DeBar, L., Wilson, G. T., May, A., & Kraemer, H. C. (2009, July). Gender difference in the prevalence of eating disorder symptoms. *International Journal of Eating Disorders, 42*(5), 471-4. DOI: 10.1002/eat.20625. PMID: 19107833; PMCID: PMC2696560.

Stroud, L. R., Salovey, P., & Epel, E.S. (2002, Aug.). Sex differences in stress responses: social rejection versus achievement stress. *Biological Psychiatry, 15;52*(4), 318-27. DOI: 10.1016/s0006-3223(02)01333-1. PMID: 12208639.

Sullivan, H. S., Perry, H. S., Gawel, M. L., & Gibbon, M. (Eds.). (1956). *Clinical studies in psychiatry*. New York, NY: Norton.

Sullivan, R. (2021). What rules will the Taliban impose on women in Afghanistan? Retrieved from https://www.independent.co.uk/asia/south-asia/taliban-afghan-women-children-rules-b1903373.html.

Suraci, P. (2011). Sybil in her own words. Abandoned Ladder Press. [Amazon Kindle]

Swatt, B. (2011). Themis: Goddess of Justice. Washington, DC: University of Washington School of Law Library. Retrieved from https://lib.law.uw.edu/ref/themis.html#1

Tabassum, N. J. (2013). Tattoo subculture: Creating a personal identity in the context of social stigma. [MSc Thesis] Fargo, ND: North Dakota State University Graduate School. Retrieved

515

from
https://library.ndsu.edu/ir/bitstream/handle/10365/26888/Tatto
o%20Subculture%20Creating%20a%20Personal%20Identity
%20in%20the%20Context%20of%20Social%20Stigma.pdf?se
quence=3

Tagliacozzi, G. (1597). De curtorum chirurgia per insitionem, Venezia,
Italy. Retrieved from
https://books.google.com/books?id=5qg1lwTm79cC&pg=PA8
4#v=onepage&q&f=false

Tanaka, T., Hayashida, K., & Morioka, S. (2022, Apr. 25). Verbal
suggestion modulates the sense of ownership and heat pain
threshold during the "injured" rubber hand illusion. *Frontiers
in Human Neuroscience*, 4. Lausanne.

Tasca, G. A., & Balfour, L. (2014). Eating disorders and attachment: a
contemporary psychodynamic perspective. *Psychodynamic
Psychiatry, 42*(2), 257–76.

Taylor, A. E. (2015). Aristotle. London, UK: Dodge Publishing, Co.
Retrieved from https://www.gutenberg.org/files/48002/48002-
h/48002-h.html

Taylor, J. (Ed.). (1958). Selected writings of John Hughlings Jackson
(2 Volumes--Complete). Vol. 1: Epilepsy and epileptiform
convulsions. Vol. 2: Evolution and dissolution of the nervous
system speech. Various papers, addresses and lectures. New
York, NY: Basic Books, Inc.

Taylor, S. E., Klein, L. C., Lewis, B. P., Gruenewald, T. L., Gurung, R.
A., & Updegraff, J. A. (2000, July). Biobehavioral responses
to stress in females: tend-and-befriend, not fight-or-flight.
Psychological Review, 107(3), 411-29. DOI: 10.1037/0033-
295x.107.3.411. PMID: 10941275.

Tebbe, E. A., & Budge, S. L. (2022). Factors that drive mental health
disparities and promote well-being in transgender and
nonbinary people. *Nature Reviews Psychology, 1*, 694 - 707.

Techakasem, P., & Kolkijkovin, V. (2001). Comparison between
physical and sexual abuse of children in BMA medical college
and Vajira hospital. *International Medical Journal, 8*(4), 293–
298.

Temoshok, L. (1987). Personality, coping style, emotion and cancer:
Towards an integrative model. *Cancer Surveys, 6*(3), 545–567.

Temoshok, L. R. (1990). On attempting to articulate the
biopsychosocial model: Psychological–psychophysiological
homeostasis. In H. Friedman (Ed.), *Personality and Disease*
(pp. 203–225). John Wiley and Sons.

Temoshok, L. R. (2003). Type C coping and cancer progression. In R. Fernandez-Ballesteros (Ed.), *The Encyclopedia of Psychological Assessment* (Vol. 2, pp. 1052–1056). Sage.

Temoshok, L., & Dreher, H. (1992). The type C connection: The behavioral links to cancer and your health. Random House.

Teo, I., Novy, D. M., Chang, D. W., Cox, M. G., & Fingeret, M. C. (2015, Nov.). Examining pain, body image, and depressive symptoms in patients with lymphedema secondary to breast cancer. *Psychooncology, 24*(11), 1377-83. DOI: 10.1002/pon.3745. Epub 2015 Jan 20. PMID: 25601235.

The Met. (2014). Cubism: The Leonard A. Lauder collection. Retrieved from https://www.metmuseum.org/press/exhibitions/2014/cubism-the-leonard-lauder-collection.

Thompson, J. K. (1995). Assessment of body image. In D.B. Allison, (Ed.), *Handbook of Assessment Methods for Eating Behaviors and Weight Related Problems* (pp. 119–144). Thousand Oaks, CA: Sage.

Thompson, J. K., Schaefer, L. M., & Cash, T. F. (2019, Dec.). A multidimensional innovator in the measurement of body image: Some lessons learned and some lessons for the future of the field. *Body Image, 31*, 198-203. DOI: 10.1016/j.bodyim.2019.08.006. Epub 2019 Aug 30. PMID: 31477440; PMCID: PMC6897500.

Thompson, J. K. & Spana, R. E. (1988). The adjustable light beam method for the assessment of size estimation accuracy: Description, psychometric, and normative data. *International Journal of Eating Disorders, 7*(4), 521-526.

Thompson, J. K., & Van Den Berg, P. (2004). Measuring body image attitudes among adolescents and adults. In T. F. Cash and T. Pruzinsky (Eds.), *Body Image: A Handbook of Theory, Research, and Clinical Practice* (pp. 142-154). New York, NY: The Guilford Press.

Thornhill, T. (2015, Nov.). Teenage girl killed herself after becoming obsessed with having a perfect celebrity figure and taking thousands of pictures of her body. Retrieved from https://www.dailymail.co.uk/news/article-3332113/Teenage-girl-killed-obsessed-having-perfect-celebrity-figure-taking-thousands-pictures-body.html

Tichý, P. (1996, Aug.). Falopletysmografické nálezy u pachatelů pedofilně exhibicionistických deliktů [Phalloplethysmography findings in pedophilia and exhibitionism offenders]. *Casopis*

Lekaru Ceskych, 135(16), 521-4. [Original, in Czech]. PMID: 8964065.

Tiggemann M., & McGill, B. (2004). The role of social comparison in the effect of magazine advertisements on women's mood and body dissatisfaction. *Journal of Social and Clinical Psychology, 2004*(23), 23-44. DOI: http://dx.doi.org/10.1521/jscp.23.1.23.26991

Tillas, A., & Vosgerau, G. (2015). Perception, action and the notion of grounding. Retrieved from https://www.researchgate.net/publication/267577013_Percepti on_Action_and_the_Notion_of_Grounding 10.1007/978-3-319-26485-1_27.

Todd, J., Aspell, J. E. Barron, D., & Swami, V. (2019, June). Multiple Dimensions of Interoceptive Awareness are Associated with Facets of Body Image in British Adults. *Body Image 29*, 6-16. DOI: 10.1016/j.bodyim.2019.02.003

Tognotti, C. (2017). Men struggle with eating issues too: Here is my story. Retrieved from https://www.huffpost.com/entry/positive-body image_b_5193674

Tomas-Aragones, L., & Cerbuna, C. P. (2016). Body image and body dysmorphic concerns. *Acta Dermato Venereologica, 2016*(Suppl 217), 47–50.

Topolski, T. D., Edwards, T. C., & Patrick, D. (2004, March 17). Understanding quality of life among adolescents with craniofacial differences. Paper presented at American Cleft Palate-Caniofacial Annual Meeting. Chicago, IL.

Jacob A. Torres, J. A., Kruger, S. L., Broderick, C., Amarlkhagva, T., Agrawal, S., Dodam, J. R., Mrug, M., Lyons, L. A., & Weimbs, T. (2019, Dec. 3). Ketosis ameliorates renal cyst growth in polycystic kidney disease. *Cell Metabolism, 30*, 1007–1023. Elsevier Inc.

Tovian, S. M. (2002). Body image and urological disorders. In T. F. Cash and T. Pruzinsky (Eds.), *Body Image: A Handbook of Theory, Research, and Clinical Practice* (pp. 361–369). New York, NY: The Guilford Press.

Traub, A. C., & Orbach, J. J. (1964). Psychophysical studies of body image: I. The adjustable body-distorting mirror. *Archives of General Psychiatry, 11*(1) (1964), 53-66. https://doi.org/10.1001/archpsyc.1964.01720250055007

Treuer, T., Koperdak, M., Rozsa, S., & Furedi, J. (2005). The impact of physical and sexual abuse on body image in eating disorders. *European Eating Disorders Review, 13*, 106–111.

518

Trottier, K., Monson, C. M., Wonderlich, S.A., & Crosby, R.D. (2022). Results of the first randomized controlled trial of integrated cognitive-behavioral therapy for eating disorders and posttraumatic stress disorder. *Psychological Medicine 52*, 587–596. https://doi.org/10.1017/S0033291721004967

Turner, M. (2017). Really, I come here for the food: Sex as a BFOQ for restaurant servers. *The Industrial-Organizational Psychologist, 54*(3). Retrieved from https://www.siop.org/Research-Publications/TIP/TIP-Back-Issues/2017/January/ArtMID/20301/ArticleID/1624/Really-I-Come-Here-for-The-Food-Sex-as-a-BFOQ-for-Restaurant-Servers

Turner, V. (1974, July). Liminal to liminoid, in play, flow, and ritual: An essay in comparative symbology. *Rice Institute Pamphlet - Rice University Studies, 60*(3). HDL:1911/63159. S2CID 55545819

Ullman, S. E., & Brecklin, L. R. (2003). Sexual assault history and health related outcomes in a national sample of women. *Psychology of Women Quarterly, 27*, 46–57.

Undurraga, E. A., Zebrowitz, L., Eisenberg, D. T., Reyes-García, V., TAPS Bolivia Study Team, & Godoy, R. A. (2012). The perceived benefits of height: Strength, dominance, social concern, and knowledge among Bolivian native Amazonians. *Public Library of Sicence One, 7*(5), e35391. DOI: 10.1371/journal.pone.0035391. Epub 2012 May 4. PMID: 22574118; PMCID: PMC3344832.

USAfacts. (2021). US population by year, race, age, ethnicity, & more. Retrieved from https://usafacts.org/data/topics/people-society/population-and-demographics/our-changing-population?utm_source=bing&utm_medium=cpc&utm_campaign=ND-DemPop&msclkid=5817a3a1645d1500c08bc7bdd460447b

USA.gov. (2023). Life in the U.S. Retrieved from https://www.usa.gov/life-in-the-us#item-36017

Van der Hart, O., Nijenhuis, E., & Steele, K. (2006). The haunted self: Structural dissociation and the treatment of chronic traumatization. New York, NY: Norton.

Van der Hart, O., Steele, K., Boon, S., & Brown, P. (1993). The treatment of traumatic memories: Synthesis, realization, and integration. *Dissociation, 2*(2), 162-180.

Vandereycken, W., & Van Humbeeck, I. (2008). Denial and concealment of eating disorders: a retrospective survey.

European Eating Disorders Review, 16, 109–114. DOI: 10.1002/erv.857

Varga, M., & Máté, G. (2009, Oct. 22–24). The relationship of profession and tendency to orthorexia nervosa in a Hungarian sample. The 17th International Conference on Eating Disorders. (Congress Centrum Alpbach, Tirol, Austria).

Veale, D. (2001). Cognitive-behavioural therapy for body dysmorphic disorder. *Advances in Psychiatric Treatment, 2001*(7), 125–132.

Veblen, T. (2007/1899). The theory of the leisure class. Oxford, UK: Oxford University Press.

Vera Cruz, G. (2013). Cross-cultural study of facial beauty. *Journal of Psychology in Africa, 23*(1), 87-89 http://dx.doi.org/10.1080/14330237.2013.10820597

Vignemont, F. (2020). What phenomenal contrast for bodily ownership? *Journal of the American Philosophical Association 2020*, 117-137. DOI: 10.1017/APA.2019.34

Vossbeck-Elsebusch, A. N., Waldorf, M., Legenbauer, T., Bauer, A., Cordes, M., & Vocks, S. (2014, June). German version of the Multidimensional Body-Self Relations Questionnaire - Appearance Scales (MBSRQ-AS): Confirmatory factor analysis and validation. *Body Image, 11*(3), 191-200. DOI: 10.1016/j.bodyim.2014.02.002. Epub 2014 Mar 28. PMID: 24958652.

Wade, N. J. (2009). Beyond body experiences: phantom limbs, pain and the locus of sensation. *Cortex, 45*(2), 243-55. PMID: 18621367; DOI: 10.1016/j.cortex.2007.06.006

Waite, A. E. (1886). The mysteries of magic: A digest of the writings of Eliphas Lévi. London, UK: George Redway.

Waldinger, R. J., Swett, C., Frank, A., & Miller, K. (1994). Levels of dissociation and histories of reported abuse among women outpatients. *Journal of Nervous and Mental Disease, 182*, 625–630.

Waldman, A., Loomes, R., Mountford, V.A. et al. (2013). Attitudinal and perceptual factors in body image distortion: An exploratory study in patients with anorexia nervosa. *Journal of Eating Disorders, 1(17)*. https://doi.org/10.1186/2050-2974-1-17

Waling, A., Roberts, T. A., Cornelius, R., & Winn, L. (2020). Self-objectification and cognitive performance: A systematic review of literature. *Frontiers in Psychology, 11*(20), 1-13. DOI: 10.3389/fpsyg.2020.00020.

Walker, F. O. (2007). Huntington's disease. *Lancet, 369*(9557), 218–228. DOI: 10.1016/s0140-6736(07)60111-1 PMID: 17240289

Walsh, B. W., & Rosen, P. M. (1988). Self-mutilation: Theory, research and treatment. New York, NY: Guilford Press.

Wang, J., Korczykowski, M., Rao, H., Fan, Y., Pluta, J., Gur, R. C., McEwen, B. S., & Detre, J. A. (2007, Sept.). Gender difference in neural response to psychological stress. *Social Cognitive and Affective Neuroscience, 2*(3), 227-39. DOI: 10.1093/scan/nsm018. PMID: 17873968; PMCID: PMC1974871.

Wason, P. C. (1960). On the failure to eliminate hypotheses in a conceptual task. *Quarterly Journal of Experimental Psychology, 12*, 129–140.

Wason, P. C. (1968). Reasoning about a rule. *Quarterly Journal of Experimental Psychology, 20*, 273–281.

Waters, F., Allen, P., Aleman, A., Fernyhough, C., Woodward, T. S., Badcock, J. C., Barkus, E., Johns, L., Varese, F., Menon, M., Vercammen, A., & Laroi, F. (2012). Auditory hallucinations in schizophrenia and nonschizophrenia populations: A review and integrated model of cognitive mechanisms. *Schizophrenia Bulletin, 38*(4), 683–93.

Watson, A. (2014). Who am I? The self/subject according to psychoanalytic theory. *SAGE Open 4*(3). DOI:10.1177/2158244014545971 http://nrs.harvard.edu/urn-3:HUL.InstRepos:12328212

Watson, H. J. , Yilmaz, Z. , Thornton, L. M. , Hübel, C. , Coleman, J. R. I. , Gaspar, H. A. , … Bulik, C. M. (2019). Genome-wide association study identifies eight risk loci and implicates metabo-psychiatric origins for anorexia nervosa. *Nature Genetics, 51*(8), 1207–1214. 10.1038/s41588-019-0439-2

Watt, N., & Kannampilly, A. (2010, Jan.). Is Da Vinci's Mona Lisa a self-portrait? *ABC News.* Retrieved from: https://abcnews.go.com/GMA/leonardo-da-vincis-mona-lisa-self-portrait/story?id=9662394.

Waugh, J. (2015). The Mona Lisa Code: It's a self-portrait in drag! Retrieved from https://www.jessewaugh.com/blog/2015/4/3/the-mona-lisa-code-its-a-self-portrait-in-drag.

Weber, M. (2002). The Protestant ethic and the spirit of capitalism. (3rd Roxbury Edition). Stephen Kalberg, Transl. (Originally published in 1920).

Weinberger, N. A., Kersting, A., Riedel-Heller, S. G., & Luck-Sikorski, C. (2016). Body dissatisfaction in individuals with obesity compared to normal-weight individuals: A systematic review and meta-analysis. *Obesity Facts, 9*(6), 424-441. DOI: 10.1159/000454837. Epub 2016 Dec 24. PMID: 28013298; PMCID: PMC5644896.

Weinstein, B. (2009). Understanding emotional pain: A preliminary investigation. *Graduate Theses, Dissertations, and Problem Reports, 4549*. Retrieved from https://researchrepository.wvu.edu/etd/4549

Weston-Thomas, P. (2018). Beauty is shape: Beauty history of body-shaping. Retrieved from https://fashion-era.com/beauty_is_shape.htm

Wheeler, M. (2020, Fall). Martin Heidegger. In Edward N. Zalta (Ed.), *The Stanford encyclopedia of philosophy*. Retrieved from https://plato.stanford.edu/archives/fall2020/entries/heidegger/.

Whitfield, C. L., Anda, R. F., Dube, S. R., & Felitti, V. J. (2003). Violent childhood experiences and the risk of intimate partner violence in adults: Assessment in a large health maintenance organization. *Journal of Interpersonal Violence, 18*, 166–186.

White, C. A. (2000). Body image dimensions and cancer: A heuristic cognitive behavioral model. *Psycho-Oncology, 9*, 183-192.

White, C. A. (2004). Body images in oncology. In T. F. Cash and T. Pruzinsky, T. (Eds.) (2002, 2004). *Body Image: A Handbook of Theory, Research, and Clinical Practice* (pp. 379-386). New York, NY: The Guilford Press.

Whitebread, D., & Bingham, S. (2013). Habit formation and learning in young children. Cambridge, England: Cambridge University Press.

Wichstrøm L. (1995, May). Social, psychological and physical correlates of eating problems: A study of the general adolescent population in Norway. *Psychological Medicine, 25*(3), 567-79. DOI: 10.1017/s0033291700033481. PMID: 7480437.

Wiederman, M. W & Hurst, S. R. (1998, Aug). Body size, physical attractiveness, and body image among young adult women: Relationships to sexual experience and sexual esteem. *The Journal of Sex Research, 35*(3), 272.

Wilson, B. A. (2004). The sexual behavior sequelae of childhood sexual abuse in college women. *Dissertation Abstracts International: Section B: The Sciences and Engineering, 65*(3-B), 1566.

Wilson, C. (2000). The mammoth encyclopedia of the unsolved. New York, NY: Carroll & Graf Publishers.

Wilson, M. (2022). Gainsborough's Blue Boy, the Private Life of a Masterpiece. Retrieved from https://www.bbc.com/culture/article/20220120-gainsboroughs-blue-boy-the-private-life-of-a-masterpiece#:~:text=An%20article%20in%20the%20London %20Times%20claimed%20that,of%20high%20culture%20an d%20the%20noble%20British%20character.

Wilson, W. (1984). The Los Angeles Times book of California museums. New York, NY: Harry Abrams, Inc.

Wohlrab, S., Fink, B., Kappeler, P., & Brewer, G. (2009). Differences in personality attributes toward tattooed and nontattooed virtual human characters. *Journal of Individual Differences, 30*, 1-5. DOI: 10.1027/1614-0001.30.1.1

Wohlrab, S., Stahl, J., & Kappeler, P. (2007a). Modifying the body: Motivations for getting tattooed and pierced. *Body Image, 4*, 87-95. DOI: 10.1016/j.bodyim.2006.12.001

Wohlrab, S., Stahl, J., Rammsayer, T., & Kappeler, P. (2007b). Differences in personality characteristics between body-modified and non-modified individuals: Associations with individual personality traits and their possible evolutionary implications. *European Journal of Personality, 21*, 931-951. DOI: 10.1002/per.642

Wolf, N. (2002). The beauty myth: How images of beauty are used against women. New York, NY: Harper Perennial, HarperCollins Inc.

Wood, R.I., Armstrong, A., Fridkin, V., Shah, V., Najafi, A., & Jakowec, M. (2013, Feb.). Roid rage in rats? Testosterone effects on aggressive motivation, impulsivity and tyrosine hydroxylase. *Physiologcial Behavior, 2013*(Feb 17), 110-111, 6-12. DOI: 10.1016/j.physbeh.2012.12.005. Epub 2012 Dec 22. PMID: 23266798; PMCID: PMC3615053.

Woolfolk, A. (2013). Educational psychology (12th ed.). Upper Saddle River, NJ: Pearson.

Wrigley, R. (1997). Transformations of a revolutionary emblem: The liberty cap in the French revolution. *French History, 11*(2).

Wykes, M., & Gunter, B. (2005). The media and body image. Thousand Oaks, CA: SAGE.

Xie, B., Unger, J. B., Gallaher, P., Johnson, C. A., Wu, Q., & Chou, C. (2010). Overweight, body image and depression in Asian and Hispanic adolescents. *American Journal of Health Behavior, 34*, 476–488.

Yager, J., Devlin, M. J., Halmi, K. A., Herzog, D. B., Mitchell, J. E., Powers, P., & Zerbe, K. J. (2006). The practice guideline for the treatment of patients with eating disorders (3rd ed.). APA. Psychiatryonline.org

Yamamiya, Y., Cash, T. F., & Thompson, J. K. (2006). Sexual experiences among college women: The differential effects of general versus contextual body images on sexuality. *Sex Roles, 55*, 421–427. 10.1007/s11199-006-9096-x

Yamamotova, A., Bulant, J., Bocek, V., & Papezova, H. (2017) Dissatisfaction with own body makes patients with eating disorders more sensitive to pain. Journal of Pain Research, 10, 1667-1675. PMCID: PMC5522677 PMID: 28761371

Yochai A. (2019, March). When the body stands in the way: Complex posttraumatic stress disorder, depersonalization, and schizophrenia. *Philosophy, Psychiatry & Psychology, 26*(1), 19-31.

Younes, A. K., & Younes N. K. (2017, Oct.). Recovery of steroid induced adrenal insufficiency. *Translational Pediatrics, 6*(4), pp. 269-273. DOI: 10.21037/tp.2017.10.01. PMID: 29184808; PMCID: PMC5682381.

Young, J. E. (1999). Cognitive therapy for personality disorders: A schema-focused approach (2nd Ed.). Sarasota, FL: Professional Resource Press.

Young, V. L., & Watson, M. E. (2006). Breast reduction. In Sarwer et al. (Eds.), *Psychological Aspects of Reconstructive and Cosmetic Plastic Surgery: Clinical, Empirical, and Ethical Perspectives* (pp. 189-206). Baltimore: MD, Lippincott Williams & Wilkins.

Zacks, J. M., Kurby, C. A., Eisenberg, M. L., & Haroutunian, N. (2011). Prediction error associated with the perceptual segmentation of naturalistic events. *Journal of Cognitive Neuroscience, 23*(12), 4057–4066. DOI:10.1162/jocn_a_00078

Zacks, J. M., Speer, N. K., Swallow, K. M., Braver, T. S., & Reynolds, J. R. (2007). Event perception: A mind-brain perspective. *Psychological Bulletin, 133*(2), 273–293. DOI:10.1037/0033-2909.133.2.273

Zacks, J. M., Tversky, B., & Iyer, G. (2001). Perceiving, remembering, and communicating structure in events. *Journal of Experimental Psychology: General, 130*(1), 29–58.

Zaidi, Z. F. (2010). Gender differences in human brain: A review. *The Open Anatomy Journal, 2010*(2), 37-55. Bentham Open.

Zepinic, V. (2017). Trauma-focused dynamic therapy model in treating complex psychological trauma. *Psychology, 8*(13), 2059-2101. DOI: 10.4236/psych.2017.813132.

Zeyl, D., & Sattler, B. (2019, Summer). Plato's Timaeus. In Edward N. Zalta, *The Stanford Encyclopedia of Philosophy*. Retrieved from https://plato.stanford.edu/archives/sum2019/entries/plato-timaeus/

Zheng, W., Chih-Hung, Y., Wei-Hung, C., & Yen-Chun, J. W. (2016). Profile pictures on social media: Gender and regional differences. *Computers in Human Behavior, 63*, 891–98. https://doi.org/10.1016/j.chb.2016.06.041

Zhitny, V.P., Iftekhar, N., & Sombilon, E.V. (2021). History, folklore, and current significance of facial tattooing. *Dermatology, 237*, 79-80.

Zhou, J. N., Hofman, M. A., Gooren, L. J. G., et al. (1995). A sex difference in the human brain and its relation to transsexuality. *Nature, 378*(1995), 68-70. http://dx.doi.org/10.1038/378068a0

Ziferstein, I. (1995). Psychoanalysis and psychiatry: Paul Ferdinand Schilder, 1886-1940. In: Martin. Grotjahn & Samuel Eisenstein Eisenstein (Eds.), *Psychoanalytic pioneers*. New York, NY: Transaction Publishers.

Zimmer, P., Baumann, F. T., Oberste, M., et al. (2018, June). Influence of personalized exercise recommendations during rehabilitation on the sustainability of objectively measured physical activity levels, fatigue, and fatigue-related biomarkers in patients with breast cancer. *Integrative Cancer Therapies, 17*(2), 306–311. https://doi.org/10.1177/1534735417713301 PMID: 28617135

Zimmerman, K. A., & McKelvie, C. (2022). American culture: Traditions and customs of the United States. Retrieved from https://www.livescience.com/28945-american-culture.html

Zoorob, R. J., & Cender, D. (1998). A different look at corticosteroids. *American Family Physician, 58*(2), 443-450.

Zubricky, R. D., & Das, M. J. (2022). Neuroanatomy, superior colliculus. [Updated 2022 Jul 25]. In: StatPearls [Internet]. Treasure Island (FL): StatPearls Publishing; 2022 Jan-. Retrieved from https://www.ncbi.nlm.nih.gov/books/NBK544224/

Zyga, L. (2010). Signs of dark matter may point to mirror matter candidate. Retrieved from https://phys.org/news/2010-04-dark-mirror-candidate.html

Glossary
Technical Terms and Phrases Used in the Text

Acculturation: cultural modification of an individual, group, or people by adapting to or borrowing traits from another culture; also: merging of cultures as a result of prolonged contact; and: the process by which a human being acquires the culture of a particular society from infancy (MerriamWebster, 2023a).

Adjuvant Therapy: defined as "additional cancer treatment," is provided after the primary treatment, in order to lower the risk of comeback; adjuvant therapy may include chemotherapy, radiation therapy, hormone therapy, targeted therapy, or biological therapy (National Cancer Institute, 2023, par. 1).

Adonis Complex: anxiety and insecurity experienced by boys and men about their appearance or body images. In extreme cases, the complex can meet the criteria of body dysmorphic disorder. The term was introduced in 2000 by the US psychiatrist Harrison G. Pope, Jr (born 1947) in the title of his book, *The Adonis Complex: The Secret Crisis of Male Body Obsession.*

Alexithymia: coined in 1972 by Peter Sifneos, this term literally means "having no words for emotions" (a=lack, lexis=word, thymos=emotions). It is not a diagnosis, but a construct useful for characterizing patients who do not understand and cannot describe their feelings.

Alloesthesia: a condition in which a sensory stimulus, given on one side of the body, is perceived to be at the corresponding area on the opposite side, produced in patients with cerebral as well as spinal cord lesions, classified as a "disturbance of sensory pathways, not a higher cortical dysfunction" (Fukutake et al., 1993).

Allopsyche: a general term characterizing the "assignment or projection of one's own thoughts or ideas to people or events in the outside world. In an allopsychic delusion or hallucination the patient projects his own feelings into other people (*alio-* means other, or different). If he is jealous, he believes his wife is jealous; if he is hostile, he believes other people are aggressive or conspiring against him; if he wishes to cheat others, he becomes convinced that they are out to cheat him. The term *allopsychosis* has been used by Wernicke to denote a psychosis marked by disorganization of the perceptive powers for the outside world (hallucinations and illusions) but without disorder of the motor powers such as speech or action" (Sam, 2023).

Alopecia Areata: an autoimmune disorder which causes one's hair to fall out. It may affect only certain places or spots of the skin, or may be complete, all over the head (Alopecia Areata Totalis), and even the body (Alopecia Areata Universalis). Causes are unknown but it is presumed to be genetically caused, with increased propensity in certain conditions, such as asthma, thyroid disease, anemia, thyroid disease, vitiligo, and others.

Aniseikonia: Anis- (unequal) + eikőn Gk. "image" (cf. icon). A defect of binocular vision in which the two retinal images of an object differ in size. The term was invented by American ophthalmologist Walter B. Lancaster (1863-1951).

Anosognosia: lack of insight – a patient is unable to understand his or her problem, or is denying his or her diagnosis and symptomatology.

Aphasia: an acquired language impairment that results from brain damage typically in the left hemisphere. Common causes of damage include stroke, brain tumors, and cortical degenerative disorders (e.g., Alzheimer's disease). Traditionally, a distinction has been made between expressive and receptive forms of aphasia, whereby individuals with the former primarily have difficulty producing spoken and written language and those with the latter primarily have difficulty comprehending spoken and written language.

Aplasic Phantoms: people who were born without a limb, yet present a complete body image as if the limb was present.

Asomatognosia: a neurological disorder in which the individual lacks to recognize one's body or a part of it (Arzy et al., 2006; Berrios & Sierra-Siegert, 1997).

Atopic Dermatitis (AD): moderate to severe eczema which follows an increase in endogenous glucocorticoids as a result of stress, trauma, or PTSD which activate body's defensive mechanisms: the release of cortisol, catecholamines, adrenocorticotropin, and β-endorphin – which disrupt the function of the skin as a protective barrier, leaving it vulnerable to inflammatory diseases (Senra & Wollenberg, 2014).

AD is a chronic, systemic disease, requiring multidisciplinary approach in treatment.

Attributive Projection: a phenomenon which causes all individuals to alter "how they see themselves" based on their "social cognition and behavior" (Cash & Fleming, 2004, p. 278). Thus, a woman who is internally convinced that she is fat will expect others to see her that way and will assume behaviors associated with heavily overweight people, such as avoidance of social contact, poor dress, reverse interpretation of compliments.

Automonosexualism: sexual behavior where the individual is sexually excited by his own body or by "simply being nude" (Aggrawal, 2015, p. 1).

Autopsyche: a general term for impulses and ideas which originate from the self and pertain to self-consciousness, forming one's personality. Autopsychic ideas occur on both normal and pathological levels. For example, the belief in one's own competence is a normal autopsychic impulse, while a delusional belief that one is Napoleon is a pathological autopsychic impulse.

Autotelic: an individual who generally does things for their own sake, rather than in order to achieve some later external goal (Csikszentmihalyi, 1990). An individual who is driven internally, rather than externally.

Body Art: changes made to the natural body performed for decorative or symbolic purposes, such as tattoos, piercings, dying of hair, make-up, and others.

Body Dysmorphic Disorder (BDD): a distressing or impairing preoccupation with "imagined or slight defects in appearance" (Singh & Veale, 2019, p. 131). It involves repetitive behaviors that focus on body image, weight, and body image associated symptomatology, resulting in high levels of distress, depression, suicidal ideation. Evidence-based treatment approaches for BDD currently involve, among others, the use of serotonin reuptake inhibitor medication and cognitive behavioral therapy. BDD can be identified by observation of behavior, such as excessive grooming and camouflaging (using lipstick/makeup, wearing a costume/mask, wearing sunglasses, or "attempting to conceal the body part the individual believes is unattractive or otherwise deformed" (Mehmood, 2023, p. 2).

Body Ego: in psychoanalytic theory, the part of the ego that develops "out of self-perceptions of the body" (APA, 2023b). It is "the first manifestation of the core of the ego around which all perceptions of the self are grouped, including individual memories, sensations, ideas, wishes, strivings, and fantasies" (Ibid.).

Body Image Disturbance (BID): involves some degree of dissatisfaction with appearance, represented as affective, cognitive, behavioral, or perceptual disturbances resulting from one's being "directly concerned with an aspect of physical appearance" (Thompson, 1995, p. 120).

Body Modification: any form of modification of the natural body, by surgical or other means (including *body art*), exclusive of modifications performed for medical reasons (e.g., mastectomy, hysterectomy, etc.).

Bounded Rationality Theory (BRT): BRT states that all individuals act rationally, by intent, and will accept a solution which satisfies their needs, although it is not perfect. No-one can make a perfect decision because no one individual can access all data and weigh all pros and cons. Thus, individuals end up *satisficed* (viz. below).

Cognitive-Behavioral Therapy (CBT): is a treatment of psychological problems grounded in how individuals think and behave. It assumes that psychological problems are acquired through learning processes and can thus be unlearned or altered. Patients are assisted in identifying and modifying their behavior patterns, in order to eradicate dysmorphic feelings and symptoms.

Cognitive Dissonance Theory: when one is obligated to choose between two similarly attractive alternatives, a psychological tension (dissonance) is created by the "desirable aspects of the unchosen alternative" and the "undesirable aspects of the chosen one" (Alós-Ferrer, C., & Shi, F., 2015, p. 34). the *Dissonance Theory* also holds that elements of knowledge (cognitions) can be "relevant or irrelevant to one another" and that if two cognitions are relevant to one another, they can then either *consonant* or *dissonant* (Harmon-Jones & Mills, 2019, p. 1). Consonant means congruent and logically connected; dissonant means either opposite or unconnected. Dissonance leads to psychological discomfort and avoidance of cognition (Festinger, 1957). This psychological discomfort increases with the magnitude of the dissonance.

Comorbidity: having more than one disease or condition at the same time, such as an eating disorder and body dysmorphic disorder and/or obsessive-compulsive disorder. The diagnosed condition is usually referred to as the "index condition" and the condition discovered during treatment for the index condition as a "comorbid condition" or "comorbidity" (Feinstein, 1970).

Confabulations: memory distortions, "characterized by the production of verbal statements or actions that are inconsistent with the patient's history and present situation" (Bartolomeo, 2017, Abstract). Right brain-damaged patients can also sometimes "confabulate about the left, neglected part of images presented in their peripersonal space, or believe to be in another place" (reduplicative paramnesia, Ibid.).

Confirmation Bias: the tendency to seek out information which supports a hypothesis or favored position while ignoring or minimizing inconsistent information (Wason, 1960, 1968).

Cortical Magnification: cortical magnification means that the sensory surfaces that are more behaviorally important (of high tactile acuity) take up larger areas in the cortex (have larger cortical projection zones).

Cutaneous Body Image (CBI): is the "individual's mental representation of his or her skin, hair, and nails" (Gupta & Gupta, 2013, p. 72). It is an important clinical factor in dermatologic disorders and their treatment. CBI is a "highly subjective construct" that can be "significantly confounded by cultural, psychosocial, and psychiatric factors" (Ibid.).

Depersonalization, Derealization Disorder: an altered state of self-awareness and identity that "results in a feeling of dissociation, or disconnection, from oneself, one's surroundings, or both" which is "often felt as a sense of unreality or detachment from one's body" (Psychologytoday, 2022). Depersonalization may be caused by extremely stressful events or overwhelming threats, and may even become chronic.

Dialogical Self Theory: a theory of disintegration of the self, commonly as a result of trauma. The self is disintegrated into different voices, each offering a perspective based on values apparently inconsistent with the individual's history (Perona-Garcelán et al., 2008, 2015).

Dorsal Vagal Complex: the brainstem integrative center that mediates the satiety reflex and relays autonomic neural responses to stress. The dorsal vagal complex "displays adult neurogenesis, intrinsic neural stem cells and a high brain-derived neurotrophic factor (BDNF) content" which comprise "effectors of plasticity that are modulated by stress in the hippocampus" (Chigr et al., 2009). The dorsal vagal complex reacts to the mother-attachment patterns in the infant, as discussed in the chapter on Body Image Fragmentation.

Dysmorphia: from Greek *dusmorphia,* where *morphia, morphe* refers to the "form." Deformity or abnormality in shape or size (of the body), such as muscle dysmorphia.

Dysmorphophobia: see Body Dysmorphic Disorder.

Dysphoria: from Greek *dysphoros*, meaning "malaise" or "discomfort" (*dys* + *phoros, pherein* – to carry, to bear: thus, "hard to bear." The word is fairly novel in the English vocabulary, first known use dated 1842. It means a feeling of unhappiness or frustration, which may be symptomatic of various mental disorders.

Eating Disorders (ED): common ED include anorexia nervosa (AN), bulimia nervosa (BN), binge-eating disorder (BED), and avoidant restrictive food intake disorder (no acronym in common use). Each of these disorders is associated with different symptoms which revolve around preoccupation with food and body image.

Empathy: the ability to "understand and share in the internal states of others" (Christov-Moore et al., 2014, p. 605). This ability includes recognizing emotions in oneself, and in others, transfer of emotions, and emotional situational priming. Empathy is traditionally divided into two categories: 1) promoting prosocial, cooperative behavior, and 2) understanding and predicting the behavior of others (Smith, 2006).

Encephalopathy: any "diffuse disease of the brain that alters brain function or structure" (NIH, 2023). Encephalopathy may be caused by infectious agents (bacteria, viruses), metabolic, or mitochondrial dysfunction, brain tumors, or increased pressure in the skull, prolonged exposure to toxic elements, chronic progressive trauma, poor nutrition, or lack of oxygen or blood flow to the brain. Encephalopathy causes an altered mental state, progressive loss of memory and cognitive abilities, subtle personality changes, inability to concentrate, lethargy, and progressive loss of consciousness.

Ethnocentrism: the opinion and viewpoint that one's own culture and ethnicity is superior to other cultures and ethnicities. It is often interpreted as hostility and contempt of other cultures, but the reasons for ethnocentrism may be more benign, such as misunderstanding, linguistic barriers, and fear (Allport, 1954).

Ethology, or Human Ethology: the study of human behavior, phylogenetic adaptations, and genetic fixed-action patterns, especially in view of acquired and culturally bound patterns of behavior.

Exhibitionism: an uncontrollable urge to exhibit one's genitals to strangers. It is classified as an obsessive compulsive paraphilic disorder. Experts use the term *peiodeiktophilia* "specifically for a male displaying an erect penis to unsuspecting females" (Aggrawal, 2015, p. 1). It may be related to BDD and other body image disorders. Silverstein (1996) speculated that exhibitionists seek attention, in order to overcome feelings of low self-esteem, shame, and inadequacy. Exposing genitals thus "becomes a sexualized form of "countershame" that tends to create feelings of power, control, and sexual arousal (Aggrawal, Ibid.).

Exospheric Apathy: a term introduced here by for the environment in which body images do not collide and do not get to be (do not become/are not) interpreted.

False Self: a "false self" arises as a form of adaptation to trauma which the "real self" is unable to deal with

(Young, 1999). The creation of a false self is a coping mechanism which, however, frequently leads to disintegration of one's true self and fragmentation of body image.

Figure Rating Scale (FRS): also known as the Stunkard Scale, FRS is a psychometric tool developed in 1983, in order to determine one's satisfaction or dissatisfaction with one's body image. The subject is presented with nine silhouettes, ranging from very thin to very large, and the participant is asked to select the one that best indicates his or her current body size and ideal body size (IBS), the ideal body image, and the opposite sex ideal body image.

Force Field Theory: this theory was developed by Kurt Lewin (1951), originally as a market analysis (the U.S. government wanted to find out why women were purchasing certain kinds of meat, as opposed to others). It consists of the analysis of restraining, and enabling forces, in order to effectuate change. Interestingly, increasing enabling forces (e.g., testing) also increases restraining forces (e.g., stress). The most effective way to achieve change is therefore by mitigation of restraining forces.

Free Choice Paradigm: Each former choice affects the latter choice in the same direction. For example, choosing painting A from between A and B, rejects painting B. Subsequent choice between paintings C and D will underscore positive qualities in A and suppress similarities with B (Brehm, 1956). (*Cf.* Cognitive Dissonance Theory, entry above.)

Fugue: in dissociative disorders, *fugue state* is a state of memory loss, loss of awareness of one's identity (Chirisa, 2006).

Gender Dysphoria (GD) is a "marked incongruence between one's biological gender and experienced gender" (Yousafzai, 2022, p. 375). Individuals with GD often face harassment, bullying, violent physical attacks, as well as discrimination in the form of decreased job opportunities, healthcare, and social activities. The "definitive treatment" for GD is sex reassignment surgery (SRS) (Ibid.).

Gymnophobia: fear or anxiety of being seen naked, "even in situations where it is socially acceptable" (Aggrawal, 2015, p. 1). Gymnophobia stems from the feelings of inadequacy or inferiority related to one's body image. It may also be linked to perception of sexual inadequacy, and fear of vulnerability. It is the opposite of exhibitionism, though their causes are not unrelated (Ibid.).

Hemiplegia: one-sided paralysis or weakness affecting either the left or the right side of the body. The cause is usually some brain or spinal cord injury or condition. Facial paralysis, weakness in the arm, inability to express oneself or slurred speech are symptoms of hemiplegia.

Inductive Learning: the process by which "patterns and regularities in the stream of experience are identified" (Whitebread & Bingham, 2013, p. 5). Inductive learning advances as individual visual and auditory systems develop (Kirkham, Siemmer and Johnson, 2002). Inductively ascertained pieces of information form patterns which are contextually applied and through which body images are mediated and interpreted.

Inferiority Complex: a basic feeling of inadequacy and insecurity, deriving from actual or imagined physical or psychological deficiency, that may result in behavioral expression ranging from the withdrawal of immobilizing timidity to the overcompensation of excessive competition and aggression (introduced in 1907 by Alfred Adler; Adler et al., 1917; APA, 2022).

Interoception: perceiving, feeling, and understanding the internal states of the body. It involves the signals relayed from the body into the brain, in particular the brainstem, thalamus, insula, somatosensory, and anterior cingulate cortices. It is important in maintaining homeostasis, forming and stabilizing one's body image, and facilitating self-awareness (Craig, 2002; Barrett & Simons, 2015; Khalsa & Lapidus, 2016).

Isomorphic Symbolism: the representation of an object (entity, organization, individual) which conforms to others in the same field or microsphere. For example, wearing the same tattoo or dress of the kin fashion may symbolize conformity to the other(s). Similar homogenization of names among institutions and organizations may bring them legitimacy (Glynn & Abzug, 2002).

Kinanthropology: study of human movement with respect to Physical Education, sport, recreation, rehabilitation and physiotherapy. The body image in motion is the proper subject of kinanthropology. It is also concerned with "values and ethics of sport as a part of the quality of life, psycho-social functions of physical activities, biological aspects of the investigation of human movement, training of top athletes, and diagnostics of movement performance predispositions" (Faculty of Physical Education and Sport, Charles University, 2023).

Mental Distortions: prejudicial errors in thinking about body image which originate in the assumptions that everything in life is founded on how one looks (Cash, 2008).

Mentalizing, Mentalization, to Mentalize: the ability to understand behavior "on the basis of mental states" (Hagelquist, 2015, par. 1). Mental states can be "feelings, thoughts, needs, goals and reasons" (Id.).

Mirroring: copying gestures and gesticulation, including speech, tone of voice, body language, etc. of another person, in order to acquire rapport. Mirroring is a "social device which helped our ancestors fit in successfully with larger groups" (Pease, A., & Pease, B., 2004, p. 250). It is the foundation of learning and social competence. It is a powerful and largely unconscious phenomenon which helps individuals to survive and adapt. It extends to "simultaneous blinking, nostril-flaring, eyebrow-raising, and even pupil dilation," micro-gestures which "cannot be consciously imitated" (Id., p. 252).

Myofibrillar Hypertrophy: increase in the number of myofibrils in the muscle, thus in actual muscle mass.

Narcissistic Personality Disorder (NPD): is a belief in one's specialness and uniqueness, accompanied by lack of empathy in relationships, and strategies to foster self-aggrandizement and inflated self-views, as well as self-serving bias and the use of social situations to advance one's status and esteem (Campbell et al., 2004).

Nativism: a policy of favoring native inhabitants as opposed to immigrants; the revival or perpetuation of an indigenous culture especially in opposition to acculturation (MerriamWebster, 2023).

Optic Agnosia: an associative defect where the stimulus, acquired through fully functional sensory-motor means of perception, fails to be meaningfully interpreted. Such a failure is characterized as *agnosia* if it is not caused by an intellectual impairment, or associated with *aphasia* (inability to describe and name things).

Orthorexia, Orthorexia Nervosa (ON): "fixation on righteous eating" (Maine and Kelly, 2005, p. 86). The term *orthorexia* is of Greek origin, from *orthos* (accurate, straight, valid, correct) and *orexis* (hunger, appetite). ON is symptomatic of being obsessed with eating healthy food. It was first defined in 1997 by Steven Bratman. Symptoms of orthorexia include: compulsive checking of ingredient lists and nutritional labels, cutting out an increasing number of food groups (all sugar, all carbs, all dairy, all meat, all animal products), an inability to eat anything but a narrow group of foods that are deemed healthy or pure (Neda, 2022).

Pacing or Vocal Pacing: intonation matching during the mirroring (viz.) stage in communication (speakers' voices are in tune and synchrony, facilitating rapport).

Partonomic Hierarchy: term coined by Zacks, Tversky, and Iyer (2001) for the hierarchy of cognitive perception of body movements. Since segmentation is "impacted by an observer's top-down expectations" (Ratcliff & Las-siter, 2007) and "his or her semantic knowledge" (Zacks, Speer, Vettel, & Jacoby, 2006), the level of cognitive development and the stability of self-image as a neural system govern and regulate the extent to which the observed conduct is memorized and acquired (Loucks et al., Ibid.).

Phantom Body Size: Glucksman and Hirsch (1969) conducted a study of obese subjects following weight loss during a period of weight maintenance and found that the subjects overestimated their own body size despite the weight loss. They concluded that these subjects manifested a *phantom body size* phenomenon, perceiving themselves "as if they had lost almost no weight" and consistently overestimating "the size of other stimuli external to themselves before, during, and following weight loss" (p. 1).

Phantom Limb: A phantom limb sensation is a nonpainful perception of the continued presence of an amputated limb. It is part of a deafferentation syndrome, in which there is loss of sensory input secondary to amputation. Phantom limb pain describes painful sensations that are perceived in the missing limb. Phantom limb sensation is more frequent than phantom limb pain, occurring in nearly all patients who undergo amputation. However, the sensation is time-limited and usually dissipates over days to weeks. On occasion, these sensations may be confused with stump pain, which is pain at the site of the amputation (Duarte & Argoff, 2009).

Placebo Effect: a well-documented medical fact that the belief that one has received a beneficial treatment results in a positive, favorable outcome, such as the putative use of carbohydrates in stamina, or the application of makeup in a job interview, or the purported (assumed) use of anabolic steroids (Ariel & Saville, 1972; Clark et al., 2000; Evans, 2003; Maganaris et al., 1999).

Priming: an effect caused by the "repeated experience of a stimulus" (Sam, 2022, par. 1). Repeated exposure to a stimulus will eventually either facilitate or inhibit the processing of data, because the stimulus will be timely identified and consequent reaction may become instinctive. Also: "The activation of social representations (e.g., traits, stereotypes, or goals) by exposure to different types of information, and the application of these activated representations in social judgments and behaviors" (Molden, 2014, p. 3).

Projection: psychological projection is one of the several defensive mechanisms postulated by Sigmund Freud (1920/1977). It states that the self fails to recognize that it possesses certain undesirable or unwanted traits, drives, or characteristics – or refuses to acknowledge them – and projects them onto others as a form of self-defense.

Proprioception: in Physiology, proprioception means the perception or awareness of the position and movement of the body. Proprioception is one of the means of forming and perceiving one's body image.

Psychiatric Morbidity: a mental illness, characterized by a behavioral or intellectual impairment in functioning which causes some distress or impairment in the life of the individual. It may arise from a single traumatic episode, but may also occur continually, or on a relapsing and remitting basis.

Psychoeducation: education in providing individuals (patients) with information about their disease or condition, etiology, therapeutic options, and prognosis. Educating patients about the physical connection to their psychological condition and emotional reactions to the BDD can be helpful in reducing the feelings of depression and their sense of isolation and social stigmatization.

Psychological Dismembering: a term created by Paul Schilder (1964) to describe the optical vs. tactile difference in perception of various body-parts, creating the notion of interchangeability of body-parts, as well as a psychological delusion in focus on one body-part at a time, which may happen when a person is obsessed with, for example, the size and shape of her nose, or the size of his biceps.

Reflexivity: Schwandt (2001) defines reflexivity as "the process of critical self-reflection on one's biases, theoretical predispositions," and "preferences" (p. 224). It includes emotional and cognitive processes related to "social reality" (Davies, 2007, p. 224). Reflexivity is a process of body image mediation in social context. Reflexive behavior is of extreme social, cultural, and ethnographic-anthropological importance (Malinowski, 1922/2005).

Regression: an unconscious defense mechanism in which the individual's ego reverts to an earlier stage of development. It is usually caused by stress, frustration, or a traumatic event (Freud, 1920/1977). Lokko and Stern (2015) list insecurity, fear, and anger among the chief causes of regression in adults. Individuals "revert to a point in their development when they felt safer and when stress was nonexistent, or when an all-powerful parent or another adult would have rescued them" (par. 4). Balint (1965) depicted regression in a more positive light, as a pathway to innocence, security, and reciprocated love (see also Jung, 1926/1992).

Revenge Body: a body improved by reducing fat and increasing muscle mass, in order to "revenge" oneself against the ex-partner or ex-lover. The "revenge body" is intended for the possessor to become the craved attraction again, at which point it will be she who rejects the one she was rejected by.

Sarcoplasmic Hypertrophy: increase in the overall volume of sarcoplasmic fluid in the muscle.

Satisficing: the process of adaptation of an organism (individual) on some level of satisfaction of specific needs (Simon, 1956). All individuals "satisfice" but do not "optimize (p. 136).

Scopophilia (also: Scoptophilia): from Gk. σκοπέω skopeō, to "look to" or "examine" + φῐλῐ́ᾱ philíā, which means "having a tendency toward" something. Sigmund Freud interpreted scopophilia as a form of obsessional neurosis, while Otto Fenichel suggested that it can be a form of psychological identification with the object. Sexually, a socophiliac derives pleasure from looking at prurient objects of eroticism, such as porn magazines, and such pleasure substitutes the real contact with a human being (Schneiderman, 1980).

Selfitis: an obsessive compulsive desire to take pictures of one's self and post them on social media, in order to increase self-esteem and to "fill a gap in intimacy" (Singh et al., 2016).

Self-Referential Analysis: analysis referring to one's self in the given environment, at the given time. In approaching body image dysfunctional conditions and feelings, one must capture the moment-in-time exactly when the body image issues arose or continue to arise. In other words, body image analysis must be self-referential, tapping into environmental triggers. The solution does not come from staring in the mirror, focusing on the self – rather, it is an analysis of what brought on the feelings (e.g., of ugliness): Social comparison with a peer? Commercial? Something someone said?...

Self-Schema: a system-process of schemata constructed by all individuals during the integration of information and experiences from their environment (Markus, 1977; Markus & Sentis, 1982). Self-schemas include one's thoughts, feelings, and experiences. They also incorporate aspects of the individual self, one's thoughts, beliefs, physical characteristics, social roles, personality traits. Self-schemas reflect a variety of behavioral domains, such as: body weight (Markus, Hamill, & Smith, 1987), exercise (Kendzierski, 1988), sex roles (Markus, Crane, Bernstein, & Siladi, 1982), independence (Markus, 1977; Stein & Markus, 1990) and academic performance (Garcia & Pintrich, 1994; Stein, 1994, 1995). Self-schemata are created by the individual in conjunction with environmental body image mediation, as well as cultural values and norms (Josephs, Markus, & Tafarodi, 1992). Since perceptions, memories, emotional and behavioral responses are included in this concept, it is much broader than that of the body image (Greenwald & Pratkanis, 1984; Markus & Wurf, 1987)

Selfobject: The term *selfobject* was coined by Heinz Kohut (1913-1981), an Austrian-born American psycho-analyst, who was primarily concerned with the analysis of the self. His original intention for the selfobject consisted of the function of the object as an extension of the person (Goldberg, 1980). The APA defines *selfobject* as "one's experience of another person (object) as part of, rather than as separate and independent from, one's self, particularly when the object's actions affirm one's narcissistic well-being" (APA, 2023a).

Semiotics: a general theory of signs and symbols, especially, the "analysis of the nature and relationship of signs in language" (Turner, 1974, p. 54). It includes syntactics, semantics, and pragmatics:

Syntactics or syntax deals with formal relationships of signs and symbols to one another, apart from their users or external reference; the organization and relationship of groups, phrases, clauses, sentences, and sentence structure.

Semantics focuses on the relationship of signs and symbols to the things to which they refer, that is, their referential meaning.

Pragmatics is primarily concerned with the relations between signs and symbols, and their users.

547

Sexual Self-Schemas: cognitive generalizations about sexual aspects of oneself that are "derived from past experience, manifest in current experience, influential in the processing of sexually relevant social information," and which "guide sexual behavior" (Andersen, & Cyranowski, 1994, p. 1079).

Short Stature Dysphoria: a deep dissatisfaction with one's height (see the story of Alex, above).

Somatic Symptom Disorder (SSD): psychological condition characterized by excessive preoccupation with one's health and well-being. The individual suffers from constant thoughts about a certain condition (such as a headache), interpreting it as a more serious condition (such as a tumor) while suffering from increasing anxiety about it, even creating other symptoms which may not be real. Sometimes, antidepressants are administered, but the treatment should focus on building trust with the physician and persuading the patient that SSD is not a serious condition.

Somatoparaphrenia (SPP): a delusional belief where a person feels that his paralyzed limb does not belong to his body. The symptom is typically associated with unilateral neglect and most frequently with anosognosia for hemiplegia (Gandola et al., 2011). SPP is a subtype of asomatognosia (viz.) and involves "delusional misidentification and confabulation" when the patient claims a part of his body belongs to someone else and confabulates an explanation why it is attached to his own body (Feinberg et al., 2010, p. 273).

Somatosensory Cortex (SC): a region of the brain "that is truly in touch with the outside world" (Nelson & Liu, 2009, p. 79). Information about things that are touched and what body part is touching them is represented in the SC. This information contributes to the formation of what could be termed a body image map.

Somatosensory Function: the ability to interpret bodily sensation. Sensation takes a number of forms, including touch, pressure, vibration, temperature, itch, tickle, and pain. The somatosensory system allows individuals to interpret sensory messages received from the body and consists of sensory receptors located in the skin, tissues, and joints; the nerve cell tracts in the body and spinal cord; and brain centers that process incoming sensory information.

Spectatoring: a technical term for "cognitive self-absorption" during an intimate contact "wherein individuals fixate on and carefully monitor personal body parts and/or the adequacy of personal sexual functioning" (Faith & Schare, 1993, p. 345).

Stigmatophilia: arousal from "stigmatization" or from a partner who is "stigmatized" (e.g., tattoos, piercings, scars).

Synesthesia: the term for a state occurring when a stimulus evokes a secondary experience not associated with it primarily. Bainssy et al. (2014) non-exhaustively list: lexical-gustatory synesthesia, when words evoke the experience of tastes; synesthetic experiences of color, taste, touch, and sound.

Synaesthetic: concomitant feeling with image, stimulation of a body-part evoking a particular sense or imagery.

Appendix A: Key Works in Psychology

- 1758: William Battie's *Treatise on Madness* published.
- 1855: Herbert Spencer's *Principles of Psychology* (referenced by Darwin, C. R. in *The Expression of the Emotions in Man and Animals* (1872).
- 1878: G. Stanley Hall becomes the first American to earn a Ph.D. in psychology.
- 1879: Wilhelm Wundt establishes the first experimental psychology lab in Leipzig, Germany dedicated to the study of the mind.
- 1883: G. Stanley Hall opens the first experimental psychology lab in the U.S. at Johns Hopkins University.
- 1885: Herman Ebbinghaus publishes his seminal *Über das Gedächtnis* ("On Memory").
- 1886: Sigmund Freud begins offering therapy to patients in Vienna, Austria.
- 1888: James McKeen Cattell becomes the first professor of psychology at the University of Pennsylvania. He would later publish *Mental Tests and Measurements*, marking the advent of psychological assessment.
- 1890: William James publishes *Principles of Psychology*. Sir Francis Galton establishes correlation techniques to better understand the relationship between variables in intelligence studies.
- 1892: G. Stanley Hall forms the American Psychological Association (APA), enlisting 26 members.
- 1896: Lightner Witmer establishes the first psychology clinic in America.
- 1898: Edward Thorndike develops the Law of Effect.
- 1900: Sigmund Freud, the *Interpretation of Dreams*.
- 1901: The British Psychological Society is established.

- 1905: Mary Whiton Calkins is elected the first woman president of the American Psychological Association. Alfred Binet introduces the intelligence test.
- 1906: Ivan Pavlov publishes his findings on classical conditioning. Carl Jung publishes *The Psychology of Dementia Praecox.*
- 1911: Edward Thorndike publishes *Animal Intelligence*, which leads to the development of the theory of operant conditioning.
- 1912: Max Wertheimer publishes *Experimental Studies of the Perception of Movement*, which leads to the development of Gestalt psychology.
- 1913: Carl Jung begins to depart from Freudian views and develop his own theories, which he refers to as analytical psychology. John B. Watson publishes *Psychology As the Behaviorist Views*, in which he establishes the concept of behaviorism.
- 1915: Freud publishes work on repression.
- 1920: Watson and Rosalie Rayner publish research on the classical conditioning of fear, highlighting the subject of their experiment, Little Albert.
- 1932: Jean Piaget becomes the foremost cognitive theorist with *The Moral Judgment of the Child.*
- 1942: Carl Rogers develops the client-centered therapy, fostering respect and positive regard for patients.
- 1952: The first *Diagnostic and Statistical Manual of Mental Disorders* is published.
- 1954: Abraham Maslow publishes *Motivation and Personality*, describing his theory of a hierarchy of needs, founding "humanistic psychology."
- 1958: Harry Harlow publishes *The Nature of Love*, which describes the importance of attachment and love in rhesus monkeys.

- 1961: Albert Bandura conducts his now-famous Bobo doll experiment, in which child behavior is described as a construct of observation, imitation, and modeling.
- 1963: Bandura first describes the concept of observational learning to explain aggression.
- 1968: The DSM-II is published.
- 1974: Stanley Milgram publishes *Obedience to Authority,* which describes the findings of his famous obedience experiments.
- 1980: The DSM-III is published.
- 1990: Noam Chomsky *On the Nature, Use, and Acquisition of Language.*
- 1991: Steven Pinker, *The Language Instinct.*
- 1994: The DSM-IV is published.
- 2003: Genetic researchers finish mapping human genes, with the aim of isolating the individual chromosomes responsible for physiological and neurological conditions.4
- 2010: Simon LeVay publishes *Gay, Straight, and the Reason Why*, which argues that sexual orientation emerges from prenatal differentiation in the brain.
- 2013: The DSM-5 is released. Among other changes, the APA removes "gender identity disorder" from the list of mental illnesses and replaces it with "gender dysphoria" to describe a person's discomfort with their assigned gender.
- 2014: John O'Keefe, May-Britt Moser, and Edvard Moser share the Nobel Prize for their discovery of cells that constitute a positioning system in the brain that is key to memory and navigation.

Appendix B: Rosenberg Self-Esteem Scale

Morris Rosenberg (1922-1992) received his M.A. (1950) and Ph.D. (1953) from Columbia University. He was an Assistant Professor of Sociology at Cornell University and Professor of Sociology at the State University of New York at Buffalo. In 1975, he joined the faculty at the University of Maryland, College Park, where he remained until his death.

Rosenberg devised his Self-Esteem Scale (RSE) as a 10-item scale to measure the self-esteem of high school students. The scale has successfully been used with adults as well. Scoring has a form of combined ratings, as follows: low self-esteem responses are "disagree" or "strongly disagree" on items 1, 3, 4, 7, 10, and "strongly agree" or "agree" on items 2, 5, 6, 8, 9. Two or three out of three correct responses to items 3, 7, and 9 are scored as one item. One or two out of two correct responses for items 4 and 5 are considered as a single item; items 1, 8, and 10 are scored as individual items; and combined correct responses (one or two out of two) to items 2 and 6 are considered to be a single item. The scale can also be scored by totaling the individual 4 point items after reverse-scoring the negatively worded items. The scale is highly reliable, showing a Guttman scale coefficient of reproducibility of .92, and only slightly lower coefficients of stability, .85 and .88 over two weeks, indicating excellent stability (Rosenberg, 1965, 1979).

Scale

Instructions:

Below is a list of statements dealing with your general feelings about yourself. Please indicate how strongly you agree or disagree with each statement.

1. On the whole, I am satisfied with myself.

Strongly Agree   Agree   Disagree   Strongly Disagree

2. At times I think I am no good at all.

Strongly Agree   Agree   Disagree   Strongly Disagree

3. I feel that I have a number of good qualities.

Strongly Agree   Agree   Disagree   Strongly Disagree

4. I am able to do things as well as most other people.

Strongly Agree   Agree   Disagree   Strongly Disagree

5. I feel I do not have much to be proud of.

Strongly Agree   Agree   Disagree   Strongly Disagree

6. I certainly feel useless at times.

Strongly Agree   Agree   Disagree   Strongly Disagree

7. I feel that I'm a person of worth, at least on an equal plane with others.

Strongly Agree   Agree   Disagree   Strongly Disagree

8. I wish I could have more respect for myself.

Strongly Agree   Agree   Disagree   Strongly Disagree

9. All in all, I am inclined to feel that I am a failure.

Strongly Agree   Agree   Disagree   Strongly Disagree

10. I take a positive attitude toward myself.

Strongly Agree   Agree   Disagree   Strongly Disagree

Scoring:

Items 2, 5, 6, 8, 9 are reverse scored. Give "Strongly Disagree" 1 point, "Disagree" 2 points, "Agree" 3 points, and "Strongly Agree" 4 points. Sum scores for all ten items. Keep scores on a continuous scale. Higher scores indicate higher self-esteem.

Regarding Self-Esteem

Baumeister et al. (2003) found that high self-esteem does not lead to good performance but, rather, that good performance is cause of high self-esteem. Efforts to boost the self-esteem of pupils "have not been shown to improve academic performance" and may even be counterproductive (Id, Abstract). Indeed, while correlation exists between the two, causal relationship is not always unidirectional, nor does it always occur in the same direction. The only exception found by Baumeister et al. was the positive causal relationship between high self-esteem and "persistence after failure" (Ibid.). High self-esteem has been positively correlated with attractiveness and likability, although the latter is a matter of subjective opinion and viewpoint. Degree of self-esteem does not predict either the duration or the quality of relationships. Nonetheless, positive body image and high self-esteem are correlated positively. Self-esteem also "has a strong relation to happiness" (Ibid.). The latter may be causally underscored, as low self-esteem is more likely to lead to depression than high self-esteem, and high self-esteem may also mitigate the negative effects of stress and various negative social affects (such as bullying and harassment). Finally, high self-esteem is no bar to drug addiction or engaging in early sex, rather the opposite is the case, as individuals with high self-esteem tend to take initiative and explore feelings of pleasure.

Although promoting self-esteem *per se* does nothing to foster learning and improve academic performance, Ciarrochi, J., Heaven, P. C. L., & Fiona, D. (2007) found that "positive thinking" (self-esteem being one variable of positive thinking) was causally positively correlated to future high school grades, teacher-rated adjustment, and students' reports of their affective states. In their longitudinal study of seven hundred eighty-four high school students (382 males and 394 females; 8 did not indicate their gender) students who were rated as having low self-esteem were more likely to be sad, fearful, and suffered from negative affect. This relationship was found to be bi-directional, that is low self-esteem causes sadness, just as sadness may produce low self-esteem. In conclusion, self-esteem "predicted decreases in sadness and increases in activated positive affect, hope predicted increases inactivated positive affect, and positive attributional style was predictive of decreases in fear and hostility" (p. 1173).

Appendix C: Body Shape Questionnaire[189]

BSQ-34

We should like to know how you have been feeling about your appearance over the **PAST FOUR WEEKS**. Please read each question and circle the appropriate number to the right. Please answer all the questions.

OVER THE PAST FOUR WEEKS:

Never
| Rarely
| | Sometimes
| | | Often
| | | | Very oft
| | | | | Alv
| | | | | |

1. Has feeling bored made you brood about your shape?........................... 1 2 3 4 5 6

2. Have you been so worried about your shape that you have been feeling you ought to diet?.. 1 2 3 4 5 6

3. Have you thought that your thighs, hips or bottom are too large for the rest of you?.. 1 2 3 4 5 6

4. Have you been afraid that you might become fat (or fatter)?................. 1 2 3 4 5 6

5. Have you worried about your flesh being not firm enough?.................. 1 2 3 4 5 6

6. Has feeling full (e.g. after eating a large meal) made you feel fat?......... 1 2 3 4 5 6

7. Have you felt so bad about your shape that you have cried?................. 1 2 3 4 5 6

8. Have you avoided running because your flesh might wobble?.............. 1 2 3 4 5 6

9. Has being with thin women made you feel self-conscious about your shape?.. 1 2 3 4 5 6

10. Have you worried about your thighs spreading out when sitting down? 1 2 3 4 5 6

11. Has eating even a small amount of food made you feel fat?.................. 1 2 3 4 5 6

12. Have you noticed the shape of other women and felt that your own shape compared unfavourably?.. 1 2 3 4 5 6

13. Has thinking about your shape interfered with your ability to concentrate (e.g. while watching television, reading, listening to conversations)?.. 1 2 3 4 5 6

14. Has being naked, such as when taking a bath, made you feel fat?.......... 1 2 3 4 5 6

15. Have you avoided wearing clothes which make you particularly aware of the shape of your body?.. 1 2 3 4 5 6

558

Never
| Rarely
| | Sometimes
| | | Often
| | | | Very often
| | | | | Alway
| | | | | |

17. Has eating sweets, cakes, or other high calorie food made you feel fat?   1   2   3   4   5   6

18. Have you not gone out to social occasions (e.g. parties) because you have felt bad about your shape?..   1   2   3   4   5   6

19. Have you felt excessively large and rounded?..   1   2   3   4   5   6

20. Have you felt ashamed of your body?...   1   2   3   4   5   6

21. Has worry about your shape made you diet?...   1   2   3   4   5   6

22. Have you felt happiest about your shape when your stomach has been empty (e.g. in the morning)?...   1   2   3   4   5   6

23. Have you thought that you are in the shape you are because you lack self-control?..   1   2   3   4   5   6

24. Have you worried about other people seeing rolls of fat around your waist or stomach?..   1   2   3   4   5   6

25. Have you felt that it is not fair that other women are thinner than you?.   1   2   3   4   5   6

26. Have you vomited in order to feel thinner?..   1   2   3   4   5   6

27. When in company have your worried about taking up too much room (e.g. sitting on a sofa, or a bus seat)?...   1   2   3   4   5   6

28. Have you worried about your flesh being dimply?.................................   1   2   3   4   5   6

29. Has seeing your reflection (e.g. in a mirror or shop window) made you feel bad about your shape?...   1   2   3   4   5   6

30. Have you pinched areas of your body to see how much fat there is?.....   1   2   3   4   5   6

31. Have you avoided situations where people could see your body (e.g. communal changing rooms or swimming baths)?...................................   1   2   3   4   5   6

32. Have you taken laxatives in order to feel thinner?................................   1   2   3   4   5   6

33. Have you been particularly self-conscious about your shape when in the company of other people?..   1   2   3   4   5   6

34. Has worry about your shape made you feel you ought to exercise?.......   1   2   3   4   5   6

Appendix D: Eating Disorders Questionnaire

In order to help determine if treatment is necessary, the Eating Disorders Foundation (EDF, 2023) offered the following questionnaire. You may suffer from an eating disorder if you have answered "yes" to any of the following questions. The EDF (Ibid.) notes that this questionnaire is not a diagnostic tool and does not substitute professional diagnosis and counsel.

1. Do you feel guilt and remorse when you eat?
2. Are you terrified of being overweight?
3. Do you isolate so that you can eat?
4. Do you avoid eating when you're hungry?
5. Do you continue to eat even after you feel full?
6. Do you take medication or exercise instead of eating a meal?
7. Do you weigh yourself at least once a day?
8. Do you evaluate yourself based on your body size and shape?
9. Do you eat large amounts of food in a brief amount of time?
10. Do you feel out of control when you eat?
11. Do you make yourself vomit to avoid gaining weight?
12. Do you regularly take laxatives or diuretics to lose weight?

13. Do you exercise no matter how tired or sick you may feel?

14. Do you skip meals in order to lose weight or to avoid gaining weight?

15. Do you diet often?

16. Do you exercise more than once a day?

17. Do you hide food?

18. Do your emotions affect your eating habits?

19. Are you preoccupied with food or your body size?

20. Do you avoid close relationships or social activities?

21. Do you feel as if food controls your life?

By the Same Author

Collections of Poetry:

- 69 with God (1996)
- Oedipus (1997)
- Electra (1998)
- Chasing Time (2000)
- Ways of a Dead Condor (2001)
- I Glimpsed the Stars of Heaven (2002)
- Butterflies (2003)
- Angels Out of Sight (2004)
- Longing (2004)
- Nights without You (2005)
- Me (2005)
- America (2005)
- Song of the Rose (2005)
- Ancient Citadels (2006)
- When the Currents Turn Awry (2006)
- Europe (2006)
- Meditations (2008)
- 101 in Missing You (2010)
- Poems of War (2010)
- America Vol. I – From Columbus to Civil War (2011)

- America Vol. II – The Civil War (2012)
- Songs of the Human Heart (2012)
- In Throes of Fleeting Shades (2012)
- Love (2013)
- Buried Dreams (2013)
- Soldier's Death (2013)
- New York: Poems about New York City and Its Great People (2013)
- Los Angeles (2014)
- Words (2014)
- My America (2014)
- Beowulf (2014)
- American Chronicles, Vol. I 2013-2014 (2015)
- American Chronicles, Vol. II 2015-2016 (2016)
- Someone Like You (2016)
- Ancient Rites (2017)
- Angel by My Side (2020)
- Auguste Rodin: Artist to Artist (2021)
- Americus: The American Epos (2021)
- Homage to New Dawn (2022)
- My Heritage (2022)
- Recollections (2022, Ed.)
- Art (2022)

Fiction (novels):

- The Hunt and Other Stories (1993)
- Marianne (1996)
- Dance of Her Life (2006)
- It Ended with Adam (2012)
- Escape (2012)
- Becoming Rich (2012)
- On the Road (2012)
- Homecoming (2013)
- Prince Tommy (2014)

Non-Fiction:

- The Game of Deposition (2012)
- Rechtliche Seite: Legal German – for Lawyers and Non-Lawyers (2012)
- Interpretation of Legal Discourse (2013)
- Advanced Swimming: Swimming Preparation and Nutrition for Masters (2014)
- Advanced Swimming: Condor on Swimming, Vol. II (2014)
- Swimming Coach's Compendium (2014)
- Swimming Workouts for Master Swimmers (2014)

- Advanced Workouts for Master Swimmers (2014)
- My Training Log (2014)
- Diet and Nutrition, with a Special Focus on Swimming and Bodybuilding (2015)
- The Official Rulebook of INBA (2015)
- Socialism and Democracy (2016)
- Educational Leadership (2018)
- Educational Administration (2018)
- Organizational Behavior in Education (2019)
- Education Financing in California (2019)
- Cultural Diversity and Immigration (2019)
- Law and Public Schools (2019)
- Bullying and Harassment (2021)

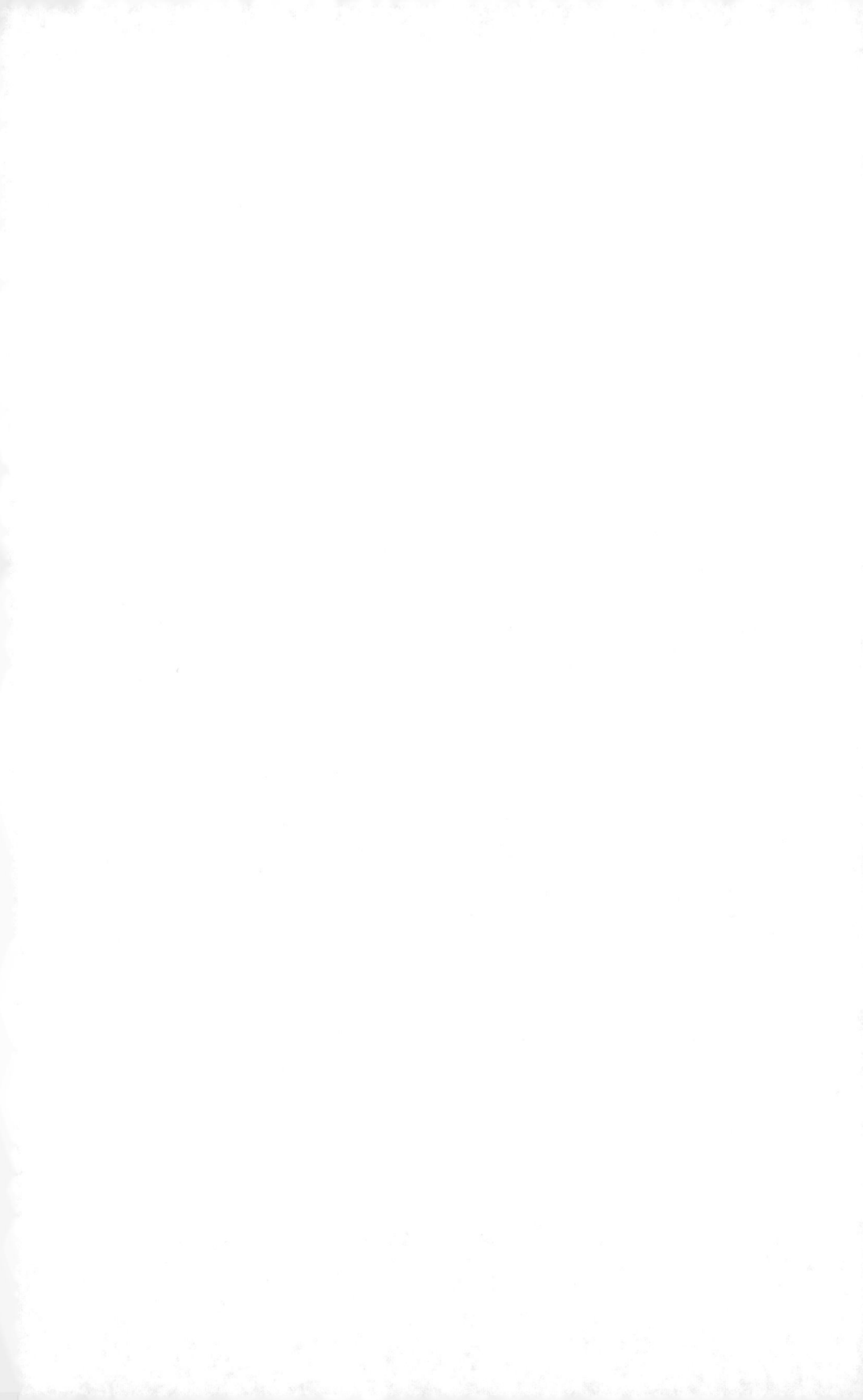

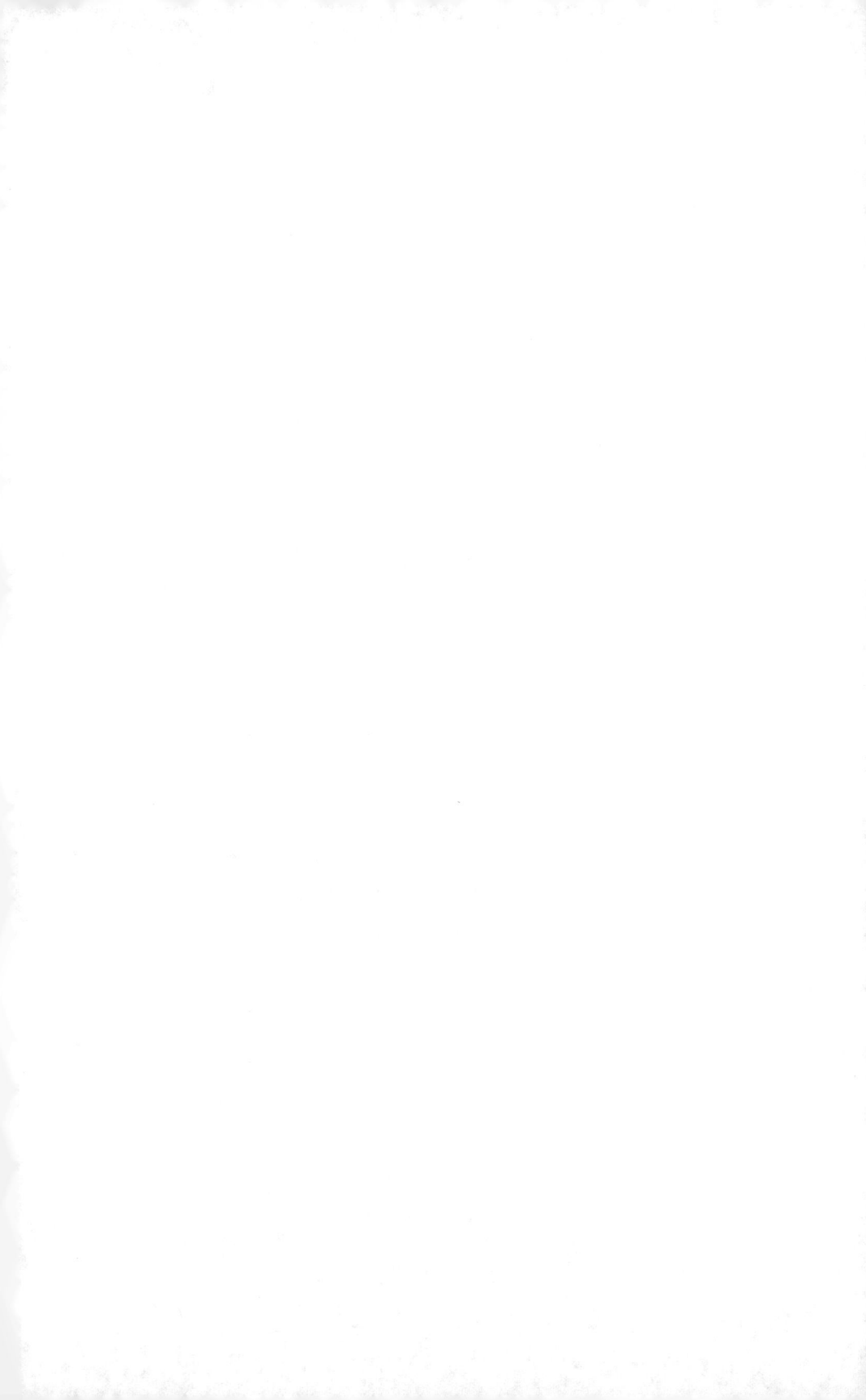